T0344713

INTERNATIONAL REVIEW OF CHILD NEUROLOGY SERIES

Central Nervous System Infections in Childhood

Edited by Pratibha Singhi, Diane E Griffin and Charles R Newton

© 2014 Mac Keith Press
6 Market Road, London N7 9PW

Editor: Hilary Hart
Managing Director: Ann-Marie Halligan
Production Manager: Udoka Ohuonu
Project Management: Pat Chappelle

The views and opinions expressed herein are those of the authors and do not necessarily represent those of
the publisher

All rights reserved. No part of this publication may be reproduced, stored in a retrieval system, or
transmitted in any form or by any means, electronic, mechanical, photocopying, recording or otherwise,
without the prior permission of the publisher

First published in this edition 2014

British Library Cataloguing-in-Publication data

A catalogue record for this book is available from the British Library

ISBN: 978-1-909962-44-6

Printed by Berforts Information Press, Eynsham, Oxford, UK

Cover design includes a photograph of a retina in a child with cerebral malaria demonstrating haemorrhages, white exudates and changes in
the colour of the vessels (courtesy of Nick Beare), and an MRI scan depicting bilateral thalamic involvement in a child with Japanese
encephalitis

INTERNATIONAL REVIEW OF CHILD NEUROLOGY SERIES

Central Nervous System Infections in Childhood

Edited by

PRATIBHA SINGHI
Professor and Chief, Pediatric Neurology and Neurodevelopment, Post
Graduate Institute of Medical Education and Research, Chandigarh, India

DIANE E GRIFFIN
University Distinguished Service Professor, Alfred and Jill Sommer Chair,
W Harry Feinstone Department of Molecular Biology and Immunology,
Johns Hopkins Bloomberg School of Public Health, Baltimore, MD, USA

and

CHARLES R NEWTON
Professor of Psychiatry, St John's College and Department of Psychiatry,
University of Oxford, UK; and Senior Clinical Researcher, Kenya Medical
Research Institute–Wellcome Trust Programme, Kilifi, Kenya

2014
Mac Keith Press

INTERNATIONAL REVIEW OF CHILD NEUROLOGY SERIES

SENIOR EDITOR

Charles RJC Newton
University of Oxford Department of Psychiatry
Oxford, UK

EMERITUS SENIOR EDITOR

Peter Procopis
The Children's Hospital at Westmead
Sydney, NSW, Australia

FOUNDING EDITOR

John Stobo Prichard

EDITORIAL BOARD

Peter Baxter
Department of Paediatric Neurology
Sheffield Children's NHS Trust,
Sheffield, UK

Paolo Curatolo
Department of Paediatric Neurology and
Psychiatry
Tor Vergata University
Rome, Italy

Lieven Lagae
Department of Paediatric Neurology
University Hospitals KU Leuven
Leuven, Belgium

Makiko Osawa
Department of Pediatrics
Tokyo Women's Medical University
Tokyo, Japan

Ingrid Tein
Division of Neurology
Hospital for Sick Children
University of Toronto
Toronto, ON, Canada

Jo M Wilmshurst
Department of Paediatric Neurology
Red Cross Children's Hospital
School of Child and Adolescent Health
University of Cape Town
Cape Town, South Africa

CONTENTS

AUTHORS' APPOINTMENTS

James F Bale, Jr Professor and Vice Chair, Pediatric Residency Program Director, Department of Pediatrics; and Professor, Division of Pediatric Neurology, Departments of Pediatrics and Neurology, The University of Utah School of Medicine, Salt Lake City, UT, USA

Ari Bitnun Associate Professor, Division of Infectious Diseases, Hospital for Sick Children, University of Toronto, Canada

Bruce J Brew Professor, Head of Department and Neurosciences Program Director, Department of Neurology, St Vincent's Hospital, St Vincent's Centre for Applied Medical Research, Peter Duncan Neurosciences Unit and University of New South Wales, Sydney, Australia

Steven C Buckingham Associate Professor and Pediatric Residency Associate Program Director, University of Tennessee Health Science Center, Memphis, TN, USA

Brian S Eley Associate Professor and Head of Paediatric Infectious Diseases, Department of Paediatrics and Child Health, Red Cross War Memorial Children's Hospital and the University of Cape Town, Cape Town, South Africa

Diane E Griffin University Distinguished Service Professor, Alfred and Jill Sommer Chair, W Harry Feinstone Department of Molecular Biology and Immunology, Johns Hopkins Bloomberg School of Public Health, Baltimore, MD, USA

Richard Idro Consultant Paediatrician/Honorary Lecturer, Mulago Hospital/Makerere University College of Health Sciences, Kampala, Uganda; and Senior Clinical Research Paediatrician, Centre for Tropical Medicine, University of Oxford, UK

Chandra Kanta Associate Professor, Department of Pediatrics, King George Medical University, Lucknow, Uttar Pradesh, India

Niranjan Khandelwal	Professor and Head, Department of Radiodiagnosis, Post Graduate Institute of Medical Education and Research, Chandigarh, India
Rashmi Kumar	Professor and Head, Department of Pediatrics, King George Medical University, Uttar Pradesh, Lucknow, India
Timothy D Minniear	Research Associate, Department of Infectious Diseases, St Jude's Children's Research Hospital, Memphis, TN, USA
Brian GR Neville	Emeritus Prince of Wales Professor of Epilepsy, Neurosciences Unit, Institute of Child Health, University College London, UK
Charles R Newton	Professor of Psychiatry, St John's College and Department of Psychiatry, University of Oxford, UK; and Senior Clinical Researcher, Kenya Medical Research Institute–Wellcome Trust Programme, Kilifi, Kenya
Susan E Richardson	Head of Microbiology, The Hospital for Sick Children, Toronto; and Senior Associate Scientist, Physiology and Experimental Medicine Research Institute, Toronto; and Associate Professor of Laboratory Medicine and Pathobiology, University of Toronto, Canada
Zoran Rumboldt	Adjunct Professor of Neuroradiology, Department of Radiology and Radiological Science, Medical University of South Carolina, Charleston, SC, USA
Johan F Schoeman	Professor in Pediatric Neurology, Department of Pediatrics and Child Health, Stellenbosch University, Tygerberg Hospital, Tygerberg, Western Cape, South Africa
Rupa R Singh	Professor, Department of Pediatrics and Adolescent Medicine; Chair, Division of Neonatology; and Head, Nepal National Unit of UNESCO Chair in Bioethics, BP Koirala Institute of Health Sciences, Dharan, Nepal
Pratibha Singhi	Professor and Chief, Pediatric Neurology and Neurodevelopment, Post Graduate Institute of Medical Education and Research, Chandigarh, India
Sunit Singhi	Professor and Head, Department of Pediatrics and Pediatric Emergency and Intensive Care, Advanced Pediatrics Centre, Post Graduate Institute of Medical Education and Research, Chandigarh, India

Authors' Appointments

John T Sladky Emeritus Professor of Pediatrics and Neurology, Dunwoody, GA, USA

Ronald van Toorn Consultant in Pediatric Neurology, Department of Pediatrics and Child Health, Stellenbosch University, Tygerberg Hospital, Western Cape, South Africa

Richard J Whitley Distinguished Professor of Pediatrics, Loeb Eminent Scholar Chair in Pediatrics, and Professor of Microbiology, Medicine and Neurosurgery, The University of Alabama at Birmingham, Birmingham, AL, USA

Hugh J Willison Professor of Neurology, Institute of Infection, Immunity and Inflammation, University of Glasgow, Scotland

Jo M Wilmshurst Professor, Head of Department and Neurosciences Program Director, Department of Neurology, St Vincent's Hospital, St Vincent's Centre for Applied Medical Research, Peter Duncan Neurosciences Unit and University of New South Wales, Sydney, Australia

FOREWORD

Infections constitute the largest group among life-threatening diseases in children particularly in resource-poor areas of the world. However, infections are also an issue in resource-rich countries where even diseases preventable by immunization, such as measles, have been causing epidemics. Moreover, increase in population mobility has facilitated spreading of infections, and imported infections in previously immunized populations are becoming more frequent.

As in other topics in medicine, our knowledge on infectious diseases has been subject to tremendous changes in the last decade: work on new vaccines, association of specific infections with specific genotypes, emerging resistance to microorganisms, and the availability of new therapeutic agents and modalities call for frequent updates for all professionals working in this specialty. A clinician can perform an extensive search on an infectious disorder using internet resources; however, it is rather time consuming and may not necessarily be holistic. While it is unrealistic to cover all developments in one volume, this book offers a concise source of the latest information on a large number of childhood central nervous system infections. Each chapter is written by a specialist with personal experience in these disorders and therefore provides pragmatic coverage of the topic. In addition to the chapters on specific infections, those on general pathogenesis and principles of management should be very useful in providing a basic understanding of the disease process and the underlying approach to management, while the chapter on neuroimaging will enlighten the clinician regarding the appropriate use of various techniques and interpretation of images to provide diagnostic clues to several central nervous system infections.

This addition to the International Review of Child Neurology series is truly an international collaborative effort and is likely to be a great contribution to the commitment of the International Child Neurology Association to education in child neurology.

Banu Anlar
Departments of Pediatrics and Pediatric Neurology
Hacettepe University
Ankara, Turkey

PREFACE

Infections of the nervous system remain an important cause of morbidity and mortality in children throughout the world. With the increase in air travel and migration of populations, many infections endemic in some parts of the world present in children attending health facilities outside these areas. Clinicians, particularly paediatric neurologists and paediatricians, need to be aware of the diverse presentations of infections of the nervous system, particularly as they can often be confused with other conditions.

This is one of the few books dedicated to infections of the nervous system in children and we hope it will be a useful successor to Bell and McCormick's excellent book *Neurologic Infections in Children*, published in 1981.*

Since then, newly recognized infections (e.g. human immunodeficiency virus) have emerged and other infections (e.g. West Nile Fever) have spread across the world. In addition, a book on this topic was requested by many members of the International Child Neurology Association when they were surveyed. Rather than providing a detailed account of all infections, we have provided an overview of the most important infections of the central nervous system, particularly their clinical manifestations, and key diagnostic tests and management decisions. The chapters have been written by clinicians who have extensive experience of the subjects of their chapters, and are well-respected authorities in their fields. We have tried to include authors from most of the continents, particularly those with expertise in infections endemic in their countries. Besides the emphasis on diagnosis and management, we have highlighted the sequelae of the infections.

It is now easier for clinicians to keep up-to-date with the rapidly changing scientific basis of infections through electronic means. Our intention is that the electronic version of this book will be updated periodically, but the print version is provided for those clinicians who prefer a hard copy and those who are unable to access the internet easily.

We hope that this book will be useful to a wide range of clinicians and health care staff who look after children with central nervous system infections, and will provide them with a basis for diagnosing and managing such infections and advising parents about the outcome.

Charles R Newton, Kilifi, Kenya
Pratibha Singhi, Chandigarh, India
Diane E Griffin, Baltimore, USA
March 2014

*Bell WE, McCormick WF (1981) *Neurologic Infections in Children, 2nd edn.* Philadelphia: WB Saunders.

ACKNOWLEDGEMENTS

We would like to thank members of the Mac Keith Press, in particular Udoka Ohuonu and Ann-Marie Halligan for their patience and support in bringing this book to completion, and James Dufficy for his work on the front cover. We also thank Pat Chappelle for his tireless copy-editing of the book. Finally, we would like to thank Professor Banu Anlar for reviewing the book and suggesting ways to improve it.

1
BURDEN OF CENTRAL NERVOUS SYSTEM INFECTIONS

Charles R Newton

The central nervous system (CNS) is particularly susceptible to infection during the period of maximum growth, from fetal life to early childhood. A variety of agents can infect and/or damage the brain during this period, leading to death or a wide range of impairments in the child. Preventive measures have reduced the incidence of infections, particularly in high-income countries, but CNS infections remain an important cause of disability in the world's children.

Viruses, bacteria and some protozoa such as malaria account for most of the burden globally, but the relative importance of the organisms varies with the region. The epidemiology of CNS infections is well documented in some areas, but in other regions, particularly resource-poor countries, the contribution of some agents, such as herpes simplex virus, is less clear. Many infections remain undetected, and thus the burden is underestimated. Determination of the incidence of CNS infections is hampered by a lack of surveillance systems to identify the fetus or child at risk or with features of infection, and by a lack of facilities to diagnose the infections.

Viral infections (Table 1.1)
Viral infections of the CNS are probably more common than bacterial infections, but the burden is much less well documented because there are more types of viruses that infect the brain, they are more difficult to diagnose, and until relatively recently there were few therapeutic options. Viruses cause meningitis and encephalitis, often occurring together as a meningoencephalitis.

Human immunodeficiency virus (HIV) is a very common viral infection of the CNS in the world. It infects the fetus, and is transmitted to the child during birth and breastfeeding. In addition, some children acquire the infection from blood, injections and sexual intercourse. In 2011, an estimated 3.4 million children were living with HIV worldwide. There were 330 000 (95% confidence intervals 280 000–380 000) new HIV infections in children and 230 000 (200 000–270 000) HIV-related deaths among children (UNAIDS 2013). It is unclear how many children have infections of the brain, but since HIV is neurotropic it is likely that many children have covert infections of the brain. Chronic CNS HIV-1 infection begins during primary systemic infection and continues in nearly all untreated seropositive individuals. In up to 18% of HIV-infected children the infection can manifest initially with

TABLE 1.1
Viruses infecting the central nervous system: distribution and routes of transmission

Virus	Distribution	Transmission
Herpes viridae		
Herpes simplex virus	Worldwide	Human to human
Varicella-zoster virus	Worldwide	Human to human
Epstein–Barr virus	Worldwide	Human to human
Cytomegalovirus	Worldwide	Human to human
Human herpesvirus 6	Worldwide	Human to human
Arboviruses		
West Nile virus	North and South America; Middle East, Africa, Europe, Australia and southern Asia (Kunjin)	Mosquito, *Culex* spp.
Japanese encephalitis virus	Asia and Southeast Asia, Australia	Mosquito, *Culex* spp.
St Louis encephalitis virus	North and South America	Mosquito, *Culex* spp.
Tick-borne encephalitis virus	Central and eastern Europe, Russia	Tick, *Ixodes* spp.
Eastern equine encephalitis virus	Eastern half of North and South America, from Canada to Argentina	Mosquito, *Culex* spp.
Western equine encephalitis virus	Western half of North and South America from Canada to Argentina	Mosquito, Culex spp.
Venezuelan equine encephalitis virus	North and South America	Mosquito, *Aedes*, *Psorophora* spp.
La Crosse virus	North America	Mosquito, *Aedes* spp.
Toscana virus	Mediterranean	Sandfly, *Phlebotomus perniciosus* and *P. perfiliewi*
Colorado tick fever virus	North America	*Dermacentor* spp.
Others		
Echovirus	Southeast Asia	Variable transmission
Rabies virus	Worldwide except western Europe, Japan	Carnivorous mammals, bat bite or scratch, licking on wounded skin or mucosae; graft transmission possible although rare
Mumps virus	Worldwide	Human to human
Measles virus	Worldwide	Human to human
Rubella virus	Worldwide	Human to human
Henipah viruses	Nipah: Malaysia, Bangladesh, India. Hendra: Australia	Probably airborne, or contact with animal faeces, from fruit bats. Pigs may be possible intermediate hosts
JC (John Cunningham) virus	Worldwide	Human to human
Enteroviruses	Worldwide	Human to human
Influenza viruses	Worldwide	Birds to human, human to human
Lymphocytic choriomeningitis virus	Worldwide	From rodents, but transmitted transplacentally and through organ transplantation

CNS involvement (Angelini et al. 2000). At least 50% of HIV-infected children display neurological signs and symptoms during the course of the disease. The CNS infections are rarely recognized, since HIV infection of the brain presents with subtle signs such as developmental delay. In untreated cohorts of individuals with perinatally acquired HIV infections, the prevalence of developmental delay is up to 56% by 18 months in the survivors (Abubakar et al. 2008). The introduction of antiretroviral drugs reduced the prevalence of the active progressive and static forms of HIV encephalopathy to 1.6% and 10% respectively (Chiriboga et al. 2005).

The incidence of the acute encephalitis syndrome is 10.5–13.8 per 100 000 per year in Western children, and is probably similar in tropical areas, despite the addition of endemic viruses such as Japanese B encephalitis (Jmor et al. 2008). The proportion of CNS viral infections with neurological sequelae varies considerably in children. Herpes simplex viruses (types 1 and 2) are probably the most common causes of the acute encephalitis syndrome (Jmor et al. 2008, Stahl et al. 2011). Human herpesviruses types 6 and 7 are common causes of seizures, but rarely cause encephalitis. Neurological complications of varicella infection occur in about 2/10 000, and the outcome is good except in the immune-compromised hosts. Epstein–Barr virus and cytomegalovirus are ubiquitous, but rarely cause CNS disease except in immune-compromised hosts.

Japanese B infections are very common in many parts of Asia, and principally affect children. The World Health Organization estimates that Japanese encephalitis is a leading cause of viral encephalitis in Asia, with 30 000–50 000 clinical cases reported annually. It is endemic in China, India, Vietnam, Thailand, the Philippines, Malaysia and Indonesia, where encephalitis occurs in young children (Campbell et al. 2011). Approximately 67 900 cases typically occur annually in the 24 countries where Japanese encephalitis is endemic, with an overall incidence of 1.8 per 100 000. In high-incidence areas with expanding vaccination programmes such as north-central and northeast India, the estimated incidence is 2.8 per 100 000 in the overall population and 5.1 per 100 000 in children under 14 years of age (Campbell et al. 2011). Japanese encephalitis is caused by infection with the mosquito-borne flavivirus. In areas where the Japanese encephalitis virus is common, the disease occurs mainly in young children because older children and adults have already been infected and are immune. Acute encephalitis occurs in about 0.001%–0.05% of infections, with death in 25% and neurological sequelae in 30% of cases. In areas of lower transmission, infections can occur year-round but intensify during the rainy season.

Recently there have been epidemics of viral infections, many with CNS involvement. The West Nile virus, although originating within Africa, has spread rapidly across the world, particularly in North America. Echovirus infections of the CNS have emerged in Eastern Asia. The epidemiology of other viral infections is largely undefined.

Bacterial infections
Bacterial meningitis remains a major cause of mortality and disability in the world, particularly in Africa and Asia (Murray et al. 2012). The best-documented CNS infections are the organisms that cause acute bacterial meningitis (ABM). The most common organisms are

Neisseria meningitidis, Streptococcus pneumoniae and until recently *Haemophilus influenzae*. Before the introduction of vaccinations, the decline in the incidence of bacterial meningitis was largely attributed to improvement in access to health care and prompt treatment of infections. Vaccinations have had a major impact on the incidence of these forms of meningitis. The introduction of the *Haemophilus* conjugate vaccine in the 1980s dramatically reduced the incidence of *Haemophilus* meningitis in both high-income and resource-poor countries. The introduction of the pneumococcal conjugate vaccines may have a more limited impact than the *Haemophilus* vaccine, since the present pneumococcal vaccines do not cover all the serotypes that may cause meningitis, and there is a risk that the serotypes that replace those prevented by the vaccine may become important causes of meningitis. Meningococcal vaccines have reduced the incidence of bacterial meningitis, but since they are not as effective as the other vaccines, there are still outbreaks of meningococcal meningitis. One of the problems is that many of the vaccines are given after the neonatal period and thus do not prevent neonatal meningitis caused by these organisms. Development of vaccines to be administered to pregnant women may influence the incidence of ABM during the neonatal period and beyond.

Neonatal sepsis or meningitis causes 5.2% of neonatal deaths (almost 393 000) globally (Liu et al. 2012). The incidence of neonatal bacterial meningitis is 0.2–1 per 1000 live births in high-income countries, constant since the 1980s. Few data are available from resource-poor countries. The incidence of meningococcal disease in Europe is 2–89/100 000/year in infants and 1–27/100 000/year in 1- to 4-year-olds. Epidemics of meningococcal meningitis in Africa may produce incidences of up to 1000/100 000/year and are usually associated with serogroup A (WHO 2011). The global incidence of pneumococcal meningitis in children under 5 years was 17/100 000/year (range 8–21), amounting to over 100 000 cases per year with the highest incidence in Africa and the lowest in Europe (O'Brien et al. 2009). The case fatality rate is 59% (range 27%–80%), but the incidence of neurological sequelae is not known. These figures are influenced by HIV infection and pneumococcal vaccination. HIV infection increases the mortality rate, but its effect on neurological outcomes is unclear. The introduction of pneumococcal vaccines has decreased pneumoccal pneumonia by 35%, but there are no accurate figures for the reduction in meningitis (O'Brien et al. 2009). The incidence of *Haemophilus* meningitis in young children was at least 21 (range 16–31)/100 000 in 2000 (Watt et al. 2009), but this has reduced markedly with the introduction of Hib vaccine. The high incidence of ABM in Africa is thought to be caused by increased transmission, poverty, malnutrition, lack of health-care facilities, shortage of antimicrobials and, in the last couple of decades, the spread of HIV causing secondary immunodeficiency.

Bacterial meningitis is a major cause of disability in the world. In a recent systematic review, the median risk of at least one major or minor sequela after hospital discharge was 19.9% (95% confidence interval 12.3%–35.3%) (Edmond et al. 2010). The risk of at least one major sequela (cognitive impairment, bilateral hearing loss, motor deficit, seizures, visual impairment or hydrocephalus) was 12.8% (7.2%–21.1%), and that of at least one minor sequela (behavioural problems, learning difficulties, unilateral hearing loss, hypotonia or diplopia) was 8.6% (4.4%–15.3%). The risk of at least one major sequela was 24.7% (16.2%–35.3%) in pneumococcal meningitis, 9.5% (7.1%–15.3%) in *Haemophilus influenzae* type b, and 7.2% (4.3%–11.2%) in meningococcal meningitis. In the meta-analysis, all-cause risk of a major sequela was twice as high in Africa (pooled risk estimate 25.1% [18.9%–32.0%]) and southeast Asia (21.6% [13.1%–31.5%]) than in Europe (9.4% [7.0%–12.3%]).

Tuberculosis is very common in some parts of the world, but the incidence of tubercular meningitis or the prevalence of tuberculomas is largely unknown. One reason is the difficulty in making the diagnosis, and the lack of laboratory techniques in many parts of the world where this infection is common. India and China together account for almost 40% of the world's tuberculosis cases. Nearly 10% of patients with tuberculosis develop CNS tuberculosis. Tubercular meningitis is one of the common chronic CNS infections in resource-poor countries that primarily affects children under 5 years of age. The spread of HIV infection has had a profound influence on the epidemiology of tuberculosis, with an increase in the incidence of acute infections including tubercular meningitis.

The epidemiology of other bacterial infections of the CNS, such as brain abscess, cerebritis and ventriculitis, is less well documented. There are no studies reporting the incidence of these complications.

Parasitic infections
Malaria and cysticercosis are the most common parasitic infections of the CNS.

Over 2 billion people are exposed to falciparum malaria. In 2010, there were 218 million clinical episodes, most of which occurred in children living in sub-Saharan Africa (White et al. 2013). *Plasmodium falciparum*-infected red blood cells sequester within the brain, even in asymptomatic infections, and thus the incidence of CNS malaria is likely to be underestimated. In malaria-endemic areas, up to 40% of admissions to local hospitals are due to malaria, and nearly half of these have overt neurological manifestations such as impaired consciousness, seizures, agitation and prostration (Idro et al. 2007). In Kenya, the incidence of neurological manifestations in hospitalized children with falciparum malaria was 1156/100 000/year. Since nearly a quarter of children will have neurocognitive impairment and/or epilepsy following severe malaria, the burden of long-term disability is significant. *P. vivax* also appears to cause CNS manifestations, but these are not as severe as with *P. falciparum* infection, and are not associated with as much neurological impairment. But given that over 1 billion children are exposed to vivax malaria, this may be a particularly important cause of neurological morbidity in children, particularly in Asia.

Neurocysticercosis caused by the helminth *Taenia solium* is the most common cause of acquired epilepsy in certain regions of the world. In Ecuador, it is estimated that neurocysticercosis is responsible for one-third of cases of adult-onset epilepsy. In children, it is a common identifiable cause of epilepsy in endemic regions such as India, although robust epidemiological studies are not available. Hospital-based studies from India show a 2%–40% prevalence of *Taenia* ova in stool samples of patients (Prasad et al. 2002). The disease is also associated with seizures, hydrocephalus, stroke and long-term neurodevelopmental sequelae. No human vaccine currently exists for *T. solium*. Vaccinating pigs in endemic regions to prevent porcine cysticercosis may be a good option to prevent taeniasis and consequently human cysticercosis.

Toxocariasis and toxoplasmosis are ubiquitous. *Toxocara* spp. may be an important cause of epilepsy in resource-poor areas, but the burden is difficult to determine since most studies have relied on measuring the exposure by antibodies. Determination of CNS involvement requires sophisticated neuroimaging, which rarely exists in the high-prevalence, resource-poor areas. Toxoplasmosis is an important CNS infection in utero and is associated with epilepsy (Palmer 2007). Since it is a common opportunistic infection in HIV-infected individuals, the incidence has increased in the last couple of decades. Despite this increase, there are no studies reporting the burden in children.

Conclusion

Infections of the CNS are common in children, but the burden is largely underestimated because of the lack of robust epidemiological studies and facilities to detect CNS involvement. Infections are among the most preventable causes of neurological disease in children, but there are significant barriers to implementing strategies for reducing transmission, to developing vaccines against many of the aetiological agents, and to the delivery of the available vaccines. Infections will remain an important cause of neurological disability in children for at least the near future.

REFERENCES

Abubakar A, Van Baar A, Van de Vijver FJ, et al. (2008) Paediatric HIV and neurodevelopment in sub-Saharan Africa: a systematic review. *Trop Med Int Health* 13: 880–7.
Angelini L, Zibordi F, Triulzi F, et al. (2000) Age-dependent neurologic manifestations of HIV infection in childhood. *Neurol Sci* 21: 135–42.
Campbell GL, Hills SL, Fischer M, et al. (2011) Estimated global incidence of Japanese encephalitis: a systematic review. *Bull World Health Organ* 89: 766–74, 774A–E.
Chiriboga CA, Fleishman S, Champion S, et al. (2005) Incidence and prevalence of HIV encephalopathy in children with HIV infection receiving highly active anti-retroviral therapy (HAART). *J Pediatr* 146: 402–7.
Edmond K, Clark A, Korczak VS, et al. (2010) Global and regional risk of disabling sequelae from bacterial meningitis: a systematic review and meta-analysis. *Lancet Infect Dis* 10: 317–28.
Idro R, Ndiritu M, Ogutu B, et al. (2007) Burden, features, and outcome of neurological involvement in acute falciparum malaria in Kenyan children. *JAMA* 297: 2232–40.
Jmor F, Emsley HC, Fischer M, et al. (2008) The incidence of acute encephalitis syndrome in Western industrialised and tropical countries. *Virol J* 5: 134.
Liu L, Johnson HL, Cousens S, et al. (2012) Global, regional, and national causes of child mortality: an updated systematic analysis for 2010 with time trends since 2000. *Lancet* 379: 2151–61. doi: 10.1016/S0140-6736(12)60560-1.
Murray CJ, Vos T, Lozano R, et al. (2012) Disability-adjusted life years (DALYs) for 291 diseases and injuries in 21 regions, 1990–2010: a systematic analysis for the Global Burden of Disease Study 2010. *Lancet* 380: 2197–223.
O'Brien KL, Wolfson LJ, Watt JP, et al. (2009) Burden of disease caused by *Streptococcus pneumoniae* in children younger than 5 years: global estimates. Lancet 374: 893–902.
Palmer BS (2007) Meta-analysis of three case controlled studies and an ecological study into the link between cryptogenic epilepsy and chronic toxoplasmosis infection. *Seizure* 16: 657–63.
Prasad KN, Chawla S, Jain D, et al. (2002) Human and porcine *Taenia solium* infection in rural north India. *Trans R Soc Trop Med Hyg* 96: 515–6.

Stahl JP, Mailles A, Dacheux L, Morand P (2011) Epidemiology of viral encephalitis in 2011. *Med Mal Infect* 41: 453–64.

UNAIDS (2013) *Global Report: UNAIDS Report on the Global AIDS Epidemic 2013. Joint United Nations Programme on HIV/AIDS (UNAIDS).* Geneva: UNAIDS (online: http://www.unaids.org/en/resources/ campaigns/globalreport2013/globalreport).

Watt JP, Wolfson LJ, O'Brien KL, et al. (2009) Burden of disease caused by *Haemophilus influenzae* type b in children younger than 5 years: global estimates. *Lancet* 374: 903–11.

White NJ, Pukrittayakamee S, Hien TT, et al. (2013) Malaria. *Lancet* Aug 14, pii: S0140-6736(13)60024.

WHO (2011) Epidemiology of meningitis caused by *Neisseria meningitidis*, *Streptococcus pneumoniae*, and *Haemophilus influenzae*. In: *Laboratory Methods for the Diagnosis of Meningitis Caused by Neisseria meningitidis, Streptococcus pneumoniae, and Haemophilus influenzae. WHO Manual, 2nd edn.* Geneva: World Health Organization (online: http://www.cdc.gov/meningitis/lab-manual/chpt02-epi.pdf).

2
PATHOGENESIS OF CENTRAL NERVOUS SYSTEM INFECTIONS

Diane E Griffin

Central nervous system (CNS) infections are generally uncommon complications of a wide variety of infectious diseases caused by viruses, bacteria, parasites and fungi. Development of CNS disease is influenced by the age and genetic background of the person infected and by the neurotropism and neurovirulence of the infecting organism. The nervous system is relatively well protected from infection by the barriers that regulate exchange between the blood, cerebrospinal fluid (CSF) and nervous system tissue. The blood–brain barrier (BBB) is a physical and functional barrier that inhibits diffusion of microbes, toxins, water-soluble molecules and cells from the blood into the parenchyma of the brain and spinal cord through a system involving specialized endothelial cells, pericytes and astrocytes (Bernacki et al. 2008, Kim 2008, Engelhardt and Sorokin 2009). The interstitial fluid of the nervous system is in communication with the CSF (Abbott et al. 2010), and the epithelial cells of the choroid plexus form a barrier between the blood and CSF (Engelhardt and Sorokin 2009). Both the BBB and blood–CSF barrier inhibit entry of pathogens into the CNS from the blood, so the ability to enter and initiate infection in the CNS (neurotropism) is an important property of pathogens that cause CNS disease.

The most frequent modes of pathogen entry are across the BBB endothelial cells into the brain parenchyma, across the permeable vessels of the choroid plexus into the CSF or from the periphery through retrograde transport by the axons that extend to muscle or skin. The first two pathways require the pathogen to enter the blood from the initial site of infection, while the third (neuronal transport) does not. There are a number of mechanisms by which infectious agents cross the BBB (Fig. 2.1) (Combes et al. 2012).

Many neurological infections demonstrate age-dependent susceptibility and tend to be more common and more severe in the young (Chang et al. 2007, Idro et al. 2007, Modlin 2007, Watt et al. 2009). This increased severity of disease in children can be due to multiple factors including lack of previous immunity, immaturity of the immune system (Siegrist and Aspinall 2009), higher pathogen replication in immature cells (Vernon and Griffin 2005) and immaturity of the BBB (Schoderboeck et al. 2009). In addition, many genetic defects in host resistance (e.g. severe combined immunodeficiency, agammaglobulinaemia, complement deficiencies) become manifest in children as they are progressively exposed to and

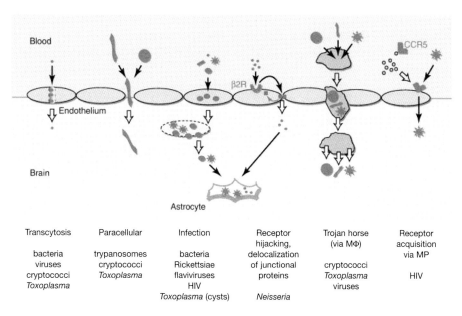

Transcytosis	Paracellular	Infection	Receptor hijacking, delocalization	Trojan horse (via MΦ)	Receptor acquisition
bacteria	trypanosomes	bacteria	of junctional		via MP
viruses	cryptococci	Rickettsiae	proteins	cryptococci	
cryptococci	*Toxoplasma*	flaviviruses		*Toxoplasma*	HIV
Toxoplasma		HIV		viruses	
		Toxoplasma (cysts)	*Neisseria*		

Fig. 2.1. Mechanisms by which pathogens cross the brain endothelial monolayer. The various biological mechanisms that can be used by pathogens to cross the blood–brain barrier are shown in black, and examples of some pathogens implementing these mechanisms are shown in red. The β2 adrenergic receptor (β2R) and the chemokine receptor, CCR5, are given as examples; several other receptors are known to serve as tools for central nervous system invasion. MP, microparticles. (Reproduced by permission from Combes et al. 2012.) A colour version of this figure is available in the plate section at the end of the book.

infected with different pathogens, some of which will cause neurological disease.

Once within the CNS, different anatomical and cellular sites can be targeted for infection, and these sites are important determinants of disease. Infection of the leptomeninges or CSF is usually accompanied by inflammation leading to meningitis. Entry into and infection of the brain parenchyma is more likely to result in encephalitis with seizures, delirium, and impairment of consciousness and cognition. Direct functional and lytic damage to cells of the CNS and the intensity of the inflammatory response often determine the severity of the symptoms (Gonzalez-Scarano and Martin-Garcia 2005, Myint et al. 2007). Much of our knowledge of the pathogenesis of nervous system infections has come from studies of experimentally infected animals.

Blood–brain and blood–cerebrospinal fluid barriers

BLOOD–BRAIN BARRIER

The BBB limits exposure of the CNS to circulating proteins, chemicals, cells and pathogens. It consists of highly specialized endothelial cells, pericytes embedded in the adjacent basement membrane and the foot processes of astrocytes. The distinct properties of BBB endothelial cells include a network of tight junctions, an intrinsic low level of pinocytosis, specialized transport mechanisms and limited expression of adhesion molecules. The tight junctions encircle the cells and consist of three types of integral membrane proteins: claudin, occluding, and junction adhesion molecules. Cytoplasmic accessory proteins (e.g. zonula occludens proteins [ZO-1, 2, 3], 7H6, cingulin) link the membrane proteins to the actin cytoskeleton. Adherens junction proteins (e.g. cadherin, β-catenin) help to regulate tight junctions. Tight junctions limit paracellular diffusion of hydrophilic molecules, confer polarity to the cells and are represented morphologically as the zona occludens where membranes are fused (Bernacki et al. 2008).

The BBB is induced and maintained by astrocytes with thickened cytoplasmic appendices that form end-feet that attach to blood vessels on one side and neurons on the other. These specialized perivascular end-feet contain high densities of aquaporin 4 and the Kir4.1 K^+ channel, and are associated with an agrin-rich basal lamina that surrounds the vessels. The signals required for BBB formation and maintenance are incompletely understood (Bernacki et al. 2008).

In addition to tight junctions that restrict paracellular diffusion, cerebral endothelial cells also have very low pinocytotic activity and lack fenestrations, thus restricting transcellular passage of molecules. The functional barrier also includes permanently active specialized transport systems for entry of essential nutrients (e.g. glucose and amino acids) and receptors for endocytosis of larger molecules (e.g. insulin, transferrin). These systems exclude molecules detrimental to neural transmission (Bernacki et al. 2008, Abbott et al. 2010).

BLOOD–CEREBROSPINAL FLUID BARRIER

The morphological correlates of the BBB for the blood–CSF barrier are the apical tight junctions between choroid plexus epithelial cells that limit paracellular diffusion of water-soluble molecules. In contrast to the BBB, the choroid plexus capillaries are fenestrated and allow free movement of molecules across endothelial cells. The epithelial cells also produce the CSF. This secretory function is maintained by expression of transport systems that direct ions and nutrients into the CSF and toxic substances out (Engelhardt and Sorokin 2009).

IMMUNE RESPONSES IN THE CENTRAL NERVOUS SYSTEM

Because of the restrictions to entry of proteins and cells, the CNS has been considered an immune privileged site. In general, small, lipophilic, hydrophobic and positively charged molecules enter the CNS most readily, but protein concentrations are low compared to plasma (Griffin and Giffels 1982). For instance, the levels of immunoglobulin and complement proteins in the CSF and brain interstitial fluid are approximately 1% that of plasma. There is limited expression of adhesion molecules, but activated lymphocytes can cross into the perivascular space where pericytes, the local antigen-presenting cells, reside.

Although pericytes and other macrophage lineage cells can present antigen to primed T cells, infections of the CNS are generally initiated in the periphery, and the activation of naive T cells and B cells occurs in secondary lymphoid tissues outside the CNS (Harling-

Berg et al. 1999). The entry of circulating leukocytes into the CNS is generally restricted by the BBB, but activated T cells routinely enter the CNS as part of the normal immunological surveillance of all tissues (Wekerle et al. 1986, Irani and Griffin 1996). Activated T cells that enter the CNS are not retained in the CNS in the absence of antigen, and either leave or die in situ. However, activated T cells are retained in the CNS when the relevant antigen is present and associated with appropriate MHC (major histocompatibility complex) molecules (Irani and Griffin 1996).

BARRIER CHANGES DURING INFECTION
The BBB is a dynamic system, and dysfunction that accompanies many CNS infections can range from mild transient tight-junction opening to chronic barrier breakdown (Abbott et al. 2010). The expression, subcellular distribution and post-translational modification of tight-junction proteins can change in response to cell signalling and infection (Persidsky et al. 2006a, Chaudhuri et al. 2008). During a systemic immune response, even in the absence of infection in the CNS, circulating cytokines upregulate expression of adhesion molecules by CNS endothelial cells, and surveillance of the CNS by activated T cells is increased (Hickey 2001). During CNS inflammation, local production of cytokines and chemokines can produce a loss of tight junctions and further increase expression of adhesion molecules by endothelial cells. These changes enhance the entry of activated cells into the CNS (Alt et al. 2002) and result in higher levels of protein in the CSF and brain parenchyma (Verma et al. 2010).

Entry of pathogens into the central nervous system
Pathogens may cross into the CNS through the BBB endothelial cells transcellularly or paracellularly, as cell-free organisms or within infected cells. Pathogens that frequently infect the CNS generally have specialized mechanisms for entry, but for many organisms these mechanisms are not fully understood.

VIRUSES
Viruses are obligate intracellular parasites, and the type of cell in which replication occurs is an important determinant of neurovirulence and of the mode of entry into the CNS. For viruses that enter the CNS from the blood, replication at the initial site of infection must be sufficiently robust to deliver either cell-free infectious virus or virus-infected cells to the bloodstream in amounts that facilitate interaction with the CNS. For viruses that enter by retrograde axonal transport, specialized mechanisms for neuronal synaptic uptake and transport to the cell body for replication are necessary. These pathways can be used simultaneously and are not mutually exclusive.

PLASMA VIRAEMIA
Enterovirus and arbovirus infections are associated with plasma viraemias, and these viruses are most likely to enter the CNS from the blood. Initial replication for the neurotropic enteroviruses (e.g. poliovirus, Coxsackie virus, echovirus, enterovirus 71) is in the gastrointestinal

tract. Initial replication for the arthropod-borne flaviviruses (e.g. West Nile virus, Japanese encephalitis virus, tick-borne encephalitis virus) and alphaviruses (e.g. eastern, western and Venezuelan equine encephalitis viruses) occurs at or near the site of the bite of the infecting insect. Amplification often occurs in local lymphoid tissue, muscle or brown fat. For each of these viruses, spread to the CNS correlates with the height of viraemia (Samuel and Diamond 2006, Griffin 2007). The presence of neutralizing antibody in plasma from residual maternal antibody, vaccination or previous infection is effective at preventing CNS infection and disease.

Some viruses that enter the CNS from the blood can infect the luminal surface of brain endothelial cells, replicate and be released toward the parenchyma to initiate infection of neurons or glial cells (Dropulic and Masters 1990, Verma et al. 2009). Virus particles may also be able to pass through endothelial cells without replicating (Dropulic and Masters 1990). Poliovirus entry into cerebrovascular endothelial cells is mediated by virus interaction with an adhesion molecule that is the poliovirus receptor (CD155). This interaction triggers both a conformational change in the virus that leads to release of viral RNA, and receptor-induced activation of a signalling pathway that results in actin rearrangement and endocytosis of the virion (Coyne et al. 2007). West Nile virus infection of cerebrovascular endothelial cells induces expression of cell adhesion molecules important for entry of immune cells into the CNS (Verma et al. 2009). Although endothelial cell infection is assumed to be the route of entry for many enteroviruses and arboviruses, infected endothelial cells are rarely seen in CNS tissue sections at autopsy (German et al. 2006). This may be due to the transient nature of virus replication in endothelial cells that leaves minimal evidence of infection at the time of clinical disease (Verma et al. 2009).

CELL-ASSOCIATED VIRAEMIA

For some viruses that infect the CNS (e.g. measles virus, cytomegalovirus, human immunodeficiency virus [HIV]), entry into the CNS is most likely to be in concert with the entry of infected cells ('Trojan horse' approach) (Mahadevan et al. 2007). These viruses infect leukocytes and activated lymphocytes, and monocytes that are often more susceptible to infection than resting cells (Yanagi et al. 2006, Haller and Fackler 2008). Activated cells can cross the normal BBB as part of normal surveillance mechanisms (Wekerle et al. 1991, Irani and Griffin 1996), facilitating spread of infection to the CNS.

AXONAL TRANSPORT

Axonal transport systems are important for movement of trophic factors, vesicles and organelles to and from the neuron cell body and the periphery. These transport systems can be hijacked by pathogens, prion proteins and toxins (e.g. tetanus toxin) for entry into the CNS (Butowt and von Bartheld 2003, von Bartheld 2004). Transport is accomplished by the microtubule-dependent motors dynein and kinesin (Goldstein and Yang 2000). Dynein drives retrograde transport of cargo-laden vesicles, including neurotrophins, from the periphery to the cell body (Butowt and von Bartheld 2003, Cosker et al. 2008). The dynein motor-domain protein associates with a complex of intermediate chains, light intermediate chains, light chains and a dynactin complex for transport of cargo. Cargo-transport speci-ficity and direction can be influenced by post-translational modification of the cargo. These mechanisms also facilitate transfer of trophic factors, toxins and pathogens within the nervous system across multiple synapses (von Bartheld 2004).

Viruses for which axonal transport is the most important route of entry into the CNS include rabies virus and the herpesviruses (e.g. herpes simplex and varicella-zoster viruses) (Diefenbach et al. 2008). Other viruses that infect neurons, including poliovirus and West Nile virus, may use both viraemic and neural transport routes for entry (Samuel et al. 2007). For retrograde transported viruses there is local replication at the site of inoculation and then interaction with axons either at neuromuscular junctions or at sites of sensory innervation (McGraw and Friedman 2009). Receptor-mediated endocytosis that leads to neuronal uptake of virions occurs at axon terminals. A variation on this theme is the ability of some organisms to be transported from the nasal epithelium to the CNS by olfactory neurons (Charles et al. 1995).

Rabies virus undergoes limited replication in local muscle after the bite of a rabid ani-mal and is then taken up by motor neurons for transport to the CNS. A number of rabies virus receptors present at the neuromuscular junction have been identified and include the nicotinic acetylcholine receptor, the neurotrophin receptor p75, the NR1 NMDA receptor and neural cell adhesion molecule (NCAM) (Butowt and von Bartheld 2003, Ugolini 2008). The relative importance of individual receptors in vivo is not clear. The rabies virus phosphoprotein interacts with the dynein light-chain LC8, important both for microtubule-directed organelle transport and actin-based vesicle transport in axons, and represents a possible mode of transport. After arrival in the nervous system, rabies virus moves trans-synaptically along neuronal pathways.

For herpes simplex virus, retrograde transport is from skin or mucosal sites of primary infection. After entering sensory nerve terminals, the surface glycoproteins are left behind in the cell membrane, many outer tegument proteins (proteins lining the space between the envelope and nucleocapsid) are phosphorylated and dissociate from the virion (Morrison et al. 1998), and the capsid, along with a few tegument proteins, binds to dynein motors for transport to the cell body (Cunningham et al. 2006). The capsid protein pUL35 binds the dynein light-chain Tctex-1, but transport is facilitated by interaction of a tegument protein with the motor complex (Diefenbach et al. 2008).

For poliovirus, the cytoplasmic domain of the cellular receptor, CD155, interacts with the dynein light-chain Tctex-1 of the retrograde motor complex. This provides a mechanism for virus-containing vesicles to be transported to the motor neuron cell body (Mueller et al. 2002).

Bacteria

Meningitis is the most common CNS bacterial infection of children. Organisms generally gain access to the subarachnoid space from the blood, although occasionally there can be contiguous spread from a focal site of infection (e.g. otitis media, mastoiditis, sinusitis) or a direct connection between the subarachnoid space and the external environment, e.g. fistula or myelomeningocele. Development of bacteraemia begins with colonization of the nasopharyngeal mucosa, followed by tissue invasion, and then survival and multiplication in the blood.

COLONIZATION AND INVASION

Colonization of the respiratory tract requires adherence to epithelial cells and evasion of local host defense mechanisms. Adherence is mediated by bacterial fimbriae (e.g. *Neisseria meningitidis*) or cell-wall components, such as choline-binding proteins (e.g. *Streptococcus pneumoniae*). Meningococcal pili bind to integrins or CD46 on nonciliated columnar epithelial cells and proliferate on the cell surface. Pseudopodia are induced that engulf the bacteria for internalization into a membranous vacuole and transcytosis for eventual dissemination into the bloodstream (Stephens 2009).

To evade the effects of secretory IgA, colonizing *N. meningitidis*, *S. pneumoniae* and *Haemophilus influenzae* secrete endopeptidases that cleave the heavy chain of IgA1 at the hinge region. This separates the antigen recognition (Fab) function from the effector (Fc) function and the released Fab fragments bind to the bacteria and prevent subsequent recognition by intact antibodies (Poulsen et al. 1989, Kilian et al. 1996).

The major barrier to invasion is the ciliated respiratory mucosa, so anything that compromises the function of this barrier (e.g. previous viral infection of the respiratory tract) will increase susceptibility. Bacteria can penetrate the mucosa through (e.g. *N. meningitidis*) or between (e.g. *H. influenzae*) epithelial cells. Bacterial factors that facilitate mucosal invasion include those that degrade the extracellular matrix (e.g. hyaluronidase produced by *S. pneumoniae*) (Jedrzejas 2004).

BACTERAEMIA

The primary virulence factor for survival and multiplication in the blood stream is the polysaccharide capsule (Kim et al. 1992, Stephens 2009). Bacterial capsules prevent complement-mediated lysis and neutrophil phagocytosis. Capsules also reduce activation of the alternative complement pathway that deposits C3b on the bacterial surface by expression of sialic acid to resemble host polysaccharides and binding of serum factors that regulate complement activation. These properties contribute to the induction of a high degree of bacteraemia. The best host defense against these antiphagocytic properties of the bacterial capsule is the presence of antibodies to capsular polysaccharides that facilitate efficient phagocytosis and are the basis for vaccine-induced protection.

CENTRAL NERVOUS SYSTEM ENTRY

The magnitude of the bacteraemia is correlated with the likelihood of meningeal infection (Kim et al. 1992, Kim 2003, Xie et al. 2004). Infection requires attachment to endothelial cells and can be initiated at vessels in the brain, leptomeninges or the highly vascular choroid plexus. Several bacterial pathogens that cause meningitis in children (e.g. *Escherichia coli* K1, group B streptococcus, *S. pneumoniae*, *Listeria*, *N. meningitidis*, *Mycobacterium tuberculosis*) can attach to endothelial cells through specific receptor–ligand interactions and directly traverse the BBB without evidence of disruption of intercellular tight junctions (Xie et al. 2004, Kim 2008, Pulzova et al. 2009). This process of transcytosis of nonphagocytic cells requires bacterial attachment and penetration of the cells. Multiple bacterial proteins may participate in this process. For instance, the FimH and OmpA *E. coli* K1 proteins are involved in binding to brain endothelial cells, and CNF1 (cytotoxic necrotizing factor 1) is important for invasion (Kim 2003). Cell-wall phosphorylcholine is important for the pneumococcus, internalin B for *Listeria*, and outer membrane protein Opc for the meningococcus.

Bacterial attachment to cellular receptors triggers rearrangements of the host-cell actin cytoskeleton. For *E. coli* K1, OmpA binding of gp96 results in activation of focal adhesion kinase and PI3 kinase, while CNF1 interacts with the 37kDa laminin receptor precursor to activate RhoA. Specific receptors and ligands used vary with the pathogens, but exhibit some overlap (Kim 2008). Pneumococcal phosphorylcholine interacts with the platelet-activating factor receptor, and *Listeria* internalin B (InlB) interacts with the complement component receptor gC1q-r and with Met tyrosine kinase (Kim 2006). *Streptococcus agalactiae* binds endothelial cells through the laminin-binding protein (Lmb), fibrinogen-binding protein (FbsA) and invasion-associated gene (IagA). Endothelial cell invasion by *Listeria* depends on src kinases. Cytokines such as tumour necrosis factor alpha (TNFα) and transforming growth factor beta (TGFβ) can modulate expression of cellular receptors and influence microbial entry into the CNS. Cell protrusions are formed at sites of contact with the bacteria and internalization is through a zipper mechanism. Once inside the cell, the bacteria are in membrane-bound vacuoles that do not fuse with lysosomes and thus avoid degradation and result in live delivery to the CNS (Kim 2008).

In addition to transcytosis, spirochaetes may be able to use a paracellular route of entry. Intracellular pathogens (e.g. *M. tuberculosis*, *Listeria*) can also cross into the CNS within infected phagocytes, as well as across endothelial cells (Kim 2008).

Parasites

Trypanosomes cause sleeping sickness by penetrating the brain from the blood. These large extracellular organisms may penetrate the CSF by paracellular penetration of BBB endothelial cells (Pulzova et al. 2009) or through areas where the BBB is poorly formed, e.g. choroid plexus. Interferon-γ plays an important role in regulating entry by making the endothelial cells resistant to penetration.

The pathogenesis of cerebral malaria is complicated and not well understood. Parasitized erythrocytes adhere to a number of ligands on microvascular endothelium, e.g. gC1q-r, but do not invade the brain. Attachment activates NFkB inflammatory pathways and induces adhesion molecule expression on the endothelial cells (Tripathi et al. 2007, 2009). Sequestration of parasitized red blood cells within postcapillary venules, along with cytokine induction and BBB damage, results in vascular obstruction, impaired perfusion and hypoxia, leading to seizures and coma (Idro et al. 2010).

Fungi

Fungaemia precedes invasion of the CNS by *Cryptococcus neoformans*, and the site of entry appears to be cerebral capillaries rather than the choroid plexus. Binding to CD44 on endothelial cells requires the *CPS1* gene. Transcellular traversal of brain endothelial cells has been reported both for *Candida albicans* and *C. neoformans*, suggesting that this may be an important mechanism by which these organisms enter the CNS (Chang et al. 2004, Kim 2006).

Development of disease: pathogen replication and inflammation in the central nervous system

INFLAMMATION

Once the pathogen has entered the CNS, innate intracellular and/or extracellular host pathways of pathogen recognition (e.g. toll-like receptors, RNA helicases, NOD receptors, mannose receptor, etc.) will be activated to induce local cytokine (e.g. interferon, IL-1β, TNFα, IL-6) and chemokine (e.g. IL-8, MCP-1, IP-10) production (Mogensen et al. 2006). These mediators attract inflammatory cells to the site of infection and increase adhesion molecule expression on endothelial cells. For bacteria these signalling pathways are distinct from those used for transcytosis of endothelial cells (Kim 2008).

Interaction of neutrophils and monocytes with endothelial cells induces a signalling cascade that increases intracellular Ca^{++} and activation of endothelial-cell Rho GTPases to modulate the actin cytoskeleton and induce the degradation of junction components to enhance paracellular leukocyte migration and increase BBB permeability (Persidsky et al. 2006b). Bacterial infections tend to attract neutrophils, while viral infections tend to attract lymphocytes and monocytes to the CNS.

VIRAL MENINGITIS AND ENCEPHALOMYELITIS

Once within the CNS, the cellular tropism of the virus will be an important determinant of the disease. Most common, particularly for enteroviruses, is infection of the leptomeninges to cause aseptic meningitis. Poliovirus, enterovirus 71, herpesviruses, and the encephalitic alphaviruses and flaviviruses can cause meningitis, but have a predilection for infection of neurons (Johnson et al. 1985, German et al. 2006). Different types of neurons may be targeted and infection can induce dysfunction or death. When motor neurons of the spinal cord are infected (e.g. poliovirus, West Nile virus), infection can cause flaccid paralysis. If neurons of the basal ganglia are infected, parkinsonian symptoms may result. Neuronal infection also tends to lead to seizures and cognitive impairment. Neurological sequelae are common.

BACTERIAL MENINGITIS

Because of the restrictions of the BBB, the subarachnoid space is deficient in the antibacterial host defenses found in blood with low levels of antibody, complement and phagocytic cells. Therefore, once bacteria reach the CSF, they multiply efficiently and can extend into the brain parenchyma along penetrating blood vessels. Infection leads to induction of cytokines, chemokines, matrix metalloproteinases and arachadonic acid metabolites, and breakdown of the BBB with an influx of neutrophils into the subarachnoid space. The consequences of these pathological processes can be vascular occlusion, decreased cerebral blood flow, release of excitotoxic amino acids and reactive oxygen species, oedema, increased intracranial pressure and neuronal damage (Kim 2003).

Summary

Infections of the CNS involve a complicated interplay between host and pathogen to allow entry and replication of viruses, bacteria, parasites or fungi in the nervous system. Infection must first be established at the site of pathogen infection in the periphery, and then enter the CNS either via the blood or by retrograde axonal transport. The CNS is protected from invasion from the bloodstream by the blood–brain and blood–CSF barriers. Organisms have developed attachment and transport mechanisms for passing through or around these barriers. Once within the CNS, host defenses are less available than in the periphery, and infection can result in severe consequences for the host.

REFERENCES

Abbott NJ, Patabendige AA, Dolman DE, et al. (2010) Structure and function of the blood–brain barrier. *Neurobiol Dis* 37: 13–25.
Alt C, Laschinger M, Engelhardt B (2002) Functional expression of the lymphoid chemokines CCL19 (ELC) and CCL 21 (SLC) at the blood–brain barrier suggests their involvement in G-protein-dependent lymphocyte recruitment into the central nervous system during experimental autoimmune encephalomyelitis. *Eur J Immunol* 32: 2133–44.
Bernacki J, Dobrowolska A, Nierwinska K, Malecki A (2008) Physiology and pharmacological role of the blood–brain barrier. *Pharmacol Rep* 60: 600–22.
Butowt R, von Bartheld CS (2003) Connecting the dots: trafficking of neurotrophins, lectins and diverse pathogens by binding to the neurotrophin receptor p75NTR. *Eur J Neurosci* 17: 673–80.
Chang LY, Huang LM, Gau SS, et al. (2007) Neurodevelopment and cognition in children after enterovirus 71 infection. *N Engl J Med* 356: 1226–34.
Chang YC, Stins MF, McCaffery MJ, et al. (2004) Cryptococcal yeast cells invade the central nervous system via transcellular penetration of the blood–brain barrier. *Infect Immun* 72: 4985–95.
Charles PC, Walters E, Margolis F, Johnston RE (1995) Mechanism of neuroinvasion of Venezuelan equine encephalitis virus in the mouse. *Virology* 208: 662–71.
Chaudhuri A, Yang B, Gendelman HE, et al. (2008) STAT1 signaling modulates HIV-1-induced inflammatory responses and leukocyte transmigration across the blood–brain barrier. *Blood* 111: 2062–72.
Combes V, Guillemin GI, Chan-Ling T, et al. (2012) The crossroads of neuroinflammation in infectious diseases: endothelial cells and astrocytes. *Trends Parasitol* 28: 311–9.
Cosker KE, Courchesne SL, Segal RA (2008) Action in the axon: generation and transport of signaling endosomes. *Curr Opin Neurobiol* 18: 270–5.
Coyne CB, Kim KS, Bergelson JM (2007) Poliovirus entry into human brain microvascular cells requires receptor-induced activation of SHP-2. *EMBO J* 26: 4016–28.
Cunningham AL, Diefenbach RJ, Miranda-Saksena M, et al. (2006) The cycle of human herpes simplex virus infection: virus transport and immune control. *J Infect Dis* 194 Suppl 1: S11–8.
Diefenbach RJ, Miranda-Saksena M, Douglas MW, Cunningham AL (2008) Transport and egress of herpes simplex virus in neurons. *Rev Med Virol* 18: 35–51.
Dropulic B, Masters CL (1990) Entry of neurotropic arbovirus into the central nervous system: an in vitro study using mouse brain endothelium. *J Infect Dis* 161: 685–91.
Engelhardt B, Sorokin L (2009) The blood–brain and the blood–cerebrospinal fluid barriers: function and dysfunction. *Semin Immunopathol* 31: 497–511.
German AC, Myint KS, Mai NT, et al. (2006) A preliminary neuropathological study of Japanese encephalitis in humans and a mouse model. *Trans R Soc Trop Med Hyg* 100: 1135–45.

Goldstein LS, Yang Z (2000) Microtubule-based transport systems in neurons: the roles of kinesins and dyneins. *Annu Rev Neurosci* 23: 39–71.

Gonzalez-Scarano F, Martin-Garcia J (2005) The neuropathogenesis of AIDS. *Nat Rev Immunol* 5: 69–81.

Griffin DE (2007) Alphaviruses. In: Knipe DL, Howley PM, Griffin DE, et al., eds. *Field's Virology.* Philadelphia: Lippincott Williams & Wilkins, pp. 1023–67.

Griffin DE, Giffels J (1982) Study of protein characteristics that influence entry into cerebrospinal fluid of normal mice and mice with encephalitis. *J Clin Invest* 70: 289–95.

Haller C, Fackler OT (2008) HIV-1 at the immunological and T-lymphocytic virological synapse. *Biol Chem* 389: 1253–60.

Harling-Berg CJ, Park TJ, Knopf PM (1999) Role of the cervical lymphatics in the Th2-type hierarchy of CNS immune regulation. *J Neuroimmunol* 101: 111–27.

Hickey WF (2001) Basic principles of immunological surveillance of the normal central nervous system. *Glia* 36: 118–24.

Idro R, Ndiritu M, Ogutu B, et al. (2007) Burden, features, and outcome of neurological involvement in acute falciparum malaria in Kenyan children. *JAMA* 297: 2232–40.

Idro R, Marsh K, John CC, Newton CRJ (2010) Cerebral malaria: mechanisms of brain injury and strategies for improved neuro-cognitive outcome. *Pediatr Res* 68: 267–74; doi: 10.1203/PDR.0b013e3181eee738.

Irani DN, Griffin DE (1996) Regulation of lymphocyte homing into the brain during viral encephalitis at various states of infection. *J Immunol* 156: 3850–7.

Jedrzejas MJ (2004) Extracellular virulence factors of *Streptococcus pneumoniae*. *Front Biosci* 9: 891–914.

Johnson RT, Burke DS, Elwell M, et al. (1985) Japanese encephalitis: immunocytochemical studies of viral antigen and inflammatory cells in fatal cases. *Ann Neurol* 18: 567–73.

Kilian M, Reinholdt J, Lomholt H, et al. (1996) Biological significance of IgA1 proteases in bacterial colonization and pathogenesis: critical evaluation of experimental evidence. *APMIS* 104: 321–38.

Kim KS (2003) Pathogenesis of bacterial meningitis: from bacteraemia to neuronal injury. *Nat Rev Neurosci* 4: 376–85.

Kim KS (2006) Microbial translocation of the blood–brain barrier. *Int J Parasitol* 36: 607–14.

Kim KS (2008) Mechanisms of microbial traversal of the blood–brain barrier. *Nat Rev Microbiol* 6: 625–34.

Kim KS, Itabashi H, Gemski P, et al. (1992) The K1 capsule is the critical determinant in the development of Escherichia coli meningitis in the rat. *J Clin Invest* 90: 897–905.

Mahadevan A, Shankar SK, Satishchandra P, et al. (2007) Characterization of human immunodeficiency virus (HIV)-infected cells in infiltrates associated with CNS opportunistic infections in patients with HIV clade C infection. *J Neuropathol Exp Neurol* 66: 799–808.

McGraw HM, Friedman HM (2009) Herpes simplex virus type 1 glycoprotein E mediates retrograde spread from epithelial cells to neurites. *J Virol* 83: 4791–9.

Modlin JF (2007) Enterovirus déjà vu. *N Engl J Med* 356: 1204–5.

Mogensen TH, Paludan SR, Kilian M, Ostergaard L (2006) Live *Streptococcus pneumoniae, Haemophilus influenzae*, and *Neisseria meningitidis* activate the inflammatory response through Toll-like receptors 2, 4, and 9 in species-specific patterns. *J Leukoc Biol* 80: 267–77.

Morrison EE, Wang YF, Meredith DM (1998) Phosphorylation of structural components promotes dissociation of the herpes simplex virus type 1 tegument. *J Virol* 72: 7108–14.

Mueller S, Cao X, Welker R, Wimmer E (2002) Interaction of the poliovirus receptor CD155 with the dynein light chain Tctex-1 and its implication for poliovirus pathogenesis. *J Biol Chem* 277: 7897–904.

Myint KS, Gibbons RV, Perng GC, Solomon T (2007) Unravelling the neuropathogenesis of Japanese encephalitis. *Trans R Soc Trop Med Hyg* 101: 955–6.

Persidsky Y, Heilman D, Haorah J, et al. (2006a) Rho-mediated regulation of tight junctions during monocyte migration across the blood–brain barrier in HIV-1 encephalitis (HIVE). *Blood* 107: 4770–80.

Persidsky Y, Ramirez SH, Haorah J, Kanmogne GD (2006b) Blood–brain barrier: structural components and function under physiologic and pathologic conditions. *J Neuroimmun Pharmacol* 1: 223–36.

Poulsen K, Brandt J, Hjorth JP, et al. (1989) Cloning and sequencing of the immunoglobulin A1 protease gene (iga) of *Haemophilus influenzae* serotype b. *Infect Immun* 57: 3097–105.

Pulzova L, Bhide MR, Andrej K (2009) Pathogen translocation across the blood–brain barrier. *FEMS Immunol Med Microbiol* 57: 203–13.

Samuel MA, Diamond MS (2006) Pathogenesis of West Nile Virus infection: a balance between virulence, innate and adaptive immunity, and viral evasion. *J Virol* 80: 9349–60.

Samuel MA, Wang H, Siddharthan V, et al. (2007) Axonal transport mediates West Nile virus entry into the central nervous system and induces acute flaccid paralysis. *Proc Natl Acad Sci U S A* 104: 17140–5.

Schoderboeck L, Adzemovic M, Nicolussi EM, et al. (2009) The "window of susceptibility" for inflammation in the immature central nervous system is characterized by a leaky blood–brain barrier and the local expression of inflammatory chemokines. *Neurobiol Dis* 35: 368–75.

Siegrist CA, Aspinall R (2009) B-cell responses to vaccination at the extremes of age. *Nat Rev Immunol* 9: 185–94.

Stephens DS (2009) Biology and pathogenesis of the evolutionarily successful, obligate human bacterium *Neisseria meningitidis*. *Vaccine* 27 Suppl 2: B71–7.

Tripathi AK, Sullivan DJ, Stins MF (2007) Plasmodium falciparum-infected erythrocytes decrease the integrity of human blood–brain barrier endothelial cell monolayers. *J Infect Dis* 195: 942–50.

Tripathi AK, Sha W, Shulaev V, et al. (2009) *Plasmodium falciparum*-infected erythrocytes induce NF-kappaB regulated inflammatory pathways in human cerebral endothelium. *Blood* 114: 4243–52.

Ugolini G (2008) Use of rabies virus as a transneuronal tracer of neuronal connections: implications for the understanding of rabies pathogenesis. *Dev Biol (Basel)* 131: 493–506.

Verma S, Lo Y, Chapagain M, et al. (2009) West Nile virus infection modulates human brain microvascular endothelial cells tight junction proteins and cell adhesion molecules: transmigration across the in vitro blood–brain barrier. *Virology* 385: 425–33.

Verma S, Kumar M, Gurjav U, et al. (2010) Reversal of West Nile virus-induced blood–brain barrier disruption and tight junction proteins degradation by matrix metalloproteinases inhibitor. *Virology* 397: 130–8. doi: 10.1016/j.virol.2009.10.036.

Vernon PS, Griffin DE (2005) Characterization of an in vitro model of alphavirus infection of immature and mature neurons. *J Virol* 79: 3438–47.

von Bartheld CS (2004) Axonal transport and neuronal transcytosis of trophic factors, tracers, and pathogens. *J Neurobiol* 58: 295–314.

Watt JP, Wolfson LJ, O'Brien KL, et al. (2009) Burden of disease caused by Haemophilus influenzae type b in children younger than 5 years: global estimates. *Lancet* 374: 903–11.

Wekerle H, Linington C, Lassman H, Meyermann R (1986) Cellular immune reactivity within the CNS. *Trends Neurosci* 9: 271–7.

Wekerle H, Engelhardt B, Risau W, Meyerman R (1991) Interaction of T lymphocytes with cerebral endothelial cells in vitro. *Brain Pathol* 1: 107–14.

Xie Y, Kim KJ, Kim KS (2004) Current concepts on *Escherichia coli* K1 translocation of the blood–brain barrier. *FEMS Immunol Med Microbiol* 42: 271–9.

Yanagi Y, Takeda M, Ohno S (2006) Measles virus: cellular receptors, tropism and pathogenesis. *J Gen Virol* 87: 2767–79.

3
THE PRINCIPLES OF MANAGEMENT OF CENTRAL NERVOUS SYSTEM INFECTIONS

Sunit Singhi

Infections of the central nervous system (CNS) can be caused by several micro-organisms. However, regardless of aetiology, most children with CNS infection have similar clinical presentations and complications, and therefore many of the principles of management are common.

Reduction in mortality and long-term morbidity from CNS infection is critically dependent on rapid diagnosis, prompt initiation of appropriate antimicrobials and of supportive and adjunctive therapy, and management of complications that occur early (e.g. raised intracranial pressure, seizures and status epilepticus) and late (e.g. hydrocephalus, focal neurological deficits, psychomotor delay and sensorineural hearing loss). These are challenging goals, because of non-specific initial symptoms, limitation in obtaining cerebrospinal fluid (CSF) for diagnosis, pharmacokinetic barriers in achieving effective concentrations of antimicrobials in the CNS, emerging resistance to available antimicrobials, limited availability of effective antiviral drugs, and lack of adjunctive therapies to block the pathophysiological mechanisms and prevent complications. These issues are even more challenging in resource-poor settings due to infrastructural or administrative limitations.

Evaluation and diagnosis
The evaluation of a patient suspected of having a CNS infection aims to arrive at an aetiological diagnosis based on clinical features, CSF analysis, neuroimaging and serological tests. Clinical features seldom help in distinguishing between bacterial meningitis and the viral encephalitides. However, no isolated clinical feature is diagnostic, and it is not clear which combination of clinical features can provide the most accurate diagnosis (Best and Hughes 2008, Curtis et al. 2010). Some viruses can have characteristic presentations, such as parotitis associated with mumps, and aero- and hydrophobia associated with rabies. Characteristic clinical signs associated with different viral encephalitides in children are listed in Table 3.1.

CEREBROSPINAL FLUID ANALYSIS
CSF analysis is the cornerstone of definitive diagnosis of CNS infection, and a lumbar puncture must be done as early as possible in a suspected case of meningitis unless contra-

TABLE 3.1
Clinical clues to viral encephalitis

Symptoms/signs	Probable causative virus
Rash	Entero, adeno, measles
Conjunctivitis	Adeno, measles, entero70
Parotitis	Mumps, entero, Epstein–Barr, HIV
Pharyngitis	Adeno, entero, Epstein–Barr. Other respiratory viruses
Adenopathy	Epstein–Barr, CMV
Pneumonia	Measles, adeno, influenza, measles, varicella, CMV, dengue
Enteritis	Entero
Hepatitis	Adeno, CMV, varicella, Epstein–Barr
Aero- and hydrophobia	Rabies
Behaviour changes, temporal lobe seizures	Herpes simplex

HIV, human immunodeficiency virus; CMV, cytomegalovirus.

TABLE 3.2
Contraindications for lumbar puncture

1 Signs of elevated intracranial pressure (ICP) secondary to a suspected mass lesion of the brain or spinal cord (fundus examination for papilloedema, and head CT to rule out raised ICP are mandatory before proceeding with a lumbar puncture in such cases)

2 Symptoms and signs of pending cerebral herniation (decerebrate or decorticate posture, abnormal pupil size and reaction, ocular palsies, absence of the oculocephalic response and fixed oculomotor deviation of the eyes, and respiratory abnormalities)

3 Critically ill/moribund patient: bradycardia or irregular respirations (lumbar puncture is temporarily withheld because the procedure may precipitate cardiorespiratory arrest)

4 Focal neurological deficits

5 Sedation or muscle paralysis

6 Skin infection at the site of the lumbar puncture

7 Significant thrombocytopenia (platelet count <20 000/mm^3 may cause uncontrolled bleeding in the subarachnoid or subdural space)

indicated (Table 3.2). Analysis of CSF should include white cell count and differential, glucose and protein concentrations along with Gram stain and cultures, and depending upon suspected underlying infections, stain for acid-fast bacilli and other studies. Simultaneously the blood glucose level needs to be measured. Routine computerized tomography (CT) of the head before lumbar puncture is not necessary and may delay the commencement of antimicrobial therapy. CT before lumbar puncture is required in patients with clinical features suggestive of an intracranial mass lesion or elevated intracranial pressure such as those with a rapidly deteriorating level of consciousness, coma, focal neurological deficits, seizures,

TABLE 3.3

Typical cerebrospinal fluid assay findings in various central nervous system infections

CNS infection	Opening pressure (mmH$_2$O)	White blood cell count (cells/mm^3)	Protein (mg/dL)	Glucose (mg/dL)
Normal	50–80	Neonates: usually up to 5; may be 20–30 / Children: 0–5; ≥75% lymphocytes	Neonates: up to 120, falls by 3 months / Children: 10–40	>50 (or 60% blood glucose)
Bacterial meningitis	Usually high (100–300)	Elevated (100–10000 or more), usually 200–2000; PMNs predominate	Usually 100–500	Decreased, usually <40 (or <50% blood glucose)
Partially treated bacterial meningitis	Normal or high	5–10000; PMNs usual but mononuclear cells may predominate if treated for long period of time	Usually 100–500	Normal or decreased
Viral meningitis or meningoencephalitis	Normal or slightly high (80–150)	10–500; lymphocytes predominate, sometimes PMNs in early phase	Usually 50–200	Generally normal; may be decreased <40 in mumps (15%–20% of cases)
Tubercular meningitis	Usually high	Normal to elevated (10–500); PMNs early but lymphocytes predominate rest of the course	100–3000; may be higher in presence of block	<50 in most cases; decreases with time if not treated
Fungal meningitis	Usually high	Normal to elevated (5–500); lymphocytes predominate	25–500	<50 in most cases; decreases with time if not treated
Brain abscess	Usually high (100–300)	Normal to elevated (5–200); rarely acellular; lymphocytes predominate	75–500	Normal unless ruptures into ventricular system
Ventriculitis	Usually high	Elevated (100–5000); PMNs predominate	Elevated	Decreased
Subdural empyema	Usually high (100–300)	100–5000; PMNs predominate	100–500	Normal

PMN, polymorphonuclear leukocyte.

22

papilloedema, and brainstem signs (bradycardia or irregular respiratory pattern). In such patients antimicrobials are started empirically before neuroimaging is obtained.

Normal CSF in children has 0–5 mononuclear cells/mm^3; neutrophils are seen very rarely. Presence of even a single neutrophil in the clinical setting of meningitis should be considered significant. Normal neonatal CSF contains up to five white blood cells/mm^3. Mild pleocytosis can be found in infants with non-specific symptoms without CNS infection (Martín-Ancel et al. 2006). A CSF absolute neutrophil cell count above 1000/mm^3 is highly predictive of bacterial meningitis (Berkley et al. 2001, Lussiana et al. 2011). CSF lympho-cytosis is seen in aseptic meningitis, tubercular and fungal meningitis, demyelinating disease, brain or spinal cord tumour, and immunological disorders including collagen vascular disease. CSF pleocytosis may be absent in patients with severe overwhelming sepsis and meningitis, and in immune-compromised and severely undernourished children, and is a poor prognostic sign. Typical CSF findings in various forms of CNS infections are shown in Table 3.3.

In viral CNS infection there is normal-to-mild increase of opening CSF pressure, CSF lymphocytosis (neutrophils if tested early), a white cell count of 50–2000/mm^3, normal glucose and mildly elevated protein. Herpes simplex (HSV-1) encephalitis is often associated with elevated CSF red cell count, typically 10–15 erythrocytes per high-power field. The presence of more erythrocytes in CSF indicates a traumatic tap or a subarachnoid haemorrhage. Progressive clearing of blood from CSF during collection and clear supernatant of centrifuged CSF specimen suggests a traumatic tap. A xanthochromic supernatant without progressive clearing indicates subarachnoid haemorrhage. The presence of crenated red blood cells does not differentiate a traumatic tap from a subarachnoid haemorrhage.

The normal ratio of CSF to blood glucose is above 0.6 in term neonates and above 0.4 in children. A lowering of CSF glucose (hypoglycorrhachia) is seen in diffuse meningeal disease, particularly bacterial or tubercular meningitis, and in metabolic conditions. It may also occur in subarachnoid haemorrhage, fungal meningitis, and occasionally aseptic meningitis. A reduced absolute CSF glucose (<40mg/dL or <2.2mmol/L) is highly sensitive and specific for bacterial meningitis (Berkley et al. 2001). Smears for Gram stain should be obtained from centrifuged sediment; however, if the CSF is cloudy, fresh uncentrifuged specimen can be used. Gram stain is positive in a large majority of cases of meningitis caused by *Streptococcus pneumoniae*, *Haemophilus influenzae* and *Neisseria meningitidis*, and in about 50% of those caused by gram-negative bacilli. False-positive Gram stain may occur rarely from reagent or skin flora contamination.

Culture of the CSF gives a specific diagnosis in over 80% of patients with bacterial meningitis. Inadequate facilities for collection, storage and transport of CSF may be a cause of the low positivity rates seen in resource-poor countries. In cases with negative culture of CSF, attention must be paid to a positive blood culture.

Previous antimicrobial therapy may decrease the likelihood of getting a positive bacterial culture but it does not significantly affect CSF white blood cell count, percentage of lymphocytes and neutrophils, or frequency of positive Gram stains up to 24 hours (Nigrovic et al. 2008).

Bacterial antigen detection tests such as the latex agglutination test (LAT) may be useful for patients pretreated with antimicrobials in whom the CSF Gram stain is negative; LAT is positive in 50%–100% of cases depending on the organism; it has a specificity of 96% and 100% in *S. pneumoniae* and *N. meningitidis* respectively, but a lower sensitivity, varying from 69% to 100% for *S. pneumoniae* and from 37% to 70% for *N. meningitidis*. Routine use of LAT in CNS infections has been questioned (Nigrovic et al. 2004). A negative LAT result does not exclude the specific infection and therefore does not appear to modify the decision to give antibiotics. Elevated serum procalcitonin (>5µg/L) (Dubos et al. 2008), CSF lactate above 35mg/dL, and serum C-reactive protein above 50mg/dL may be useful to differentiate between bacterial and aseptic meningitis. A low C-reactive protein (<10mg/dL) has a high negative predictive value for bacterial meningitis.

Bacterial and viral DNA detection by polymerase chain reaction (PCR) for common organisms is available and is undergoing refinement. Broad-range real-time bacterial DNA detection PCR, multiplex PCR and DNA sequencing for diagnosis of bacterial meningitis allow detection of virtually all pathogenic bacteria, with a sensitivity of 86%–100% and a specificity of 98% (Wang et al. 2012). Similarly, multiplex PCR DNA microarray has been found useful for diagnosis of viral CNS infections (Leveque et al. 2011).

NEUROIMAGING STUDIES

Neuroimaging studies are imperative for the diagnosis of many CNS infections and their complications; the subject is discussed in Chapter 4. CT is most commonly used because it is widely available. It is useful for diagnosis of tubercular meningitis and granulomas, and for detection of complications of bacterial meningitis. Magnetic resonance imaging (MRI) is sensitive for early detection of parenchymal involvement and for differentiating various types of encephalitis that have characteristic neuroimaging patterns (such as herpes simplex and Japanese encephalitis), as well as for the diagnosis of acute disseminated encephalitis. The use of sophisticated MRI techniques helps in distinguishing bacterial, fungal and tubercular abscesses. Magnetic resonance venography is indicated in suspected cerebral venous sinus thrombosis. Spinal MRI should be performed urgently in patients with suspected myelopathy, especially transverse myelitis and spinal epidural abscess. It may also help in the diagnosis of rabies.

Familiarity with the clinical course and imaging appearances of various CNS diseases is helpful in making correct differential diagnoses and in prompting timely treatment.

Emergency management

AIRWAY AND BREATHING

In unconscious patients, airway patency should be ensured by proper positioning of the head and suctioning of oral secretions to prevent hypoxaemia and hypercapnia. Oro- or nasopharyngeal airways can be used; forceful opening of clenched jaws should be avoided. The stomach should be decompressed by early insertion of nasogastric tube to prevent aspiration.

Oxygen can be started with a non-rebreathing mask, and if needed, bag-valve mask ventilation, to ensure adequate oxygenation. Children with a Glasgow Coma Scale (GCS) score of 8 or under often have significant pharyngeal hypotonia, poor gag reflex and loss of swallowing reflex, all of which can lead to upper-airway obstruction and aspiration. If there are signs of inadequate ventilation and oxygenation, such as irregular respiratory efforts, inadequate chest movements, poor air entry, respiratory distress, central cyanosis or peripheral oxygen staturation of 92% or less, endotracheal intubation should be done. An endotracheal tube may be necessary even in situations where ventilation is adequate.

Rapid sequence induction accompanied by cricoid pressure (Sellick manoeuvre) is preferred for emergency intubation to prevent aspiration and sudden surge in intracranial pressure (ICP). Thiopental, lidocaine or a short-acting non-depolarizing neuromuscular blocking agent (e.g. vecuronium, atracurium) can be used for such induction.

HAEMODYNAMIC STABILIZATION AND MANAGEMENT

Vascular access should be immediately established for administration of fluids, anticonvulsants and antibiotics. Patients with signs of poor perfusion or hypotension should receive a bolus of normal saline (20mL/kg) before continuing with the rest of the assessment and management. Rapid rehydration should be avoided. All emergency medication and fluids that are given intravenously can be administered by intraosseous route if needed, especially in children below 6 years of age.

HYPERTENSION

Increase in blood pressure is common in acute CNS infections. The causes include pain, agitation, and Cushing response to raised ICP (i.e. widening of pulse pressure with an increase in systolic blood pressure, bradycardia and irregular breathing). Systemic hypertension may increase cerebral blood flow and ICP when autoregulation is impaired, which may promote cerebral oedema. Moderate elevation of blood pressure in the acute stage often resolves with sedation and does not require antihypertensive medication. Treatment is indicated in patients with impending congestive cardiac failure, those with evidence of rapidly worsening brain oedema on CT, or an extreme surge in blood pressure, which may persist. Nonetheless, the decision to use antihypertensive medication has to be individualized. Vasodilators, such as nitroprusside, nitroglycerine and nifedipine, should be avoided as they can increase ICP. Beta-blockers or central acting α-receptor agonists are preferred because they reduce blood pressure without worsening ICP.

After stabilization in the emergency room, patients should be assessed and those in need of intensive care should be transferred to an intensive care unit. Clinical signs that suggest the need for admission to an intensive care unit are shown in Table 3.4.

Specific treatment

All patients suspected of having bacterial meningitis are started on antibiotics as soon as possible. Ceftriaxone is the initial choice in immunocompetent children beyond neonatal age. Prompt administration of antimalarials is required for children with severe malaria in endemic areas.

TABLE 3.4
Clinical signs that suggest need for admission to the intensive care unit

1 Glasgow Coma Scale score ≤8	9 Abnormal posturing
2 Airway instability	10 Impaired papillary response
3 Poor/irregular respiratory effort	11 Abnormal doll-eye response
4 Respiratory distress	12 Abnormal motor response
5 Hyperventilation	13 Focal neurodeficits
6 Poor perfusion/hypotension	14 Cranial nerve palsy
7 Oliguria/anuria	15 Seizures
8 Hypertension/bradycardia	16 Bleeding diathesis

Herpes simplex viral encephalitis is treated with aciclovir; cytomegalovirus and human herpesvirus 6 encephalitis with a combination of ganciclovir and foscarnet; and severe adenovirus infections with cidofovir or ribavirin. Life-threatening enterovirus infections have been treated successfully with pleconaril.

General supportive care

NURSING CARE
Clinical evaluation and monitoring of patients includes assessment of level of consciousness, and the detection of new neurological signs, seizures, agitation and pain. Changes in neurological condition may be subtle. Important nursing care components include mouth, skin and eye care; checking urinary catheters, nasogastric tubes and intravascular catheters; dressing changes for monitoring devices; appropriate body positioning; and respiratory care.

POSITIONING OF COMATOSE PATIENTS
A neutral or side-lying position should be adopted, with a pillow between the legs to prevent internal rotation, adduction and inversion of the upper leg. It is important to guard against compression at the elbows to protect the ulnar nerve. 'Proper alignment' of the patient includes a dorsal (supine) position, the head in neutral position, arms flexed at the elbow with the hands resting at the side of the abdomen, knees slightly flexed, with rolls of padding folded under the greater trochanter–hip joint area to reduce pressure on the peroneal nerve at the fibula head, the feet at 70–90° to the legs, and the toes pointing upward.

Comatose patients with marked extensor posturing are difficult to position. Footboards and splints are not useful, because they apply stretch and potentially further increase the tone. In patients with hemiparesis the head and neck should be in midline. A pillow is placed in the axilla to counter the tendency of the arm to adduct and rotate internally. The paralysed arm is supported on a pillow with the elbow partially flexed. Trochanter rolls are used to prevent external rotation at the hip joint. In the lateral position, patients should be turned on the unaffected side without flexion of the trunk/spine. Extension, adduction and internal rotation of the shoulder should be avoided.

SEDATION AND ANALGESIA

Children with acute CNS infections are often uncomfortable or agitated, particularly if they are mechanically ventilated. Pain is expressed not only by moaning, crying, grimacing and extreme restlessness, but also by profuse sweating, tachycardia, fluctuating blood pressure and dilated pupils. Agitation, pain and anxiety increase the cerebral metabolic rate and ICP, and should be prevented with appropriate sedation and adequate analgesia. Use of distractors (music, television, family) can reduce pain.

There are no specific protocols or randomized studies to indicate the best choice of medication or dosing in children with acute neurological injury. Opioid analgesics (morphine 0.1mg/kg, 4–6 hourly) remain the mainstay of pain management, especially in patients for whom sedation is unacceptable. Nonsteroidal anti-inflammatory agents are useful in patients with severe headaches. An appropriate sedative should have minimum effect on blood pressure and ICP, and recovery from sedation should be rapid. Drugs that cause hypotension and raised ICP (e.g. ketamine) are contraindicated. Benzodiazepines are commonly used sedatives. Selection of shorter-acting agent midazolam (0.2mg/kg bolus followed by infusion at a rate of 2–3µg/kg/min) or propofol (0.1mg/kg/min with incremental doses at 5min intervals until reasonable sedation) in older children may have the advantage of allowing brief interruption of sedation to examine neurological status. Effect of midazolam can also be rapidly reversed with flumazenil (0.2–0.4mg IV over 15 seconds). Hypovolaemia should be corrected before administering sedatives.

Fluid, electrolytes and nutrition

Most children with CNS infections have alteration in their fluid and electrolyte homeostasis that needs correction. Fever, diminished intake and vomiting may lead to dehydration and hypovolaemia; sepsis-induced capillary leak can further worsen the situation. Dehydration often unveils in the form of a sudden fall in blood pressure when patients are placed on a mechanical ventilator.

The main goals of fluid therapy are to maintain euvolaemia and normoglycaemia, and to prevent hyponatraemia. Empirical fluid restriction to two-thirds of normal maintenance has been practised by many paediatricians under the assumption that hyponatraemia in most children with CNS infections results from the syndrome of inappropriate secretion of antidiuretic hormone (SIADH). It has been argued that SIADH may lead to free water retention, hypo-osmolarity and hyponatraemia, which worsen cerebral oedema and raised ICP in these children. However, available evidence does not justify this practice. In a prospective study in children with acute meningitis, high ADH levels returned to normal on fluid administration, suggesting that elevation of ADH is an appropriate response to hypovolaemia (Powell et al. 1990). In animal models of bacterial meningitis, fluid restriction did not improve brain oedema but caused lowering of blood pressure and cerebral blood flow, and led to cerebral ischaemia (Tureen et al. 1992). In randomized controlled clinical trials, fluid restriction did

TABLE 3.5
Differential diagnosis of hyponatraemia in central nervous system disease

	Cerebral salt wasting	Syndrome of inappropriate antidiuretic hormone secretion
Intravascular volume	↓	↑ or normal
Salt balance	Negative	Variable
Water balance	Negative	↑ or normal
Signs and symptoms of dehydration	Present	Absent
Central venous pressure	↓	↑ or normal
Serum osmolality	↓	↓
Haematocrit	↑ or normal	Unchanged
Plasma creatinine	↑ or normal	↓
Urine sodium	↑↑	↑
Urine volume	↑↑	↓ or normal
Treatment	Normal saline, hypertonic saline, fludrocortisone	Fluid restriction. hypertonic saline, democycline, furosemide

not improve the outcome of acute meningitis in children (Singhi et al. 1995).

A Cochrane database systematic review concluded that, at least for settings with high mortality rates and where patients present late, evidence supports giving normal maintenance intravenous fluids rather than fluid restriction in the first 48 hours (Maconochie et al. 2008). Therefore, daily maintenance plus replacement fluids aimed at maintaining normovolaemia, normal urine output (>1mL/kg/h) and normal blood pressure, and thereby adequate cerebral perfusion, are recommended. All fluids should be isotonic; hypotonic fluids should be avoided.

Approximately 25% of patients with bacterial meningitis develop hyponatraemia. The aetiology can be multifactorial, such as salt wasting, SIADH, aggressive hydration or adrenal insufficiency. Hyponatraemia should be identified early and corrected slowly over 36–48 hours to maintain serum sodium at 135–140mmol/L, with serial monitoring of serum electrolytes. It is important to differentiate SIADH from cerebral wasting (Table 3.5), since the management is different.

Hypokalaemia may occur secondary to gastrointestinal losses, haemodilution, osmotherapy, diuretic therapy and associated septicaemia, and requires prompt correction. Both hyperglycaemia and hypoglycaemia should be avoided.

Rarely, acute CNS infection may lead to diabetes insipidus because of hypothalamic and/or pituitary involvement; it is generally associated with poor prognosis.

Enteral feeding is preferably started within 72 hours of hospital admission. Early enteral feeding is associated with a dramatic decrease in duration of stay in the intensive care unit and complications. Children with acute neurological injury have caloric needs 30%–60% greater than their basal metabolic rate, and should be supplemented accordingly.

Seizures and status epilepticus

Seizures are common in CNS infections. They may be generalized or focal, and may progress to status epilepticus in a substantial proportion of children especially those under 2 years of age. This could be detrimental to the already compromised brain, because it increases oxygen and metabolic demand, and leads to increased cerebral blood flow and cerebral blood volume, which can worsen the raised ICP.

Early, aggressive and prompt treatment of seizures and status epilepticus is essential for prevention of secondary brain injury. A pre-designed protocol helps in a methodical management (Fig. 3.1). Immediate termination of seizures is achieved with intravenous administration of benzodiazepines. Intravenous lorazepam, diazepam or midazolam can be used; all three drugs have onset of action within 1–3 minutes of administration and they are equally effective. However, since the duration of action of lorazepam is much longer (24–48 hours) as compared to diazepam (15–30 minutes), lorazepam is often preferred. The dose can be repeated after 5–10 minutes if seizures persist.

If seizures continue, phenytoin or fosphenytoin infusion is used with cardiac monitoring to avoid hypotension and cardiac arrhythmia. Maintenance dose of 5–8mg/kg/d should be given in two divided doses after 12–24 hours of initial loading dose.

Phenobarbital (loading dose 15–20mg/kg) is generally preferred over phenytoin in neonates and in status epilepticus associated with fever that has not responded to benzodiazepines. However, there is no evidence to substantiate this preference.

Persistence of seizures even after adequate treatment with benzodiazepines and phenytoin and/or phenobarbital, is referred to as refractory status epilepticus. It is common in CNS infections, but there is little consensus regarding the standard protocol for management of refractory status epilepticus.

BARBITURATE COMA

About 10% of children with CNS infection may need thiopental infusion to control refractory status epilepticus (Singhi et al. 2004). Facility for mechanical ventilation and invasive arterial blood pressure monitoring should be available if thiopental infusion is planned. The initial dose is 3–4mg/kg IV over 2 minutes, followed by infusion of 0.2mg/kg/min. The rate is increased every 3–5 minutes by 0.1mg/kg/min until status epilepticus is controlled or a burst–suppression EEG recording is obtained. The infusion is continued for about 6 hours after seizures are controlled. Complications such as respiratory depression, hypotension, delayed recovery and risk of ventilator-associated pneumonia are the major limitations of thiopental infusion.

Intravenous sodium valproate, levetiracetam, midazolam, diazepam and propofol infusions have been used before going on to thiopental infusion. We use sodium valproate as it is free of adverse effects such as respiratory depression and hypotension and is therefore useful in a resource-limited setting where facilities for ventilation and intensive care are not easily available (Mehta et al. 2007). It has a rapid onset of action and there is no time lag between peak serum and peak brain concentration. Levetiracetam also does not cause respiratory depression and hypotension, and may be a good alternative to valproate. However,

Child with seizures 0–5 minutes

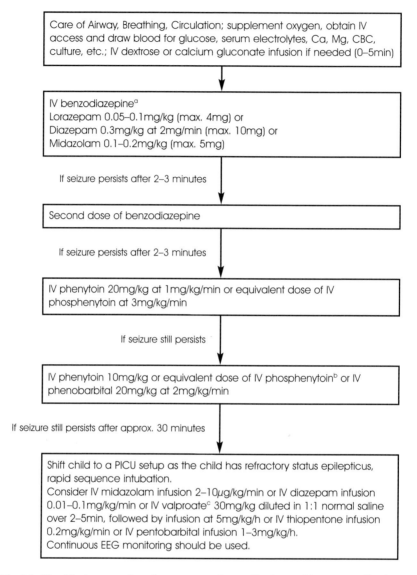

Fig. 3.1. Algorithmic approach to the treatment of generalized convulsive status epilepticus.
[a]If IV access is not immediately available; intramuscular midazolam, intranasal lorazepam and rectal diazepam are the alternatives. Intraosseous route may also be used.
[b]If IV access is not available, phosphenytoin may be given intramuscularly.
[c]Used particularly when ventilation facilities are not available; avoid in children with suspected metabolic or hepatic disorders.
IV, intravenous; CBC, complete blood count; PICU, paediatric intensive care unit; EEG, electroencephalography.

further studies are needed to establish the efficacy of both these drugs in different settings.

Etomidate, lidocaine and ketamine infusions have also been used for resistant seizures. However, these drugs have side-effects, and randomized trials are needed to recommend their use in paediatric age-groups.

Raised intracranial pressure

The majority of hospitalized patients with CNS infection have intracranial hypertension at initial presentation or develop it within 48 hours of admission. Raised ICP is an important cause of mortality. The pathogenesis in CNS infection is multifactorial. Early increase in ICP is primarily due to inflammatory cytotoxic oedema, infarction, and increased capillary permeability in brain parenchyma (vasogenic oedema) and subarachnoid space, and rarely because of early hydrocephalus. Later, raised ICP is contributed by ventriculitis, subdural effusion, basal exudates and obstructed or communicating hydrocephalus, especially in purulent meningitis and tubercular meningitis.

Raised ICP compromises cerebral blood flow (CBF) and causes ischaemic injury to the brain, leading to progressive brain injury. With impaired autoregulation, CBF becomes a direct function of cerebral perfusion pressure (CPP) and highly sensitive to rise in ICP or fall in mean arterial blood pressure. In a study on bacterial meningitis, decreased CBF was seen in 80% of infants in the first 48 hours. The decrease was 30%–70% in one-third of patients, predominantly in subcortical white matter, and was associated with poor outcome (Menamin and Volpe 1984).

The management goals in patients with raised ICP are to prevent brain herniation, break the vicious cycle of raised ICP and cerebral ischaemia at the earliest, and maintain an adequate CPP. Normal CPP values for children are not clearly established, but generally accepted minimum CPP values are 50–60mmHg in older children and 40–50mmHg in infants and toddlers. Much of this data is extrapolated from studies on patients with traumatic brain injury, but some corroboration comes from studies in children with CNS infection and raised ICP (Shetty et al. 2008, Singhi et al. 2014). Protocols for the management of raised ICP are presented in Figure 3.2.

INTRACRANIAL PRESSURE MONITORING

Clinical symptoms of increased ICP such as headache, nausea and vomiting are impossible to elicit in comatose patients. Papilloedema is uncommon in acute infections, even in patients with documented elevated ICP. Clinical signs that are helpful indicators of raised ICP are abnormal posturing, pupillary dilatation, fluctuating heart rate (bradycardia) and hypertension, abnormal respiratory pattern (periodic breathing, hyperventilation) and a GCS score below 8; these correlate well with raised ICP and decreased CPP, but occur late. CT findings of brain swelling and compressed basal cisterns are predictive of increased ICP, but intracranial hypertension can occur without these findings. Therefore, ICP monitoring for the initial 24–48 hours, where feasible, can be helpful in maintaining adequate CBF and CPP in children with CNS infection who have a GCS score of 8 or less or abnormal CT findings (Singhi et al. 2011). The goals of ICP monitoring are to maintain ICP below

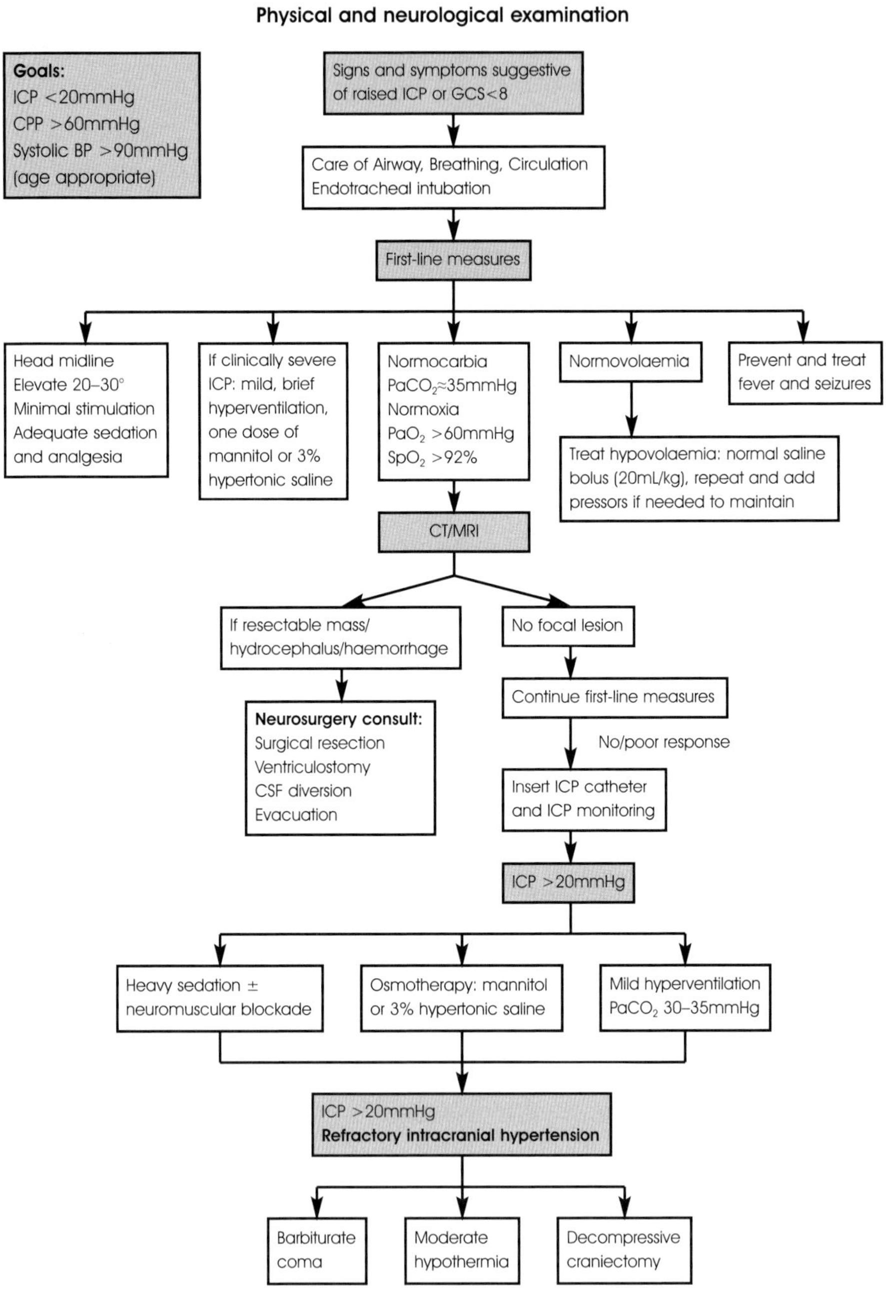

Physical and neurological examination

Goals:
ICP <20mmHg
CPP >60mmHg
Systolic BP >90mmHg
(age appropriate)

Signs and symptoms suggestive
of raised ICP or GCS<8

Care of Airway, Breathing, Circulation
Endotracheal intubation

First-line measures

Head midline
Elevate 20–30°
Minimal stimulation
Adequate sedation
and analgesia

If clinically severe
ICP: mild, brief
hyperventilation,
one dose of
mannitol or 3%
hypertonic saline

Normocarbia
PaCO₂≈35mmHg
Normoxia
PaO₂ >60mmHg
SpO₂ >92%

Normovolaemia

Prevent and treat
fever and seizures

Treat hypovolaemia: normal saline
bolus (20mL/kg), repeat and add
pressors if needed to maintain

CT/MRI

If resectable mass/
hydrocephalus/haemorrhage

No focal lesion

Neurosurgery consult:
Surgical resection
Ventriculostomy
CSF diversion
Evacuation

Continue first-line measures

No/poor response

Insert ICP catheter
and ICP monitoring

ICP >20mmHg

Heavy sedation ±
neuromuscular blockade

Osmotherapy: mannitol
or 3% hypertonic saline

Mild hyperventilation
PaCO₂ 30–35mmHg

ICP >20mmHg
Refractory intracranial hypertension

Barbiturate
coma

Moderate
hypothermia

Decompressive
craniectomy

Fig. 3.2. Management of raised intracranial pressure (ICP).
CPP, cerebral perfusion pressure; BP, blood pressure; GCS, Glasgow Coma Score; CT, computerized tomography; MRI, magnetic resonance imaging; CSF, cerebrospinal fluid.

20mmHg and CPP above 50–60mmHg by manipulating blood pressure and ICP, and to keep in check the factors that aggravate or precipitate elevated ICP.

GENERAL MEASURES

Prevention or treatment of factors that may aggravate ICP is essential. These include pain, agitation, hypoxia, hypercapnia, fever, severe hypertension, hyponatraemia, anaemia and seizures. A patent airway and normal blood pressure should be maintained in all patients. In intubated patients suctioning should be done only if necessary, using a bolus of lidocaine (1mg/kg IV) before suction to dampen the ICP surge.

Positioning

The patient should lie comfortably with the head elevated 20–30° and kept in midline to promote venous drainage via the external jugular veins. When head elevation is used, the pressure transducers for blood pressure and ICP must be zeroed at the same level.

Fever

Fever increases metabolic rate by 10%–13% per degree Celsius and induces dilation of cerebral vessels with increase in CBF and ICP. Fever should be controlled with antipyretics (IV or rectal paracetamol) and tepid sponging.

Anaemia

Severe anaemia contributes to increased ICP through increase in CBF and relative hypoxia. The common practice is to maintain haemoglobin concentration around 10g/dL. However, optimal haemoglobin concentration in patients with raised ICP needs further study (Kramer and Zygun 2009).

Prevention of seizures

Seizures occur commonly in association with raised ICP, irrespective of underlying aetiology, and worsen the raised ICP. In comatose patients with raised ICP it is advisable to start continuous EEG monitoring for nonconvulsive seizures; phenytoin prophylaxis (5–8kg/d) is used by some.

HYPEROSMOLAR THERAPY

Mannitol

Mannitol is widely used for reduction of cerebral oedema. The usual dose is 0.25–0.5g/kg administered over 10–15 minutes repeated every 4–6 hours for 48–72 hours. For urgent reduction of ICP an initial dose up to 1g/kg may be given. Mannitol creates an ongoing osmotic gradient that reduces cerebral oedema and decreases intracranial volume. Mannitol also transiently expands intravascular volume and reduces viscosity and thereby improves CBF. When using mannitol, volume status needs to be carefully monitored because mannitol-induced diuresis can cause profound hypovolaemia and can adversely affect the outcome.

In our experience the use of mannitol in acute meningitis and clinically evident raised ICP was associated with increased risk of mortality among those who had polyuria (urine output exceeding 3mL/kg/h) (unpublished data). Serum osmolarity must be kept under 320mOsm/L; and serum sodium below 160meq/L. Higher osmolarity increases the risk of acute tubular necrosis and renal failure. Use of mannitol may also lead to rebound intracranial hypertension.

Hypertonic saline
The mechanism of action of hypertonic saline (3.0%–23.4%) is not fully clear, but it is likely that it has an osmotic effect similar to mannitol. We use 3% saline, in a loading dose of 10mL/kg over 30 minutes followed by 0.1–1mL/kg/h as continuous infusion. Serum osmolarity must be monitored and kept under 350mOsm/L. Hypertonic saline has been shown to achieve a greater reduction in ICP as compared to other hyperosmolar therapies in CNS infections (Gwer et al. 2010), although further studies are needed to confirm this.

HYPERVENTILATION
A short burst of hyperventilation, using bag-valve mask, is good enough for emergency reduction of raised ICP in children who present with signs of imminent or impending herniation. Prolonged hyperventilation can result in vasoconstriction, reduced CBF and increased risk of ischaemia. Hyperventilation lasting more than an hour has been associated with poor long-term outcome. However, mild hyperventilation ($PaCO_2$ 32–35mmHg) can be used when other measures to decrease ICP are not effective. This is done mainly by increasing respiratory rate, while maintaining normal tidal volume (8–10mL/kg). End-tidal CO_2 can be used to monitor CO_2 and to guard against sudden reduction in pCO_2. Weaning from hyperventilation is done gradually to prevent rebound rise of ICP.

HEAVY SEDATION AND PARALYSIS
A commonly used regimen is morphine and lorazepam for analgesia and sedation, and cisatracurium or vecuronium as a muscle relaxant, with dose titrated by twitch response to stimulation. The major problem with this therapy is that the neurological examination cannot be monitored closely because the neuromuscular block eliminates motor activity. These children should have continuous EEG monitoring.

BARBITURATE COMA
Barbiturates reduce the cerebral metabolic rate and lower ICP. However, they can also cause significant hypotension threatening cerebral perfusion. High-dose therapy is an option in haemodynamically stable patients with intracranial hypertension refractory to other interventions. Thiopental is given in a loading dose of 5mg/kg over 30 minutes followed by infusion of 1–5mg/kg/h until EEG shows a burst–suppression pattern. There is no evidence to support the use of barbiturates for prophylactic neuroprotection or for prevention of the development of intracranial hypertension in children with acute neurological injury.

CEREBROSPINAL FLUID DRAINAGE

This can be done if a ventriculostomy is present. Lumbar drains are effective in reducing ICP in adults and children, but should be used only when the basal cisterns are visible on imaging. In a two-centre study, in paediatric traumatic brain injury, continuous CSF drainage was associated with higher CSF volume drainage and lower ICP than was seen with intermittent drainage (Shore et al. 2004).

DECOMPRESSIVE CRANIECTOMY

This may be needed for control of raised ICP refractory to medical treatment, in patients with fulminant cerebral oedema such as in severe viral encephalitis (Adamo and Deshaies 2008).

CONTINUOUS PERFUSION PRESSURE VERSUS INTRACRANIAL PRESSURE TARGETED PROTOCOLS

In cases where ICP monitoring is done, CPP targeted therapy aimed at maintaining CPP above 50mmHg may be useful (Shetty et al. 2008); a CPP below 40mmHg is associated with a high risk of death.

Adjunctive therapy

CORTICOSTEROIDS

Bacterial meningitis

The routine use of corticosteroids in meningitis is debated. Several studies from resource-rich countries have shown a reduction of audiological and neurological sequelae in patients who received dexamethasone, particularly in *Haemophilus* meningitis, and to some extent in pneumococcal meningitis. The American Academy of Pediatrics (2003) recommended empiric use of dexamethasone, 0.15mg/kg every 6 hours for 48 hours in bacterial meningitis if the organism is *H. influenzae* type, with the first dose given 15 minutes before the first dose of antibiotic. No beneficial effect of corticosteroid therapy has been found in resource-poor countries (Sankar et al. 2007, Brouwer et al. 2013). A meta-analysis of individual patient data from five trials including 2029 patients concluded that adjunctive dexamethasone does not significantly reduce death or neurological disability (van de Beek et al. 2010). The benefit of empiric use of dexamethasone needs to be reconsidered with the drastic reduction in *Haemophilus* type b meningitis in the USA and Europe following the widespread use of vaccination, and the emergence of pneumococcus as the dominant aetiological agent. Available evidence does not support the routine use of steroids in children with bacterial meningitis in resource-poor countries. Also, there are no data to support the use of adjunctive steroids in patients who have (1) nosocomial meningitis, (2) CSF shunt infection-related meningitis, (3) post-neurosurgical meningitis, or (4) neonatal bacterial meningitis.

Tubercular meningitis (see Chapter 14)

The use of adjunctive corticosteroid treatment in tubercular meningitis has been recommended for more than 50 years. There have been concerns that steroids reduce the penetration of antitubercular drugs into the CNS, cause gastrointestinal bleeding and, although they might save lives, increase the number of survivors with residual impairments; these concerns remain unsubstantiated. A recent Cochrane systematic review and meta-analysis of seven randomized controlled trials involving 1140 participants (with 411 deaths) concluded that corticosteroids reduced the risk of death or disabling residual neurological deficit in HIV-negative children and adults with tubercular meningitis (Prasad and Singh 2008). Adverse events included gastrointestinal bleeding, bacterial and fungal infections and hyperglycaemia, but these were mild and treatable. The benefit of corticosteroid treatment in tubercular meningitis in HIV-positive children remains uncertain.

Corticosteroids are advocated in patients with intracranial tuberculomas without meningitis or spinal-cord tuberculosis even though no controlled trials have examined their efficacy in this setting.

ORAL GLYCEROL

Glycerol has been used in reducing ICP in various neurosurgical and neurological disorders. A large double-blind randomized trial from six Latin American countries that involved 654 patients with bacterial meningitis between 2 months and 16 years of age found that oral glycerol (6g/kg/d) 6 hourly for 2 days, reduced severe neurological sequelae (Peltola et al. 2007). Oral glycerol increases plasma osmolarity in children with bacterial meningitis for the first 12–24 hours of treatment, which can reduce cerebral oedema and enhance cerebral circulation by reducing CSF formation (Singhi et al. 2008). A recent trial of oral glycerol in adults with bacterial meningitis in Malawi (a resource-poor setting with a high HIV prevalence) did not find any benefit of glycerol in reducing death or disability (Ajdukiewicz et al. 2011). A recent Cochrane analysis concluded that while glycerol may reduce audiological sequelae, it should not be used routinely during the treatment of acute bacterial meningitis (Wall et al. 2013). Further studies are needed to establish the role of glycerol.

ANTI-INFLAMMATORY THERAPY (STRATEGIES TO PREVENT NEURONAL DAMAGE)

Ongoing research into the pathophysiology of brain damage in bacterial meningitis (see Chapter 12) aims at providing the scientific basis for future development of more efficient adjunctive options. The pathogenetic mechanisms identified as targets for adjuvant therapy are as follows.

1 Bacterial killing coupled with prevention of associated release of bacterial components: bacteriolytic antibiotics (rifamycins, rifampicin, macrolides, clindamycin, ketolides, daptomycin and quinolones) combined with antibiotics that inhibit RNA/protein synthesis or DNA replication, reduce bacterial lysis.
2 Recognition of bacterial components, and modulation of the inflammatory reaction by adjuvant therapy to reduce leukocyte recruitment in the CSF.
3 Inhibition of inflammatory and/or neurotoxic mediators (antioxidants, trylizad-mesylate, matrix metalloproteinase inhibition, tumour necrosis factors and neutralization antibodies).

4 Modulation of apoptotic pathways (caspase inhibitors, exogenous brain-derived neuro-trophic factor).

Future research in antibiotic therapy for bacterial meningitis may focus on limiting the release of bacterial components, provided that a sufficiently rapid CSF sterilization can be achieved (Woehrl et al. 2011).

Mechanical ventilation
Patients with CNS infection may need mechanical ventilation because of impaired mechanics, impaired respiratory drive (apnoea, or ataxic or cluster breathing), or aspiration pneumonia that may cause hypoxaemia or hypercarbia. Depressed level of consciousness is not an absolute indication for ventilation. Hyperventilation in these patients may be a sign of hypoxia or an early signal of the development of diencephalic herniation. Impaired respiratory mechanics can occur because of neuromuscular failure involving diaphragm/intercostal muscles due to bulbar involvement or myelopathy. The signs suggestive of imminent neuromuscular failure are restlessness, tachycardia, tachypnoea, forehead sweating, paradoxical breathing, and weakness of trapezius and neck muscles. Aspiration occurs frequently in comatose patients, and in patients with acute bulbar dysfunction, repeated seizures and/or vomiting. Aspiration is rarely witnessed; patients often develop signs of respiratory distress and cough after 4–6 hours.

Settings of mechanical ventilation depend on the indication and condition of underlying lung. Ventilation is aimed at maintaining normoxia and normocarbia ($pCO_2 \approx 35mm/Hg$). In a patient with normal lung and impaired respiratory mechanics, the ventilator is set in synchronized intermittent mandatory ventilation (SIMV) mode with rate and tidal volume (8mL/kg) that are near-normal for age. Positive end expiratory pressure (PEEP) is maintained at 3–5mmHg, and the inspiratory:expiratory time ratio at 1:2 to 1:3; FiO_2 is set at 0.4 or more to achieve normoxia (PaO_2 60–80mmHg). Control mode is used in patients with impaired respiratory drive, refractory raised ICP, herniation and status epilepticus. Once the condition improves and spontaneous efforts appear, assist control or SIMV pressure support mode is appropriate. Patients having spontaneous hyperventilation may be served better by assisted mode of ventilation with mild sedation.

High PEEP can worsen ICP by impeding venous return and increasing cerebral venous pressure. PEEP at low-to-moderate levels is used. End-tidal CO_2 monitoring is recommended in all ventilated patients to guard against inadvertent CO_2 wash out or hypercarbia; both are detrimental.

Weaning from the ventilator should be gradual. Sudden transition may be stressful. Pressure-support weaning with gradual decrement may be preferred.

Isolation and infection precautions
CNS infections require strict isolation. These include rabies, varicella, measles and haemorrhagic fevers. Patients should be cared for in a separate room having negative-pressure air flow or laminar flow. Precautions to be observed include use of masks, gowns and gloves.

Strict hand-washing should be observed between visits to patients. Gloves should be worn for anticipated contact with blood, secretions and any moist body substances (body substance isolation). Gloves should be changed immediately after patient contact.

Patients requiring contact isolation include those with adenovirus, herpes simplex (disseminated) and major staphylococcal infections. Gowns, goggles and mask should be worn when secretions, blood or body fluids are likely to soil or splash on clothing, skin or face.

The patient's family

Many patients with CNS infections are not able to communicate or are comatose, and may rapidly worsen. The physician should anticipate a very complex physician–family relationship in the first 24 hours. The main goals are (1) clarification and explanation of the acute neurological disease; (2) discussion of the level of responsiveness of the patient; and (3) the expected progression or improvement in the first few days. One should avoid a discussion on possible long-term functional outcome.

Initially the family's assessment of prognosis can be more optimistic than that of the physician. It is ill-advised to express an exaggerated sense of hope and optimism in the first 24 hours. On the other hand, acute stress reaction that an acute neurological catastrophe may cause among some family members should be dealt with calmly. When no improvement in the neurological deficit is seen and the outlook for a meaningful recovery is remote, withdrawal of treatment and support must be discussed with the family.

In brief, management of CNS infection involves the complete range of diagnostic evaluation, emergency and neurocritical care, with specific attention to adjunctive therapies, fluid and electrolyte balance, observing infectious disease precautions and counselling of the stressed family. Attention to each aspect is necessary for improving outcome.

REFERENCES

Adamo MA, Deshaies EM (2008) Emergency decompressive craniectomy for fulminating infectious encephalitis. *J Neurosurg* 108: 174–6.
Ajdukiewicz KM, Cartwright KE, Scarborough M, et al. (2011) Glycerol adjuvant therapy in adults with bacterial meningitis in a high HIV seroprevalence setting in Malawi: a double-blind, randomised controlled trial. *Lancet Infect Dis* 11: 293–300.
American Academy of Pediatrics (2003) Red Book: 2003 Report of the Committee on Infectious Diseases – Subcommittee on dexamethasone therapy for bacterial meningitis in infants and children. Elk Grove, IL: American Academy of Pediatrics.
Berkley JA, Mwangi I, Ngetsa CJ, et al. (2001) Diagnosis of acute bacterial meningitis in children at a sub-Saharan district hospital. *Lancet* 357: 1753–7.
Best J, Hughes S (2008) Evidence behind the WHO Guidelines: hospital care for children—what are the useful clinical features of bacterial meningitis found in infants and children? *J Trop Pediatr* 54: 83–6.
Brouwer MC, McIntyre P, Prasad K, van de Beek D (2013) Corticosteroids for acute bacterial meningitis. *Cochrane Database Syst Rev* 6: CD004405. doi: 10.1002/14651858.CD004405.pub4.
Curtis S, Stobart K, Vandermeer B, et al. (2010) Clinical features suggestive of meningitis in children: a systematic review of prospective data. *Pediatrics* 126: 952–60.
Dubos F, Korczowski B, Aygun DA, et al. (2008) Serum procalcitonin level and other biological markers to distinguish between bacterial and aseptic meningitis in children: a European multicenter case cohort study. *Arch Pediatr Adolesc Med* 162: 1157–63.
Gwer S, Gatakaa H, Mwai L, et al. (2010) The role for osmotic agents in children with acute encephalopathies: a systematic review. *BMC Pediatr* 10: 23.

Kramer AH, Zygun DA (2009) Anemia and red blood cell transfusion in neurocritical care. *Crit Care* 13: R89.

Leveque N, Van Haecke A, Renois F, et al. (2011) Rapid virological diagnosis of central nervous system infections by use of a multiplex reverse transcription-PCR DNA microarray. *J Clin Microbiol* 49: 3874–9.

Lussiana C, Lôa Clemente SV, Pulido Tarquino IA, Paulo I (2011) Predictors of bacterial meningitis in resource-limited contexts: an Angolan case. *PLoS One* 6: e25706. doi: 10.1371/journal.pone.0025706.

Maconochie I, Baumer H, Stewart ME (2008) Fluid therapy for acute bacterial meningitis. *Cochrane Database Syst Rev* 1: CD004786. doi: 10.1002/14651858.CD004786.pub3.

Martín-Ancel A, García-Alix A, Salas S, et al. (2006) Cerebrospinal fluid leucocyte counts in healthy neonates. *Arch Dis Child Fetal Neonatal Ed* 91: F357–8.

McMenamin JB, Volpe JJ (1984) Bacterial meningitis in infancy: effects on intracranial pressure and cerebral blood flow velocity. *Neurology* 34: 500–4.

Mehta V, Singhi P, Singhi S (2007) Intravenous sodium valproate versus diazepam infusion for the control of refractory status epilepticus in children: a randomized controlled trial. *J Child Neurol* 22: 1191–7.

Nigrovic LE, Kuppermann N, McAdam AJ, Malley R (2004) Cerebrospinal latex agglutination fails to contribute to the microbiologic diagnosis of pretreated children with meningitis. *Pediatr Infect Dis J* 23: 786–8.

Nigrovic LE, Malley R, Macias CG, et al. (2008) Effect of antibiotic pretreatment on cerebrospinal fluid profiles of children with bacterial meningitis. *Pediatrics* 122: 726–30.

Peltola H, Roine I, Fernandez J, et al. (2007) Adjuvant glycerol and/or dexamethasone to improve the outcomes of childhood bacterial meningitis: a prospective, randomized, double-blind, placebo-controlled trial. *Clin Infect Dis* 45: 1277–86.

Powell KR, Sugarman LI, Eskenazi AE, et al. (1990) Normalization of plasma arginine vasopressin concentrations when children with meningitis are given maintenance plus replacement fluid therapy. *J Pediatr* 117: 515–22.

Prasad K, Singh MB (2008) Corticosteroids for managing tuberculous meningitis. *Cochrane Database Syst Rev* 1: CD002244. doi: 10.1002/14651858.CD002244.pub3.

Sankar J, Singhi P, Bansal A, et al. (2007) Role of dexamethasone and oral glycerol in reducing hearing and neurological sequelae in children with bacterial meningitis. *Indian Pediatr* 44: 649–56.

Shetty R, Singhi S, Singhi P, Jayashree M (2008) Cerebral perfusion pressure—targeted approach in children with central nervous system infections and raised intracranial pressure: is it feasible? *J Child Neurol* 23: 192–8.

Shore PM, Thomas NJ, Clark RS, et al. (2004) Continuous versus intermittent cerebrospinal fluid drainage after severe traumatic brain injury in children: effect on biochemical markers. *J Neurotrauma* 21: 1113–22.

Singhi S, Jarvinen A, Peltola H (2008) Increase in serum osmolality is possible mechanism for the beneficial effects of glycerol in childhood bacterial meningitis. *Pediatr Infect Dis J* 27: 892–6.

Singhi SC, Singhi PD, Srinivas B, et al. (1995) Fluid restriction does not improve the outcome of acute meningitis. *Pediatr Infect Dis J* 14: 495–503.

Singhi SC, Khetarpal R, Baranwal AK, et al. (2004) Intensive care needs of children with acute bacterial meningitis: a developing country perspective. *Ann Trop Paediatr* 24: 133–40.

Singhi S, Bansal A, Kumar R, Bhatti A (2014) Randomized comparison of cerebral perfusion pressure (CPP) with intracranial pressure (ICP) targeted therapy in children with acute CNS infections. *Crit Care Med* (in press).

Tureen JH, Täuber MG, Sande MA (1992) Effect of hydration status on cerebral blood flow and cerebrospinal fluid lactic acidosis in rabbits with experimental meningitis. *J Clin Invest* 89: 947–53.

van de Beek D, Farrar JJ, de Gans J, et al. (2010) Adjunctive dexamethasone in bacterial meningitis: a meta-analysis of individual patient data. *Lancet Neurol* 9: 254–63.

Wall EC, Ajdukiewicz KM, Heyderman RS, Garner P (2013) Osmotic therapies added to antibiotics for acute bacterial meningitis. *Cochrane Database Syst Rev* 3: CD008806. doi: 10.1002/14651858.CD008806.pub2.

Wang X, Theodore MJ, Mair R, et al. (2012) Clinical validation of multiplex real-time PCR assays for detection of bacterial meningitis pathogens. *J Clin Microbiol* 50: 702–8.

Woehrl B, Klein M, Grandgirard D, et al. (2011) Bacterial meningitis: current therapy and possible future treatment options. *Expert Rev Anti Infect Ther* 9: 1053–65.

4
NEUROIMAGING

Section 1: Bacterial, Fungal, Tuberculous and Parasitic Infections

Niranjan Khandelwal

Imaging of the central nervous system (CNS) has an important role to play in the diagnosis and management of CNS infections. Employing optimum techniques and interpreting the results require an understanding of the imaging techniques, their applications and limitations. The use of advanced and research imaging techniques may provide further insights. In this chapter, an integrative imaging approach to different clinical syndromes of CNS infections is presented. The pathologies pertaining to the various CNS infections are described in the other chapters.

Imaging modalities
There are a variety of radiological techniques to examine the CNS. Although skull radiography is useful for detecting calcified lesions, it is rarely used in children, and thus will not be discussed further.

CRANIAL ULTRASOUND
Cranial ultrasound remains the most commonly used technique in the fetus and young infant (until the fontanelle closes) as it is widely available, portable, inexpensive and does not involve ionizing radiation. Thus, repeated examinations can be easily performed. A standard cranial ultrasound examination includes six coronal views, five sagittal views, and at least two additional focused views of abnormalities detected. High frequencies (>7.5MHz) give better visualization but less penetration. Convex transducers allow better visualization through smaller fontanelles than the more common phased-array transducers. Insonation through the posterior fontanelle can be used to detect abnormalities in the occipital horns of the lateral ventricles, and the posterior parts of the cerebrum and cerebellum. The mastoid fontanelle can be used as a portal to examine the cerebellum, fourth ventricle, aqueduct and cisterna magna.

COMPUTERIZED TOMOGRAPHY (CT)

CT is widely available, provides detailed images of most of the cerebrum, some of the cere-bellum, the ventricles, and destructive lesions of skull bones. It is particularly useful in detecting calcification and blood within the parenchyma. It is also helpful in detecting hydrocephalus and brain herniations. It is less useful for lesions in the temporal lobe, brain-stem or cerebellum, because of the bone-induced artefacts. The advantages in children include more rapid acquisition of images than with magnetic resonance imaging (MRI), and less noise and anxiety, requiring less sedation or anaesthesia. However, CT exposes the chil-dren to a considerable amount of radiation and provides limited resolution between different tissues of the brain. Iodine-based contrast agents may increase the sensitivity and specificity of detecting infectious lesions. Poor sensitivity of CT limits its usefulness in children with acute neurological syndromes for excluding space-occupying lesions prior to lumbar puncture, and detecting calcification.

MAGNETIC RESONANCE IMAGING

MRI is much more sensitive than CT in detecting CNS infections because it provides excel-lent contrast between tissues in all parts of the brain (Table 4.1). Most magnets in current clinical use are 1.5 Tesla, but in our experience the use of more powerful magnets (≥3.0 Tesla) along with gadolinium-based contrast increases the sensitivity of detecting CNS infections. MRI has limited availability in resource-poor settings, takes more time to acquire, is more prone to movement artefact, and can be considerably more frightening than CT. Thus children often need to be sedated or given an anaesthetic. The recommended MRI sequences for CNS infections are outlined in Table 4.2, but other established and research techniques may be helpful if available.

DIFFUSION-WEIGHTED IMAGING (DWI) AND DIFFUSION TENSOR IMAGING (DTI) (Table 4.3)

DWI is based on the principle of imaging the differences of Brownian motion of protons in normal and pathological tissues. It is the method of choice in the differentiation of pyogenic abscess from cystic or necrotic tumour. Pyogenic and tuberculous abscesses typically show reduced diffusion either due to the viscous pus within the abscess reducing free water motion, or due to the higher concentration of dead cells and proteins within the abscess hin-dering the active transport of proteins or water molecules. In contrast, the cystic and/or necrotic components of most tumours generally show increased diffusion due to cellular necrosis and increased size of intercellular space. This restriction of diffusion may be less apparent in small abscesses, possibly secondary to averaging of diffusion information from normal surrounding brain tissue (Reiche et al. 2010). DWI also helps to differentiate between cerebritis and infarction secondary to meningitis. An infarct appears bright with matched area of decreased signal on apparent diffusion coefficient map.

DTI adds directionality (anisotropy) to the diffusion properties of the molecule. The tensor is a mathematical algorithm obtained by applying diffusion gradient pulses in a min-imum of six directions. The directionality or anisotropy is measured by fractional anisotropy and the diffusion is measured by mean diffusivity by mathematical equations derived from

TABLE 4.1
Magnetic resonance imaging sequences

Modality	Basis	Clinical applications
T1-weighted imaging	Time to recover 62.3% of the longitudinal magnetization	Structural abnormalities. Assessment of brain maturation in 0- to 6-month-olds
T2-weighted imaging	Time necessary for dephasing to cause 62.3% loss of signal	Assessment of brain maturation in children >6 months old
Fluid-attenuated inversion recovery (FLAIR)	Inversion-recovery pulse sequence to nullify fluids such as cerebrospinal fluid	Accentuates the lesions, especially those at periventricular or juxtacortical location
Diffusion-weighted imaging (DWI)	Generates image contrast based upon the different mobility of water molecules in their local environment	Pus on DWI appears very hyperintense
Diffusion tensor imaging (DTI)	Differentiates between isotropic and anisotropic diffusion, and provides measurements of fractional anisotropy	Injury to white matter tracts, including vasogenic oedema
Susceptibility-weighted imaging (SWI)	Amplifies the paramagnetic effects of calcification and blood products including deoxyhaemoglobin, methaemoglobin and haemosiderin	Very sensitive for detection of calcification and haemorrhages associated with congenital infections or herpes simplex virus
Perfusion-weighted imaging (PWI)	Measures signal changes related to the first pass of a bolus of gadolinium contrast agent through the vasculature	Helps in distinguishing infections from neoplasms because in general tumours show high perfusion parameters
Proton magnetic resonance spectroscopy (MRS)	Detection of spectrum from metabolites	Malignancy, metabolic condition and certain infections

Eigen vectors, which are directional diffusion coefficients in a single given direction (Mukherjee et al. 2008). Originally applied for depiction of white matter tract pathologies and displacement/distortions of peritumoural white matter tracts, fractional anisotropy has found additional application in the evaluation of ring-enhancing lesions and brain abscesses (Gupta et al. 2005).

SUSCEPTIBILITY-WEIGHTED IMAGING (SWI)
SWI is a fully velocity-compensated gradient-echo sequence with special magnitude and phase processing that can be used in a standard clinical setting. It can differentiate between calcification and haemorrhage because on SWI-filtered phase images, paramagnetic substances such as iron and haemorrhage show negative phase (dark–hypointense) and the diamagnetic substances such as calcium show a positive phase (bright–hyperintense) (for a right-handed system).

TABLE 4.2
Imaging techniques in central nervous system infections

Standard sequences	*Established techniques*
T1-weighted sagittal, axial views	Magnetic resonance spectroscopy
T2-weighted axial, coronal views	Magnetization transfer imaging
Fluid-attenuated inversion recovery (FLAIR)	Susceptibility-weighted imaging
Post-contrast T1-weighted	3D high-resolution T2-weighted imaging
Diffusion-weighted imaging	Perfusion imaging
Post-contrast FLAIR	
– optional	*Research techniques*
Magnetic resonance angiography	Diffusion tensor imaging

TABLE 4.3
Role of diffusion-weighted imaging and diffusion tensor imaging in central nervous system infections[a]

1 Differentiation of abscesses from tumours
   (Bright lesions with low diffusion coefficients in pyogenic and tuberculous abscess on diffusion-weighted imaging. High fractional anisotropy with restricted mean diffusivity in the pyogenic abscess cavity on diffusion tensor imaging)

2 Differentiation of cerebritis from infarct
   (Brighter lesion in infarct due to reduced diffusivity)

3 Restricted diffusion in lymphoma lesions may help in differentiation from toxoplasma lesions

4 Treatment follow-up of tuberculomas and pyogenic abscesses
   (Increase in fractional anisotropy in response to treatment)

[a]Gupta et al. (2005), Haris et al. (2008).

TABLE 4.4
Role of magnetic resonance perfusion imaging in central nervous system infections

Differentiation of brain abscesses and cystic brain tumours
Assessing treatment response in tuberculoma
Differentiation of toxoplasmosis from lymphoma in immunocompromised state

MAGNETIC RESONANCE PERFUSION IMAGING (Table 4.4)
Magnetic resonance perfusion imaging is based on the measurement of the magnetic resonance signal intensity using either a T2-weighted sequence (dynamic susceptibility contrast-perfusion MRI) or a T1-weighted sequence (dynamic contrast-enhanced MRI) during the first pass of a bolus of a paramagnetic contrast agent. Additionally, arterial spin labelling techniques may be performed without any contrast media. The T2*-weighted sequences are by far the most commonly used in clinical practice.

TABLE 4.5
3D heavily T2-weighted sequences

Balanced steady-state sequences (gradient-echo based)
CISS (constructive interference in steady state)
FIESTA-C (fast imaging employing steady-state acquisition cycled phases)
Balanced FFE (fast Fourier echo)

Variable flip-angle sequences (spin-echo based)
SPACE (sampling perfection with application-optimized contrasts using different flip-angle evolutions)
3D fast spin-echo (FSE) cube
XETA (extended echo train acquisition)

TABLE 4.6
Spectral peak patterns for various metabolites

Parts per million	Spectral assignment	Short TE	Intermediate TE
0.9–1.3	Macromolecules, amino acids, lipids	+++	+
1.35	Lactate (Lac)	+	+
1.47	Alanine (Ala)	++	+
1.9	Acetate (Ace)	++	+
2.02	N-acetyl aspartate (NAA)	+	+
2.05/2.5	Glutamate + glutamine (Glx)	+	
2.4	Pyruvate (Pyr)	++	+
	Succinate (Succ)		
3.02	Creatine (Cr)	+	+
3.2	Choline (Cho)	+	+
3.6–3.8	Trehalose	+	+
3.94	Serine	+	+

TE, echo time.

HEAVILY T2-WEIGHTED HIGH-RESOLUTION SEQUENCES (Table 4.5)
The imaging sequences for heavily T2-weighted imaging can be gradient-echo based or spin-echo based. The gradient-echo based sequences use steady-state methods, whereas spin-echo based sequences employ variable flip-angles. The 3D constructive interference in steady state (CISS) sequence is widely described for this purpose. Another sequence that is used is 'sampling perfection with application-optimized contrasts using different flip-angle evolutions' (SPACE). We use this sequence in our institute for 3D heavily T2-weighted imaging to detect neurocysticercosis lesions in the CSF spaces. Intraventricular cysticercal cysts usually located in the fourth ventricle are difficult to identify on routine sequences, as they are surrounded by CSF, which has the same signal intensity as the cyst fluid. However, the cyst wall and scolex are well visualized on CISS and other similar gradient-echo and spin-echo sequences. The increased sensitivity of the 3D-CISS sequence is due to its higher contrast-to-noise ratio and may also be related to accentuation of the T2 value between the cystic fluid and the surrounding CSF (Amaral et al. 2005).

TABLE 4.7
Signs of raised intracranial pressure on computerized tomography or magnetic resonance imaging

Effaced basal cisterns
Effaced ventricles and cortical sulci
Coning: descent of cerebellar tonsils and brainstem through the foramen magnum
Cerebellar reverse sign: cerebellum appears bright as compared to the rest of the brain

MAGNETIC RESONANCE SPECTROSCOPY (MRS)

Proton MRS is a subspectrum of chemical shift imaging, a technique that allows one to study the pattern of metabolites in the brain non-invasively.

MRS provides in vivo biochemical information wherein the peaks of the spectra obtained correspond with various metabolites. The horizontal axis (abscissa) represents resonance frequency as parts per million (ppm) to the total resonance frequency. The vertical axis plots the relative signal amplitude or concentrations for various metabolites. The metabolites and their spectral pattern that can be identified with proton MRS are dependent on the echo time (Table 4.6). With a 1.5 Tesla magnet, the following metabolites can be visualized utilizing intermediate to long echo time (144–288ms): N-acetyl aspartate (NAA), choline (Cho), creatine (Cr), lactate (Lac) and alanine (Ala). Short echo-time acquisitions (TE<40ms) include the above metabolites as well as myoinositol (Myo), glutamate and glutamine (Glx), glucose, amino acids and some macromolecular proteins and lipids. MRS can be helpful in distinguishing (1) abscess from cystic lesions, (2) neurocysticercosis from tuberculoma, abscess or other mass lesions, and (3) toxoplasmosis from lymphoma. It also provides clues to the aetiology of brain abscess or fungal lesions.

Imaging clinical syndromes of central nervous system infection

Infections of the CNS present with meningeal signs, impaired consciousnesss, focal neurological deficits or convulsions. The role of the radiologist is to detect the radiological corroboration of the pathology of these symptoms and provide suggestions as to the possible aetiological agents.

MENINGITIS

In children with meningism, the aims of imaging are to exclude conditions that contraindicate lumbar puncture such as raised intracranial pressure or space-occupying lesions (Table 4.7), to detect possible complications, and to exclude other conditions (Kastrup et al. 2008). In uncomplicated meningitis, most contrast-enhanced CT scans are normal, whilst 50% of contrast-enhanced MRI scans are also normal. Both CT and MRI may demonstrate obliteration of subarachnoid spaces and basal cisterns, ventriculomegaly and meningeal enhancement (Fig. 4.1). MRI is more sensitive than CT but its sensitivity varies with the performed sequences (Hughes et al. 2010) and hyperintensity of the subarachnoid spaces may be present on fluid-attenuated inversion recovery (FLAIR) images without contrast agents.

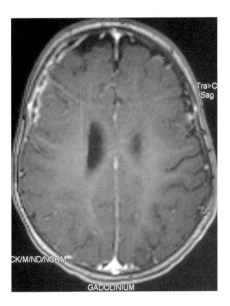

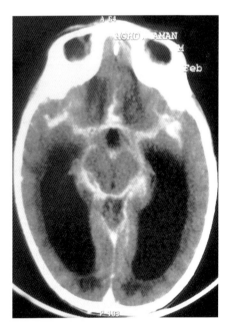

Fig. 4.1. Pyogenic meningitis. T1-weighted contrast-enhanced axial MRI shows diffuse leptomeningeal enhancement.

Fig. 4.2. Tuberculous meningitis. Contrast-enhanced CT shows extensive exudates with intense contrast enhancement in basal cisterns and in bilateral sylvian fissures, and associated hydrocephalus.

Imaging of viral, bacterial or fungal meningitis shows leptomeningeal enhancement that includes the pia mater or extends into the subarachnoid spaces of the sulci and cisterns. Pachymeningeal enhancement without leptomeningeal involvement typically occurs secondary to intracranial hypotension due to CSF leaks or with idiopathic hypertrophic pachymeningitis, and may occasionally be seen with tuberculosis, syphilis and other infections. Bacterial and viral meningitis exhibit enhancement that is typically thin and linear. In tuberculous meningitis, the enhancement is typically most pronounced in the basal cisterns, but with some degree of involvement of the meninges within the sulci over the convexities and sylvian fissures; in severe cases associated hydrocephalus is often seen (Fig. 4.2) (Table 4.8). Fungal meningitis may produce thicker, lumpy or nodular enhancement in the subarachnoid space and show thick sheet-like pachymeningeal involvement. Invasive aspergillosis shows basimeningeal enhancement contiguous to the paranasal sinuses, whereas cryptococcal meningitis shows nodular meningeal thickening along the convexities (Smirniotopoulos et al. 2007).

T1-weighted post-contrast images are more sensitive (55%–70%) than CT in demonstrating meningeal enhancement. The pial enhancement may be difficult to differentiate

TABLE 4.8
Patterns of meningeal enhancement in central nervous system infections

Agent	Pattern	Distribution
Pyogenic	Leptomeningeal	Diffuse, convexities
Tuberculous	Leptomeningeal, pachymeningeal	Basal
Viral	Leptomeningeal	Diffuse
Fungal	Leptomeningeal, pachymeningeal	*Aspergillus*: basimeninges contiguous to paranasal sinuses
		Cryptococcus: nodular thickening along convexities

from normal prominent enhancing vascular structures in children. Enhancement of the subarachnoid spaces is thought to be caused by leakage of contrast through the walls of inflamed capillaries (Ferreira et al. 2005). Controversy exists over the superiority of T1-weighted or FLAIR sequences for detecting subarachnoid space diseases (Galassi et al. 2005). Post-contrast FLAIR sequences do not show contrast enhancement in vessels with slow-flowing blood, which on T1-weighted post-contrast images can be confused with meningeal enhancement. FLAIR is more sensitive than T1-weighted images to detect low concentrations of gadolinium extravasation from pial vessels in the subarachnoid space.

Role of magnetization transfer imaging (MTI)
Post-contrast T1-weighted MTI improves the visualization of normally enhancing structures and facilitates the early diagnosis of meningitis. It also shows greater CNS involvement than is apparent on conventional spin-echo images, specifically by delineating generalized meningeal enhancement as well as focal areas of brain involvement, not seen on the conventional non-contrast T2-weighted or post-contrast T1-weighted images. Leptomeninges are usually not visible on pre-contrast conventional spin-echo images. MTI is particularly applicable to tuberculous meningitis in which meningeal enhancement has been shown in all patients on pre-contrast T1-weighted MTI. Additionally, significantly different MTI ratios were found from the meninges of patients with tuberculous meningitis from those seen in bacterial, fungal and viral meningitis (Gupta et al. 1999).

Role of imaging in recurrent bacterial meningitis
Neuroimaging has an important role in the detection of structural defects that predispose children to recurrent CNS infections (Table 4.9), especially pyogenic infections (Ginsberg 2004). Thin-section cranial CT offers a relatively easy, reliable and non-invasive method of delineating anatomical defects in recurrent meningitis. Coronal thin-section CT shows detailed anatomy of the anterior cranial fossa and identifies most skull defects, which may be missed by axial cranial CT, particularly in the basal ethmoidal area and cribriform plate. Although CT may demonstrate a bony defect and suggest the site of the CSF leakage, the additional technique of CT cisternography may be needed to confirm the leakage. CT

TABLE 4.9
Structural causes of recurrent bacterial meningitis

Ethmoidal meningocele	Persistent craniopharyngeal canal
Encephalocele	Base of skull fractures
Dermal sinus, dorsal or occipital	Post-skull base surgery
Translabyrinthine fistulae	

TABLE 4.10
Complications of meningitis

Nonvascular	*Vascular*
Hydrocephalus	Vasculopathy
Cranial nerve palsy	Infarction of parenchyma
Ventriculitis	Venous thrombosis
Cerebritis/abscess	Mycotic aneurysms
Extra-axial fluid collections	

TABLE 4.11
Recommended magnetic resonance imaging protocols for complicated meningitis (excluding cerebral abscess)

Precontrast T1-weighted (± magnetization transfer)
Precontrast T2-weighted
FLAIR (fluid-attenuated inversion recovery)
Diffusion-weighted imaging/apparent diffusion coefficient (DWI/ADC)
3D time of flight (TOF) magnetic resonance arteriography for arterial complications
Phase contrast angiography (indicated if flow artefacts, T1 effects present in TOF)
2D TOF magnetic resonance venography for venous complications
Post-contrast T1-weighted (± magnetization transfer for tuberculous meningitis and tuberculomas)
Post-contrast 2D TOF magnetic resonance venography (indicated if flow artefacts present in TOF)

cisternography is currently the most reliable technique for the accurate localization of CSF leakage, and it is more sensitive than MRI (Shetty et al. 1998). Although in recent times many MRI sequences like CISS and contrast-enhanced magnetic resonance cisternography have been employed with success, in our opinion CT cisternography is quite reliable because in addition to showing the leak, it gives high-resolution bony details of the cranial floor that may show dehiscence, thereby clinching the diagnosis. Nuclear medicine studies may be used to detect the approximate leakage site but do not demonstrate the anatomical details.

COMPLICATIONS OF MENINGITIS/ENCEPHALITIS
Neuroimaging is very useful for detecting the intracranial complications of meningitis and

encephalitis (Tables 4.10, 4.11). The imaging of cerebritis/cerebral abscess is discussed under the section on space-occupying lesions.

Nonvascular complications of complicated meningitis
• *Hydrocephalus.* Hydrocephalus is a common complication in patients with meningitis and space-occupying lesions. Most patients with meningitis have a mild and transient enlargement of the ventricles, and a few have an 'arrested hydrocephalus', in which the ventricular system never returns to normal size and requires no treatment. Ventricular enlargement in hydrocephalus is easily detected by ultrasound (in infants), CT or MRI, but it needs to be differentiated from ventricular enlargement secondary to white matter atrophy. The most reliable signs of enlargement due to hydrocephalus are commensurate enlargement of the temporal horns with the lateral ventricles, and enlargement of the anterior and posterior recesses of the third ventricle (Barkovich 2005, Ferreira et al. 2005). Other features include narrowing of the mamillo-pontine distance and ventricular angle, widening of the frontal horns and effacement of the cortical sulci (Barkovich 2005, Ferreira et al. 2005).

• *Ventriculitis.* Mild ventriculitis can occur due to severe meningitis affecting the basal cisterns, or rupture of a cerebral abscess into a ventricle. It is more common in acute bacterial meningitis than in tuberculous meningitis. MRI shows thickening and marked enhancement of the ependyma, high T2-weighted signal of ventricular walls, dilated ventricles and the presence of debris with irregular margins (unlike the well-defined straight level associated with intraventricular haemorrhage) in dependent portions of ventricles. Debris is seen as high signal intensity on FLAIR and DWI. Intraventricular exudates and septations may heal by adhesions and can lead to entrapment of portions of the ventricles and result in segmental dilatation (Hughes et al. 2010).

• *Cranial nerve palsies.* Cranial nerve palsies are common in meningitis, particularly those involving the VIIIth (vestibulocochlear), VIIth (facial) and IIIrd (oculomotor). In tuberculous and fungal meningitis, involvement of cranial nerves in the cavernous sinus and optico-chiasmatic regions is common. The imaging findings include T2 hypointense, contrast-enhancing soft tissue, lateral bulge in the cavernous sinus region, and enhancement of the optic chiasma (Barkovich 2005, Gupta et al. 2011).

• *Extra-axial fluid collections.* Extra-axial fluid collections may be sterile (effusions/hygromas) or purulent (empyemas) and may remain asymptomatic or cause pressure effects. The collections are usually subdural, but can be extradural. Subdural collections can be bilateral and occur predominantly over the frontal and temporal lobes (Fig. 4.3). They are differentiated from physiologically dilated subarachnoid spaces by the presence of veins passing through the collections on contrast-enhanced CT or MRI in the latter. Subdural sterile effusions may appear brighter than CSF on proton density and FLAIR images if they are serosanguinous with high protein content. Empyema has higher T1-weighted signal intensity than CSF and higher T2-weighted signal intensity than the underlying cortex. It has thicker

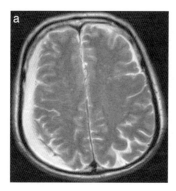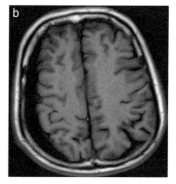

Fig. 4.3. *Haemophilus influenzae* meningitis. Axial MRI sections show (a) T2-hyperintense and (b) T1-hypointense right-sided crescent-shaped subdural effusion over the right frontoparietal convexity.

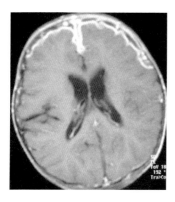

Fig. 4.4. Pyogenic meningitis. T1-weighted contrast-enhanced axial MRI shows extensive bifrontal enhancement of subdural collection suggestive of subdural empyema.

enhancing rim than sterile effusions, and internal septation (Fig. 4.4). DWI is the imaging technique of choice in the diagnosis of empyema, because empyemas show very bright signal on DWI with corresponding dark areas on the apparent diffusion coefficient (ADC) map, while sterile effusions are dark or only slightly bright on DWI and CSF-like on ADC map (Ferriera et al. 2005, Hughes et al. 2010).

Vascular complications
These can be arterial or venous. DWI has increased sensitivity in the diagnosis of arterial parenchymal infarcts and thus helps in early detection. Magnetic resonance angiography techniques are helpful in delineating the involved vessels and their extent of involvement.

• *Arterial occlusions due to vasculitis and parenchymal infarcts.* Infarction in pyogenic and tuberculous meningitis results from vasculitis (arteritis) caused by exudates surrounding the vessels, whereas direct vascular injury leading to endarteritis, aneurysm formation and

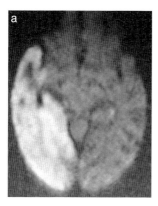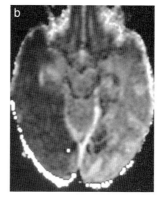

Fig. 4.5. Tuberculous meningitis with secondary vasculitis. Axial (a) diffusion-weighted MRI and (b) apparent diffusion coefficient images show restricted diffusion in right posterior cerebral artery territory suggestive of an infarct.

vascular thrombosis occurs with angioinvasive fungi. In tuberculous meningitis, exudation at the base of the brain and in the sylvian fissure causes arteritis, especially of proximal (M1) segments of the middle cerebral arteries and proximal (P1) segments of the posterior cerebral arteries (Fig. 4.5). Selective involvement of the smaller cerebral arteries, such as the lenticulostriate and the thalamo-perforating branches, is also common, leading to small infarctions in the basal ganglia, thalamus and deep white matter (Garg 2011). Similarly, angioinvasive fungi spread contiguously from sites of nasopharyngitis, oropharyngitis and sinusitis to the cavernous sinus and internal carotid artery, leading to focal thrombosis and cerebral infarction, detectable by imaging studies (Martins et al. 2010, Garg 2011). Neuro-cysticercosis can also cause lacunar infarction or large-vessel disease due to arteritis, pro-gressive midbrain syndrome, transient ischaemic attacks and brain haemorrhage. The middle and posterior cerebral arteries are most commonly affected. Multivessel involvement is noted in nearly 50% of adult patients with subarachnoid neurocysticercosis and is less common in children (Barinagarrementeria and Cantú 1998).

• *Mycotic aneurysms and subarachnoid haemorrhage.* Bacterial mycotic aneurysms tend to develop at the arterial branch points, which are the common sites of embolic impaction, particularly in the distal middle cerebral artery branches. Fungal meningoencephalitis caused by angioinvasive fungi can also be complicated by mycotic aneurysms of cavernous internal carotid artery and distal middle cerebral arteries (Phuong et al. 2002).

• *Venous complications.* Septic sinus thrombosis is a potentially fatal disorder. The dural sinuses and the emissary veins have no valves, thus blood flows in either direction accord-ing to the pressure gradients in the vascular system. This makes the cerebral venous system vulnerable to septic thrombosis resulting from spreading infections of adjacent locations.

TABLE 4.12
Imaging signs of cavernous sinus thrombosis

Direct signs
Filling defect in the cavernous sinuses
Heterogeneous enhancement within the cavernous sinuses
Enlargement and/or bulging of the lateral walls of the cavernous sinus
Hypointense signal on T2*-weighted sequences.
Intensive enhancement of the lateral wall

Indirect signs
Exophthalmos
Stranding of the retro-orbital fat
Superior ophthalmic dilatation with partial or no enhancement in case
of thrombosis extension

TABLE 4.13
**Intracranial space-occupying lesions in central nervous system
infections**

Bacterial	Fungal	Parasitic
Pyogenic abscess	Aspergillosis	Neurocysticercosis
Tuberculous abscess	Mucormycosis	Toxoplasmosis
Tuberculoma	Cryptococcosis	Hydatid disease

The cavernous sinus is the most common site of septic thrombosis in the CNS. Contrast-enhanced MRI with a focus on the cavernous sinuses is the imaging of choice (Table 4.12) (Heller et al. 2003, Kojan and Al-Jumah 2006).

CENTRAL NERVOUS SYSTEM INFECTIONS PRESENTING AS INTRACRANIAL SPACE-OCCUPYING
LESIONS
CNS infections can present with symptoms and signs of intracranial space-occupying lesions (Table 4.13), either as a result of complicated meningitis or as an isolated pathology.

Imaging: morphological imaging (computerized tomography and conventional magnetic resonance imaging)

• *Cerebritis and pyogenic abscess.* These are serious complications of bacterial meningitis, but need distinction (Table 4.14) because surgery is contraindicated in cerebritis. The ring-enhancing lesion of a cerebral abscess is classically described as having smooth inner and outer margins. Almost 90% of the abscesses demonstrate a T2-hypointense rim, and

TABLE 4.14
Imaging characteristics of pyogenic abscess

Stage of abscess	Wall characteristics	Enhancement pattern	Temporal pattern
Early cerebritis	Not discernible	Patchy enhancement	3–5 days
Late cerebritis	T1 hyperintense, T2 hypointense	Enhancement of thick rim and centre	Early second week
Early capsule formation	T1 and T2 hyperintense	Smooth rim enhancement	Late second week
Late capsule formation	T1 isointense T2 hypointense	Smooth rim enhancement	Third week to months

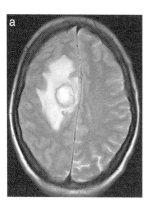 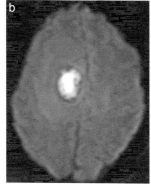 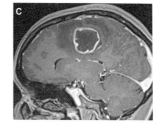

Fig. 4.6. Pyogenic abscess. Axial MRI show (a) T2-hyperintense lesion with T2-hypointense rim and perilesional oedema in right high frontal parasagittal region. (b) The lesion is bright on diffusion-weighted imaging. (c) T1-weighted sagittal section showing smooth peripheral rim enhancement of the lesion after contrast injection.

75% form a continuous rim. The thinner margin of the deep or medial aspect of the lesion is predisposed to daughter abscess formation and deep rupture of the abscess into the ventricle (Saltzman 2004, Barkovich 2005) (Fig. 4.6).

• *Fungal abscess.* Fungal abscesses are notorious for their variable imaging appearance and ability to simulate other lesions, including high-grade gliomas. The most distinct imaging characteristics of fungal abscess on CT or MRI are multiple lesions with infarction or haemorrhage in a random distribution owing to the angioinvasive nature of the fungus. *Aspergillus* abscesses are usually hypointense on T1-weighted images, but areas of high signal intensity may be seen due to the presence of iron, manganese or methaemoglobin. Haemorrhage occurs in approximately 25% of cases, and contrast enhancement is usually minimal or absent. On T2-weighted images, peripheral low-signal areas may be seen that

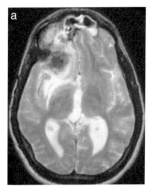
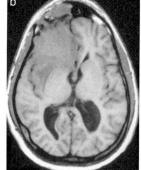
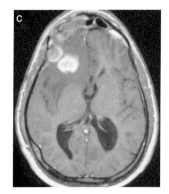

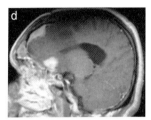

Fig. 4.7. Invasive aspergillosis. Axial MRI sections show extensive lesion in the right basifrontal lobe that is (a) T2 hypointense, and (b) T1 isointense. Contrast-enhanced T1-weighted images show (c) dense nodular and sheet-like meningeal enhancement over the adjacent right frontal pole in axial section, and (d) enhancement of sinus contents in the frontal and ethmoidal sinuses in sagittal section.

TABLE 4.15
Imaging characteristics of parenchymal tuberculomas

	T1-weighted	*T2-weighted*	*Contrast enhancement*
Tuberculoma without caseation	Hypointense centre	Hyperintense centre	Nodular
Tuberculoma with solid caseation	Hypointense/isointense centre	Hypointense centre with hypointense rim	Peripheral
Tuberculoma with liquid caseation	Hypointense centre	Hyperintense centre with hypointense rim	Peripheral

correspond to areas of haemorrhage (Khandelwal et al. 2011) (Fig. 4.7). In contrast to pyogenic abscesses, only about a half of fungal abscesses are very bright on DWI.

• *Tuberculomas and tuberculous abscesses.* On CT, tuberculomas appear as round or lobulated, contrast-enhancing, low- or high-density ring lesions with irregularly thickened wall (daRocha et al. 2005, Gupta et al. 2011). MRI features of tuberculomas depend on caseation as shown in Table 4.15 (Trivedi et al. 2009, Gupta and Kumar 2011). Tuberculous brain abscesses are relatively rare and constitute approximately 4%–7% of the total CNS tuberculosis in resource-poor countries. On MRI, these appear as large, solitary and frequently

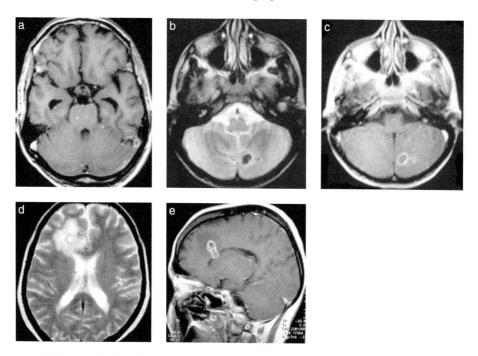

Fig. 4.8. Stages of tuberculous granulomata. (a) T1-weighted contrast-enhanced axial MRI shows non-caseating granuloma in brainstem showing nodular homogenous enhancement; (b) T2-weighted axial section shows caseating granuloma with solid caseation in the cerebellum that is T2 hypointense in the centre of the lesion; (c) peripheral contrast enhancement on T1-weighted image; (d) T2-weighted axial section shows caseating granuloma with liquid caseation and central T2 hyperintensity; and (e) peripheral post-contrast enhancement on T1-weighted image.

multiloculated ring-enhancing lesions with surrounding oedema and mass effect (Morgado and Ruivo 2005, Gupta and Kumar 2011) (Fig. 4.8).

Parasitic infections

• *Neurocysticercosis (NCC).* The imaging characteristics of the cysts in NCC vary according to their pathological forms in the brain (Barkovich 2005, da Rocha et al. 2005):

(1) Parenchymal cysticerci. (a) Vesicular: clearly marginated, non-enhancing cyst with CSF-isointense cyst fluid and a discrete, eccentrically placed scolex. (b) Colloidal vesicular: slightly T1-hyperintense and markedly T2-hyperintense lesion, with contrast enhancement of cyst wall and perilesional oedema (Fig. 4.9). (c) Granular nodular: nodular or a thick small ring-like enhancement. Occasionally, a target or bull's-eye appearance is seen with the calcified scolex in the centre of the mass. (4) Nodular calcified: small calcified nodule without mass effect on non-contrast CT.

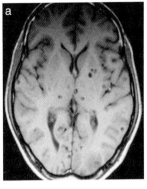
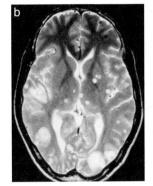
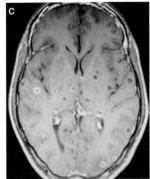

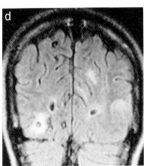

Fig. 4.9. Diffuse intraparenchymal neurocysticercosis. (a) T1-weighted, (b) T2-weighted, and (c) T1-weighted contrast-enhanced axial MRI sections show multiple cystic lesions in bilateral cerebral hemispheres. The lesions in the basal ganglia are not associated with either perilesional oedema or enhancement suggestive of vesicular stage of neurocysticercosis. The lesions in the bilateral occipital lobes are cystic in signal intensity and show perilesional oedema and post-contrast enhancement suggestive of colloid vesicular stage of neurocysticercosis. (d) Coronal fluid-attenuated inversion recovery (FLAIR) image shows presence of scolex as eccentric hyperintense nodular focus.

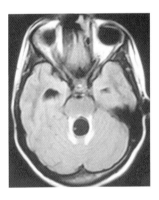

Fig. 4.10. Intraventricular neurocysticercosis. Axial fluid-attenuated inversion recovery (FLAIR) image reveals presence of dilated supratentorial ventricular system and cystic lesion in the fourth ventricle with an eccentric nodule suggestive of scolex.

(2) Leptomeningitis: soft tissue filling the basal cisterns with marked enhancement of the subarachnoid space in the involved areas. Hydrocephalus and vasculitis are common (Razek et al. 2011).

(3) Intraventricular cysts are most commonly seen in the fourth ventricle, followed by the

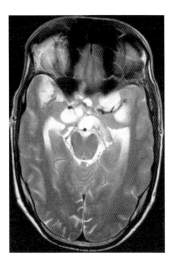

Fig. 4.11. Racemose neurocysticercosis. Axial T2-weighted MRI shows conglomerate cystic lesions in bilateral sylvian fissures and anterior interhemispheric fissure and suprasellar cistern.

lateral and third ventricles (Fig. 4.10). They can move from one ventricle to another and can be trapped in the sylvian aqueduct to cause acute hydrocephalus. MRI is superior to CT in identifying these lesions. T1-weighted images (≤3mm) optimize detection of the scolex. The use of steady-state sequences such as CISS can also be useful in detecting intraventricular or cisternal cystic lesions. Saggital and coronal sections allow better views of fourth ventricular lesions (Razek et al. 2011).

(4) Racemose cysts are multilobular and nonviable (therefore lack scolex), and are commonly located in the subarachnoid space over the cerebellopontine angle, the suprasellar region, the sylvian fissures and the basilar cisterns, which may be contrast enhancing (Fig. 4.11). On MRI, they appear as grape-like clusters of multiple cysts of varying size, with leptomeningeal enhancement. These features strongly indicate racemose cysticercus, especially in endemic areas. A chronic leptomeningitis and arteritis may accompany these cysts (Barkovich 2005, Razek et al. 2011). Another helpful technique is FLAIR sequence following supplemental administration of 100% oxygen, by which the cysts stay dark and CSF becomes bright (Amaral et al. 2005).

In endemic areas, the most common differential diagnosis of NCC is tuberculoma, assessed on the basis of the neuroimaging features listed in Table 4.16.

Hydatid disease
Cerebral hydatid cysts are usually solitary, supratentorial, with non-enhancing T2-hypointense wall and no significant perilesional oedema (Fig. 4.12). They show succinate peak on MRS. Uncommonly, the lesions have multicystic appearance (honeycomb appearance), floating detached membrane (water lily sign) and calcification (Razek et al. 2011).

TABLE 4.16
Differences between neurocysticercosis (NCC) and tuberculoma

	NCC	*Tuberculoma*
Pathognomonic features	Eccentric scolex	None
Meningeal enhancement	Rarely	More common
Location	Parietal, frontal, temporal, occipital	Basal
Number	Multiple but conglomeration not common	When multiple, conglomeration of lesion more likely
Size	Small	>20mm
Wall	Smooth	Thicker and irregular
Cystic features	Particularly early lesions	None
Prominent mass effect	No	May occur

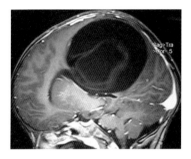

Fig. 4.12. Supratentorial hydatid cyst. Sagittal T2-weighted MRI shows large intra-axial cystic lesion.

Toxoplasmosis
Non-contrast CT may show multiple, well-localized hypo-attenuating or iso-attenuating lesions with surrounding hypodense oedema (Fig. 4.13a). The liquefied centre of the lesions is commonly T2 hyperintense and bright on ADC map. These lesions have a propensity for the basal ganglia, corticomedullary junction and periventricular white matter. There may be variable contrast enhancement. T2-weighted MRI shows typically hypo- to iso-intense multiple lesions surrounded by high signal intensity vasogenic oedema (Fig. 4.13). Ring enhancement with an eccentric nodule forms the 'target sign' highly specific for toxoplasmosis, but present in only about a third of the lesions. Toxoplasmosis needs to be differentiated from lymphoma, since both occur in immunocompromised children. Hyperdense lesions on non-contrast CT and their dark appearance on ADC map are characteristic of lymphoma (Smith and Rushing 2008).

DIFFERENTIAL DIAGNOSIS OF RING-ENHANCING LESIONS
In addition to the infectious causes of ring-enhancing lesions discussed earlier, there are certain non-infectious pathologies with similar presentation such as demyelination, subacute infarct, haemorrhage, high-grade glioma, lymphoma and metastasis.

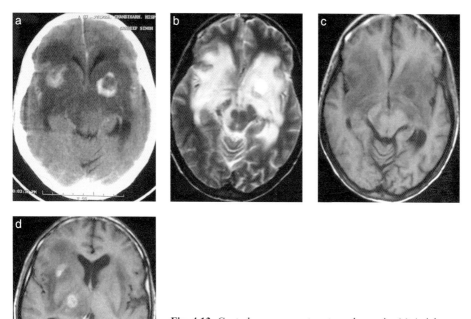

Fig. 4.13. Central nervous system toxoplasmosis. (a) Axial contrast-enhanced CT shows ring-enhancing lesions in bilateral basal ganglia with perilesional oedema. MRI axial sections show (b) T2-isointense and (c) T1-isointense wall, with (d) intense contrast enhancement with associated perilesional oedema on T1-weighted image.

Use of special imaging sequences for aetiological diagnosis of ring-enhancing lesions

• *Susceptibility-weighted imaging (SWI).* The ability of SWI to identify calcification in MRI helps differentiate ring-enhancing degenerated cyst of neurocysticercosis from tuberculoma. Presence of haemorrhages at the advancing edge of the lesion is suggestive of a fungal abscess (Saini et al. 2010). Demonstration of haemorrhages by SWI within the lesions as seen in malignancy differentiates it from infectious aetiology (Holmes et al. 2004) (Table 4.17).

• *Magnetization transfer imaging* has specific findings in intracranial tuberculosis. Tuberculomas with or without caseation have a characteristic bright rim due to low magnetization transfer ratio. Similar findings are seen in the wall of a tuberculous abscess, which are helpful in differentiating it from fungal and pyogenic abscess (Gupta and Kumar 2011).

• *Spectral characteristics of ring lesions.* The spectrum of pyogenic abscesses is characterized by the absence of N-acetyl aspartate, choline and creatinine, and the presence of

TABLE 4.17
Role of susceptibility-weighted imaging in ring-enhancing lesions

Depiction of haemorrhages in wall of the lesions in fungal lesions
Detection of calcific foci in degenerated cyst of neurocysticercosis
Detection of haemorrhages in toxoplasmosis
Differentiation of haemorrhagic gliomas from giant tuberculoma

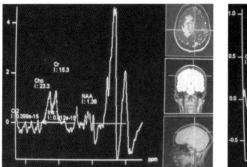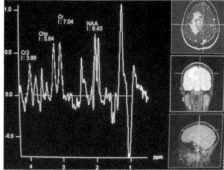

Fig. 4.14. Multi-voxel magnetic resonance spectroscopy images of pyogenic abscess at echo times of (left) 30ms and (right) 135ms show peaks of lipid lactate (1.3ppm), acetate (2.3ppm) and succinate (2.5ppm). A colour version of this figure is available in the plate section at the end of the book.

cytosolic amino acids (leucine, isoleucine and valine) and lactate, acetate, succinate and alanine, and occasionally lipids (mostly short-chain fatty acids such as butyric, isobutyric, caproic, propionic, valeric and isovaleric acids) (Garg et al. 2004) (Fig. 4.14; Table 4.18).

Discrimination between lipids (usually detected at 0.8–1.2ppm) and cytosolic amino acids (usually detected at 0.9ppm) is important because lipids may exist both in necrotic glial tumours and abscesses. Inversion of amino acid peaks at an echo-time of 135ms and splitting of peak components (J coupling) can help differentiate cytosolic amino acids from lipids. Reduction/absence of these amino acids in pyogenic brain abscess is attributed to the prolonged antibiotic therapy, as well as in the abscess due to *Staphylococcus aureus* (Garg et al. 2004). Cytosolic amino acids have been detected in spectra obtained from neurocysticercosis lesions. The presence of succinate alone or increased amounts of both succinate and acetate indicates the presence of degenerating cysticerci and differentiates them from anaerobic or tuberculous abscesses (Agarwal et al. 2004, Pretell et al. 2005). Tuberculous abscesses show only lactate and lipid signals (at 0.9 and 1.3ppm), without any evidence of cytosolic amino acids (Fig. 4.15). A similar pattern may also be seen in staphylococcal abscess. Caseating tuberculomas have lipid and lactate peaks, and sometimes serine peaks between 3.7 and 3.9ppm (Gupta and Kumar 2011, Santy et al. 2011). Fungal abscesses show cytosolic amino acids, lipids and lactate similar to pyogenic abscesses; however, the pres-

TABLE 4.18
Role of magnetic resonance spectroscopy in evaluation of ring-enhancing lesions

Lesions	Magnetic resonance spectroscopy findings
Pyogenic anaerobic	Cytosolic amino acids, lipids, alanine, acetate, succinate
Pyogenic aerobic	Lactate, cytosolic amino acids, lipids
Pyogenic streptococcal	Lactate
Pyogenic staphylococcal	Lipids and lactate
Tuberculous	Lipids and phosphoserine
Fungal	Lipids, lactate, trehalose
Nocardia	Cytosolic amino acids and lactate
Cysticercus	Cytosolic amino acids, lactate, alanine, acetate, succinate and choline

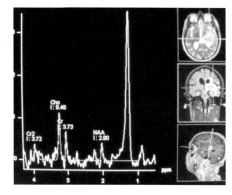

Fig. 4.15. Tuberculoma. Magnetic resonance spectroscopy at echo time 30ms showing lipid peak at 1.3ppm. A colour version of this figure is available in the plate section at the end of the book.

ence of multiple signals seen between 3.6 and 3.8ppm because of the disaccharide trehalose is a distinguishable feature of fungal abscesses (Luthra et al. 2007). MRS in toxoplasmosis reveals elevated lipid and lactate peaks, consistent with an anaerobic acellular environment within an abscess.

• *Magnetic resonance perfusion.* Distinguishing brain abscesses from cystic and necrotic brain tumours is challenging in some cases, since both of them produce ring enhancement on conventional MRI due to destruction of the blood–brain barrier. Perfusion MRI, on the other hand, directly shows the vascular proliferation within the lesion using relative cerebral blood volume (rCBV) map images. While the capsular portions of abscesses are hypovascular, causing a marked decrease in rCBV ratios, the peripheral portions of malignant cystic tumours have higher vascularization and higher rCBV ratios than those of abscesses.

Dynamic contrast-enhanced MRI in characterization of brain tuberculoma showed that the rCBV of the cellular portion significantly correlated with the microvascular density, and vascular endothelial growth factor of the excised tuberculomas (Gupta et al. 2007). The rise in perfusion parameters is suggested as a measure of angiogenesis in the cellular fraction of the brain tuberculoma or can be used as a surrogate marker of blood–brain barrier disruption in assessing therapeutic response in tuberculomas (Haris et al. 2008). Perfusion MRI shows reduced rCBV in *Toxoplasma* lesions attributable to a lack of vasculature and increased rCBV in lymphoma due to the hypervascularity of the tumour (Barcelo et al. 2010).

• *3D heavily T2-weighted imaging.* Identification of the scolex on MRI establishes the diagnosis. This scolex may be missed on routine sequences, but may be detected with 3D heavily T2-weighted high-resolution imaging.

Section 2: Viral Infections

Zoran Rumboldt

Neuroimaging constitutes an important component in the diagnostic process of viral CNS infections, along with the history, physical examination and CSF analysis. Over 100 different invading viruses, including the more common ones such as herpes simplex, herpes zoster, arboviruses and enteroviruses, have been identified as causative agents of encephalitis. Viruses gain access through haematogenous dissemination or, less frequently, along the peripheral nerves. Many have predilection for the cortical, deep or intramedullary grey matter (Fig. 4.16). Others such as human immunodeficiency virus (HIV) and John Cunningham (JC) virus preferentially affect the white matter (Rumboldt et al. 2007, Rumboldt 2008) (Table 4.19). Acute viral encephalitis produces parenchymal infiltration with inflammatory cells, leading to neuronal injury and at times extensive necrosis. The imaging findings reflect these pathological changes, generally visualized as areas of low attenuation on CT, and low T1 and high T2 signal intensity on MRI. DWI has been shown to be superior to conventional MRI for the detection of early signal abnormalities in encephalitis (Rumboldt et al. 2007, Rumboldt 2008). A number of viral infectious agents characteristically lead to specific localization and/or imaging appearance of lesions in the CNS such as increased signal on T2-weighted images in the bilateral thalami and basal ganglia (Fig. 4.17). Viral infections should particularly be taken into consideration with bilateral deep nuclei lesions in an appropriate clinical setting (Rumboldt 2008). However, viral CNS infections may have non-specific or pleomorphic radiological presentations; other infections and non-infectious diseases, including anti-NMDA (N-methyl-D-aspartate) receptor encephalitis, may simulate their characteristic imaging presentation. For instance, transient T2-weighted hyperintense signal and decreased diffusion in the splenium of the corpus callosum has been documented

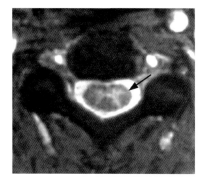

Fig. 4.16. Varicella-zoster myelitis. Axial gradient-echo T2-weighted MRI shows abnormal hyperintensity involving the grey matter on the left side (arrow).

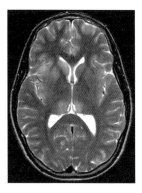

Fig. 4.17. Epstein–Barr virus encephalitis. Axial fast spin-echo T2-weighted MRI shows hyperintense abnormalities involving bilateral thalami, right basal ganglia and right insula without significant mass effect.

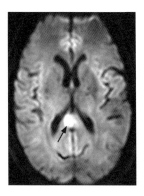

Fig. 4.18. Influenza encephalitis. Axial diffusion-weighted MRI shows a focal hyperintense lesion (arrow) in the splenium of the corpus callosum.

not only with influenza, adenovirus and rotavirus encephalitides (Fig. 4.18), but also with *E. coli* infection, antiepileptic medication withdrawal, hypoglycaemia, osmotic myelinolysis and other disease processes (Rumboldt 2008). This review includes only selected common viral encephalitides with characteristic imaging appearance. The chronology of changes in viral CNS infections on MRI is shown in Table 4.20.

TABLE 4.19
Characteristic sites of involvement in various viral central nervous system infections

Site of involvement	Typical organism	Common organisms
Hippocampus	HSV-1, HSV-2, HHV-6, JE	Rabies, enteroviruses
Other temporal lobe (predominantly grey matter)	HSV-1, HSV-2, HHV-6	Dengue, adenoviruses, many other viruses
Other cerebral lobes, predominantly grey matter	Nipah (relapse/late onset)	Many viruses
White matter – diffuse	HIV, CMV	
White matter – focal (subcortical, periventricular)	JCV (PML), measles (SSPE), chikungunya, WNV, HIV (congenital), CMV (congenital) – periventricular calcification	Rabies
White matter – splenium of corpus callosum		Influenza, adenoviruses, rotaviruses, JCV (PML)
White matter – anterior temporal lobes	CMV (congenital) – bilateral subcortical cysts	
White matter – punctate	Nipah, chickungunya, WNV	
Thalamus	JE, WNV, EBV	Influenza A (H1N1), many other viruses
Ependyma – periventricular	CMV, adenoviruses	
Basal ganglia	EBV, HIV (congenital), measles (SSPE)	Many other viruses
Brainstem	Enteroviruses – dorsal Rabies – dorsal JEV – substantia nigra	Adenoviruses
Cerebellum	JCV (PML) – white matter	Rotaviruses, adenoviruses
Spinal cord – grey matter	Enteroviruses, VZV	Dengue
Spinal cord – white matter	HIV – dorsal columns	
Enhancement – parenchymal lesions		HSV, chikungunya, measles (SSPE)
Enhancement – leptomeningeal brain/spinal cord	CMV	Many viruses (meningoencephalitis), HSV
Enhancement – cauda equina/ nerve roots	CMV, chikungunya, WNV, TBE	Enteroviruses, EBV, JE

HSV, herpes simplex virus; HHV, human herpesvirus; JEV, Japanese encephalitis virus; CMV, cytomegalovirus; JCV, John Cunningham virus; PML, progressive multifocal leukoencephalopathy; SSPE, subacute sclerosing panencephalitis; HIV, human immunodeficiency virus; EBV, Epstein–Barr virus; VZV, varicella-zoster virus; TBE, tuberculous encephalitis.

TABLE 4.20
Chronology of changes in viral central nervous system infections on neuroimaging

Type of neuroimaging	Acute (first 48 hours)	Subacute (3 to approx. 10 days)	Chronic
DWI/ADC MRI	Decreased diffusion (bright on DWI and dark on ADC maps)	Decreased or normal (pseudonormalization)	Increased (bright on ADC maps)
FLAIR and T2W MRI	Hyperintense (bright) or normal	Hyperintense	Normal or hyperintense; CSF-like – dark on FLAIR
T2*W MRI (susceptibility)	Normal or hyperintense; or hypointense (if haemorrhage)	Hyperintense and/or very hypointense (dark) – if haemorrhage (HSV, JEV)	Very dark if prior haemorrhage (haemosiderin)
T1W MRI	Normal or subtle hypointensity	Normal or hypointense (dark), hyperintense if haemorrhage (HSV, JEV)	Normal, or hypointense – CSF-like (if malacia, or hyperintense (as Nipah after 1 month – transient)
Brain CT	Normal or hypodense (dark); hyperdense (bright) if haemorrhage	Hypodense or normal; hyperdense if haemorrhage (HSV, JEV)	Normal or very dark – CSF-like (if malacia, calcification
Contrast enhancement	Absent or present	Present or absent (more commonly present on MRI)	Absent

DWI, diffusion-weighted imaging; ADC, apparent diffusion coefficient; CSF, cerebrospinal fluid; FLAIR, fluid-attenuated inversion recovery; T1W/T2W/T2*W, T1-/T2-/T2*-weighted; HSV, herpes simplex virus; JEV, Japanese encephalitis virus.

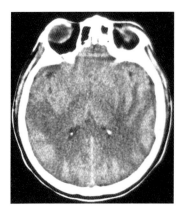

Fig. 4.19. Herpes simplex encephalitis. Axial non-enhanced CT shows bilateral hypodense areas primarily located in posterior temporal lobes.

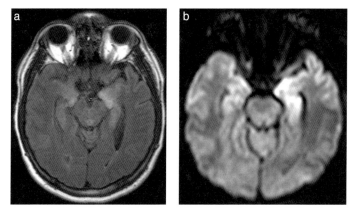

Fig. 4.20. Herpes simplex encephalitis. (a) Axial fluid-attenuated inversion recovery (FLAIR) image shows mild hyperintensity involving bilateral anteromesial temporal lobes, greater on the left than the right. (b) Corresponding diffusion-weighted imaging also reveals the abnormalities.

Herpes encephalitis

Herpes simplex virus (HSV) type 1 is the most common cause of sporadic viral encephalitis, with high mortality in untreated patients. Early diagnosis by high clinical suspicion supplemented by characteristic neuroimaging is crucial for prompt treatment and improved outcome. HSV gains entry into the brain through the sensory cranial nerves, most commonly the trigeminal nerve. This pattern of spread explains why the bilateral anterior and medial temporal lobe involvement is the hallmark of herpes simplex encephalitis (HSE). CT scans are frequently negative in the early stages of the disease; occasional areas of low attenuation may be detected in bilateral temporal lobes (Fig. 4.19). MRI is more sensitive and shows T2-hyperintense and T1-hypointense lesions. Hyperintense lesions predominantly involving the cortical grey matter are seen even earlier on FLAIR images, within 48 hours from the onset of symptoms (Demaerel et al. 1992, Rumboldt et al. 2007) (Fig. 4.20a). However, DWI may be the most sensitive imaging technique for early detection of HSE (Küker et al. 2004). Hyperintense lesions involving the cortex and adjacent white matter on DWI in acute stages of suspected viral encephalitis should be considered HSE until proven otherwise (Fig. 4.20b). Changes in diffusion abnormalities on MRI in patients with HSE also appear to correlate better with disease activity and response to treatment than conventional magnetic resonance images (Duckworth et al. 2005). Unilateral temporal lobe abnormality is not unusual, while the insula, amygdala, cingulate gyrus and orbitofrontal region are commonly involved. Contrast enhancement is usually not present early, while gyriform enhancement may be observed with disease progression (Demaerel et al. 1992, Rumboldt et al. 2007). Areas of haemorrhage may be detected. Rare chronic granulomatous HSE simulates other granulomatous disease processes, such as sarcoidosis; peripheral parenchymal enhancing lesions with associated vasogenic oedema are usually seen in the temporal lobe on MRI (Adamo et al. 2011).

Neonatal HSE is usually caused by HSV-2. The MRI features of HSV-2 encephalitis are: multifocal lesions (67%), temporal lobe involvement (67%), deep grey matter injury (58%), haemorrhage (66%), watershed pattern of ischaemic changes (40%), and occasional involvement of the brainstem and cerebellum. Early proton MRS shows elevated lactate and reduction of NAA (Vossough et al. 2008). Epstein–Barr virus, another member of the herpes family, shows tropism for deep grey nuclei with characteristic bilateral basal ganglia and thalamic involvement (Fig. 4.17) (Baskin and Hedlund 2007).

A few other conditions may also involve the temporal lobes similar to HSV on neuroimaging, most notably the paraneoplastic and human herpes virus-6 limbic encephalitis in immunocompromised patients (Provenzale et al. 2010).

Arbovirus infections

Arboviruses (arthropod-borne viruses) include three different groups of infectious agents that are transmitted by insects and ticks. *Flaviviridae* is the most prominent group that includes agents causing the Japanese, West Nile, St Louis and Murray Valley encephalitides, and tick-borne encephalitides. Dengue and chikungunya viruses have recently gained ground due to their ability to produce extensive epidemics, primarily in tropical urban centres.

JAPANESE ENCEPHALITIS

The characteristic imaging findings are bilateral thalamic (posteromedial nuclei) and brainstem (primarily substantia nigra) lesions that are of low attenuation on CT (Fig. 4.21) and of high T2 signal on MRI. Bilateral thalamic haemorrhages are considered highly specific for Japanese encephalitis (Prakash et al. 2004, Handique et al. 2006). Mesial temporal involvement limited to the hippocampus, amygdala and uncus is fairly characteristic. Concurrent involvement of the thalami and substantia nigra also allows differentiation from HSE (Handique et al. 2006). DWI helps in early diagnosis by showing characteristic hyperintensity in the bilateral thalami (Prakash et al. 2004).

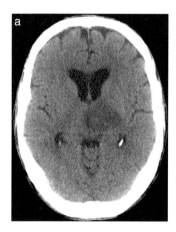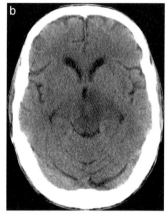

Fig. 4.21. Japanese encephalitis: computerized tomography. (a) Axial non-enhanced scan shows hypodensity in bilateral thalami with mild mass effect, much more prominent on the left side. (b) A more inferior image reveals extension into the midbrain, including the substantia nigra.

Recently, thalamic hypodensity on CT and T2 hyperintensity on MRI were evaluated for the diagnosis of Japanese encephalitis by comparison with the final serological diagnosis in children and adults with suspected CNS infections in a Japanese encephalitis-endemic area. Thalamic lesions showed low sensitivity of only 23%, but with a specificity and positive predictive value of 100% (Dung et al. 2009). Interestingly, a strong association between Japanese encephalitis and neurocysticercosis was found, suggesting that this co-infection was more than a chance occurrence (Handique et al. 2008).

The imaging findings of encephalitides caused by other *Flaviviridae* are, in general, similar to those of Japanese encephalitis. Myriad clinical and imaging features may be seen in patients infected by the West Nile virus (WNV). MRI in some patients with WNV meningo-encephalomyelitis may be normal, or show white matter DWI hyperintensities in milder cases (Ali et al. 2005), resembling vasculitis and acute demyelinating disease. More commonly it mimics Japanese encephalitis. In patients with flaccid paralysis, spinal cord T2 hyperintensity in the ventral grey matter horns and/or enhancement around the conus medullaris and cauda equina are also encountered (Petropoulou et al. 2005).

TICK-BORNE ENCEPHALITIS (TBE)
MRI of the brain may be normal, or depict T2 hyperintensity in the thalami and basal ganglia. Enhancement of the cauda equina and the anterior nerve roots of the conus has also been described (Marjelund et al. 2006).

DENGUE
Dengue virus uncommonly involves the CNS with diverse neuroimaging findings.

Hypodense lesions on CT and T2 hyperintensity on MRI may be found in unilateral or bilateral cerebral lobes (commonly temporal), pons, globus pallidi and thoracic and cervical spinal cord (Wasay et al. 2008). Meningeal enhancement and brain oedema may also be present. Although this pattern is non-specific, it does not simulate Japanese encephalitis, in contrast to most other arboviruses.

CHIKUNGUNYA

Chikungunya virus typically causes symptoms that may be indistinguishable from dengue fever, and simultaneous isolation of both dengue and chikungunya from patients has been reported (Ganesan et al. 2008). It was initially thought that the virus is non-neurotropic; however, meningoencephalitis has been reported from outbreaks in India and the Reunion Islands (Robin et al. 2008, Chandak et al. 2009). In contrast to CNS involvement in dengue, brain and spine MRI and head CT reveal pathological changes in only a minority of affected individuals (Robin et al. 2008, Chandak et al. 2009). Detailed MRI findings described in two patients were bilateral frontoparietal white matter lesions of high T2 signal with reduced diffusivity as well as contrast enhancement of the cerebral lesions and ventral cauda equina nerve roots (Ganesan et al. 2008). As with dengue encephalitis, the findings are not similar to those in Japanese encephalitis.

Enteroviruses

The enteroviruses include Coxsackie viruses A and B, poliovirus, echoviruses, and enteroviruses EV-68 to EV-71. Non-polio enteroviral encephalitis usually presents as prototypical viral encephalitis; focal cerebral involvement is uncommon, and neuroimaging is frequently normal.

Poliomyelitis caused by poliovirus has almost disappeared in resource-rich countries, thus the reports of MRI findings are very rare. MRI shows T2 hyperintensities in the central portion of the midbrain, posterior portion of the medulla oblongata and pons, bilateral dentate nuclei of the cerebellum, and bilateral ventral horns of cervical spinal cord (Fig. 4.22).

Symmetrical bilateral lesions in the dorsal brainstem and ventral horns of the cervical spinal cord are considered characteristic of enteroviral encephalomyelitis (Zeng et al. 2012, Lee et al. 2014). Spinal cord infarction typically presents with identical intramedullary imaging findings.

EV-71 may mimic polio-encephalitis and paralysis clinically, pathologically and radiologically, especially in children with hand–foot–mouth disease or herpangina. During the acute stage, T2-weighted images reveal hyperintense areas while T1-weighted images show no abnormalities, reflecting acute inflammation. Most patients recover well with appropriate management, and the lesions completely disappear within weeks to months. In patients with poor outcomes, follow-up MRI demonstrates T1 hypointensity of the lesions that remain bright on T2-weighted images, reflecting irreversible tissue destruction.

EV-71 may also present as potentially reversible unilateral acute flaccid paralysis due to radiculomyelitis. MRI characteristically shows unilateral lesions involving the anterior horns of the cervical or thoracic spinal cord and ventral root enhancement (Zeng et al. 2012,

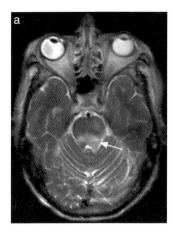
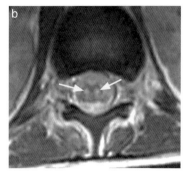

Fig. 4.22. Enterovirus encephalitis. (a) Axial single-shot T2-weighted MRI shows bilateral hyperintense abnormalities in the dorsal pons (arrow). (b) Axial fast spin-echo T2-weighted image at the lower thoracic level shows symmetrical bilateral hyperintense intramedullary lesions in the ventral portion of the spinal cord (arrows), a finding frequently referred to as 'owl's eyes'.

Lee et al. 2014). Bilateral lesions are less common and portend poor outcome. The clinical presentation and neuroimaging appearance of acute flaccid paralysis may be seen not only with enteroviruses but also with Japanese encephalitis and Epstein–Barr virus (Wong et al. 1999). Enteroviruses may also cause bilateral hippocampal encephalitis (Liow et al. 1999) and meningoencephalitis in infants that simulates periventricular leukomalacia (Verboon-Maciolek et al. 2006).

Human immunodeficiency virus and associated opportunistic viral infections
Brain infection with HIV is the most common CNS abnormality in HIV-positive patients. The most common imaging finding in acquired immunodeficiency syndrome (AIDS)–dementia complex is cerebral atrophy followed by white matter T2 hyperintensity, which is T1 isointense and without contrast enhancement or mass effect. Diffuse, bilateral and symmetrical white-matter T2 hyperintensity with relative sparing of the subcortical U-fibres is typical for HIV encephalopathy and best seen on FLAIR images (Fig. 4.23) (Post et al. 1993).

Congenital HIV infection in about half of the affected children shows symmetrical bilateral calcification of the basal ganglia and subcortical white matter of uncertain aetiology. The calcification is generally more conspicuous on CT than on MRI, usually occurs by 1 year of age and is associated with brain atrophy. Prenatal exposure to zidovudine, on the other hand, may lead to antiretroviral-induced mitochondrial dysfunction in children of HIV-infected mothers. MRI findings resemble those in congenital mitochondrial diseases and were present even in asymptomatic children (Tardieu et al. 2005).

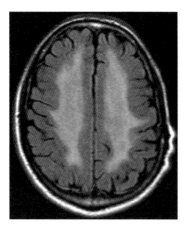

Fig. 4.23. Human immunodeficiency virus encephalitis (acquired immunodeficiency syndrome–dementia complex). Axial fluid-attenuated inversion recovery (FLAIR) image shows diffuse white matter hyperintensity with preservation of the subcortical U-fibres.

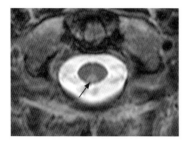

Fig. 4.24. Human immunodeficiency virus myelitis (vacuolar myelopathy). Axial fast spin-echo T2-weighted MRI at the C1–C2 spinal level in a patient with acquired immunodeficiency syndrome shows dorsal bilateral paramedial intramedullary hyperintensity (arrow), corresponding to the dorsal columns.

Vacuolar myelopathy, also known as AIDS-associated myelopathy, is pathologically characterized by posterior-dominant vacuolization in the thoracic spinal cord, strikingly similar to the myelopathy associated with vitamin B_{12} and copper deficiency (Di Rocco et al. 2002, Kumar et al. 2006). The characteristic MRI findings are bilateral symmetrical T2 hyperintensity in the dorsal columns of the spinal cord extending over multiple segments (Fig. 4.24).

Cytomegalovirus

CMV infection of the CNS usually affects immunocompromised populations, especially patients with advanced HIV infection and transplant recipients. The most common brain imaging findings in CMV encephalitis are diffuse atrophy, periventricular contrast enhancement and diffuse white matter abnormalities (Fink et al. 2010). Characteristic MRI findings of ependymal and subependymal linear periventricular hyperintensities on FLAIR images and a thin, linear contrast enhancement along the ventricular margin are suggestive but not specific of CMV infection. CMV appears to be the most common infection involving the spine in patients with AIDS. The most frequent imaging finding is diffuse leptomeningeal enhancement on contrast-enhanced T1-weighted MRI (Fig. 4.25) (Thurnher et al. 2000).

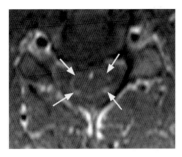

Fig. 4.25. Cytomegalovirus myelitis. Axial post-contrast T1-weighted MRI shows leptomeningeal enhancement (arrows) diffusely along the spinal cord surface.

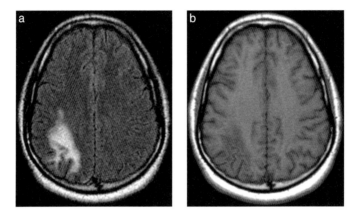

Fig. 4.26. Progressive multifocal leukoencephalopathy. (a) Fluid-attenuated inversion recovery (FLAIR) image demonstrates a focal patchy hyperintensity in the right parieto-frontal area with involvement of the subcortical U-fibres: only a thin strip of cortical grey matter is preserved. (b) Corresponding axial T1-weighted MRI shows clear hypointensity of the lesion, in contrast to the iso-intense appearance of human immunodeficiency virus encephalitis.

Congenital CMV is the most common intrauterine infection, completely unrelated to HIV. The most common imaging findings are periventricular intracranial calcification, neural migration abnormalities such as polymicrogyria, and abnormal white matter that is hypodense on CT and hyperintense on T2-weighted MRI. Subcortical T2 hyperintensity and cyst formation in bilateral anterior temporal white matter is characteristic. Ventriculomegaly, microcephaly and cerebellar hypoplasia are additional imaging findings (Fink et al. 2010).

Progressive multifocal leukoencephalopathy (PML)
In PML caused by the John Cunningham polyomavirus (JCV), multifocal white matter lesions may occur in any location, most often in the parieto-occipital region, corpus callosum and cerebellar white matter as patchy areas of T2 hyperintensities (Thurnher et al. 1997). In contrast to HIV encephalopathy, the lesions are of clearly low signal intensity on

T1-weighted images, the distribution is asymmetrical, and subcortical fibres (U-fibres) are involved (Fig. 4.26) (Thurnher et al. 1997). The mass effect is typically mild, enhancement is usually absent and haemorrhage is unusual; the grey matter may also be affected.

Immune reconstitution inflammatory syndrome (IRIS) of the CNS is a T-cell-mediated encephalitis commonly seen in HIV-infected patients receiving highly active antiretroviral therapy and in patients with multiple sclerosis treated with natalizumab. Patchy and ill-defined, usually large areas of 'lacy' contrast enhancement within cerebral white matter are the characteristic MRI appearance. There is usually associated T2 hyperintensity, low T1 signal, increased diffusivity and minimal to mild mass effect. The new imaging findings frequently occur within or adjacent to the pre-existing PML lesions, and enhancement may be absent (Rushing et al. 2008). The imaging findings are diverse and frequently atypical so that IRIS should be considered whenever an unusual MRI appearance is encountered in patients treated with antiretroviral therapy.

Other viruses

RABIES

Non-enhancing ill-defined mild hyperintensies in the brainstem, hippocampi, hypothalami, deep and subcortical white matter, as well as deep and cortical grey matter have been demonstrated on T2-weighted images (Awasthi et al. 2001, Laothamatas et al. 2011). Most commonly, the lesions are present in the dorsal brainstem, basal ganglia and hippocampi. Enhancement along the brachial plexus of the bitten arm was noted in one patient in the early phase, suggesting inflammatory reactions in response to the presence of rabies virus. Mild to moderate contrast enhancement may be seen at the hypothalami, brainstem nuclei, spinal cord grey matter and intradural cervical nerve roots during the late phase in patients with paralytic rabies (Laothamatas et al. 2011).

NIPAH

Nipah virus is a paramyxovirus with characteristic MRI findings of small, T2-hyperintense lesions initially found within the cerebral white matter and, to a lesser extent, in the grey matter, and best seen on FLAIR images (Lim et al. 2002). This is followed by the appearance of transient punctate cortical hyperintensities on T1-weighted images approximately 1 month after the infection, possibly due to an inflammatory small-vessel vasculopathy. During acute infection, some of the white matter lesions demonstrate decreased diffusion and contrast enhancement suggesting that viral infection was responsible and that these were not pre-existing lesions. There is no significant associated mass effect and cerebral oedema, even in cases with innumerable scattered lesions (Lim et al. 2002). MRI detects abnormalities in 100% of the patients and is more sensitive than blood serology, CSF examination and CSF serology. Brain CT studies remain unremarkable throughout the disease course. There is, however, a poor correlation between MRI and both disease severity and patient outcome. This is not surprising as the imaging findings primarily reflect widespread microinfarcts and ischaemia, while outcome of the patients remains mainly related to the

TABLE 4.21
Characteristic imaging findings of common viral central nervous system infections

Virus	Favoured CNS localization	Typical findings
HSV-1	Anterior and medial temporal lobe	Bright on DWI (dark on ADC maps), high T2 signal, hypodense on CT. Frequently bilateral, primarily GM. Possible haemorrhage
HSV-2 (neonatal)	Deep GM, temporal, brainstem, cerebellum	Haemorrhage, infarcts. Multifocal or limited
Epstein–Barr virus	Deep GM	Bright on DWI (dark on ADC maps), high T2 signal. Hypodense on CT
HHV-6 (immunocompromised)	Anterior and medial temporal lobe	Bright on DWI (dark on ADC maps), high T2 signal. Hypodense on CT
Cytomegalovirus (immunocompromised)	Cerebral WM, ependymal surface, spinal cord	Diffuse high T2 signal, atrophy. High T2 signal, thin linear contrast enhancement – subependymal and along the spinal cord surface
Cytomegalovirus (congenital)	Periventricular WM, temporal lobe	Periventricular chunky calcification. Subcortical bilateral anterior temporal high T2 signal and cyst formation. Cerebral WM T2 hyperintensity, hypodense on CT. Polymicrogyria
Japanese encephalitis virus	Bilateral thalami, brainstem (especially substantia nigra), mesial temporal lobe	Bright on DWI (dark on ADC maps), high T2 signal. Hypodense on CT. Frequent haemorrhage
West Nile virus	Thalami, brainstem; spinal cord ventral GM; conus medullaris and cauda equina; cerebral WM	Bright on DWI, high T2 signal. Hypodense on CT. Contrast enhancement along conus medullaris and cauda equina
Tick-borne encephalitis virus	Deep GM, conus medullaris and cauda equina	High T2 signal. Contrast enhancement along conus medullaris and cauda equina
Dengue	Temporal lobe, globus pallidus, pons, spinal cord	High T2 signal. CT hypodense
Chikungunya	Frontoparietal WM, cauda equina	Focal lesions bright on DWI, high T2 signal, contrast enhancement
Enteroviruses	Dorsal pons and medulla oblongata, central midbrain, bilateral cerebellar dentate nuclei, bilateral medullary ventral GM	High T2 signal
HIV	Cerebral WM, spinal cord posterior columns	Diffuse atrophy. High T2 signal with T1 isointensity – diffuse, bilateral and symmetrical, sparing subcortical U-fibres
JCV (PML)	WM lesions (parieto-occipital, corpus callosum, cerebellum)	Patchy asymmetrical high T2 and low T1 signal, involving subcortical U-fibres

TABLE 4.21
[continued]

Virus	Favoured CNS localization	Typical findings
Rabies	Dorsal brainstem, basal ganglia, hippocampi	Ill-defined mild T2 hyperintensity
Nipah virus	Cerebral WM	Small foci of WM high T2 signal, followed by cortical T1 hyperintensities. Normal CT
Adenoviruses (immunocompromised)	Ependymal surface, mesial temporal lobes, brainstem and cerebellum	Subependymal high T2 signal. High T2 signal, possible enhancement and mild mass effect
Influenza	Thalami, cerebral WM, splenium of corpus callosum	High T2 signal, possible haemorrhage, bright on DWI. Central splenium lesion bright on DWI
Measles virus (SSPE)	Deep GM, cerebral WM	Bilateral high T2 signal

CNS, central nervous system; HSV, herpes simplex virus; DWI, diffusion-weighted imaging; ADC, apparent diffusion coefficient; CT, computerized tomography; GM, grey matter; deep GM, basal ganglia and thalami; HHV, human herpesvirus; WM, white matter; HIV, human immunodeficiency virus; JCV, John Cunningham virus; PML, progressive multifocal leukoencephalopathy, SSPE, subacute sclerosing panencephalitis.

extent of direct neuronal involvement (Lim et al. 2002). Interestingly, MRI in asymptomatic exposed individuals reveals abnormalities similar in size, location and signal intensity to those found in encephalitis patients, suggesting that the lesions are caused by subclinical Nipah virus infection (Lim et al. 2003). The MRI findings in patients with relapse and late-onset encephalitis are markedly different from the findings of early Nipah encephalitis with distinct confluent involvement of the cortex on MRI (Lim et al. 2002).

ADENOVIRUSES

Adenoviruses are relatively rare causes of meningoencephalitis in both immunocompetent and immunocompromised individuals. Immunocompetent patients recover fully with normal neuroimaging (Dubberke et al. 2006). In immunosuppressed patients, adenovirus infection can affect multiple organ systems, including diffuse encephalitis and ependymitis similar to CMV infection and mumps (Zagardo et al. 1998). T2 hyperintensities on MRI seen in the temporal lobes and bilateral limbic systems may simulate HSE (Nagasawa et al. 2006) and in the brainstem and cerebellum may mimic *Listeria monocytogenes* rhombencephalitis (Zagardo et al. 1998). While meningoencephalitis is a rare manifestation of adenovirus infection, it should be considered when involvement of the brainstem, temporal lobes or ependymal surfaces is seen, especially in immunosuppressed patients.

The characteristic imaging findings of common viral CNS infections are summarized in Table 4.21.

Summary

Neuroimaging plays an important role in the diagnosis and management of CNS infections.

A variety of imaging techniques are now available and the appropriate ones can be chosen according to the clinical context in a particular case. CT and conventional MRI may be somewhat helpful in uncomplicated meningitis. Conventional MRI along with DWI is the investigation of choice in complicated meningitis. Many intracranial infections present as space-occupying lesions either as primary pathology or secondary to meningitis. Conventional MRI and CT can suggest the diagnosis in some of these lesions. However, multiparametric MRI using one or more advanced imaging techniques is rapidly evolving as the imaging investigation of choice. Characteristic neuroimaging findings in several viral infections provide important aetiological clues in appropriate clinical settings.

REFERENCES

Adamo MA, Abraham L, Pollack IF (2011) Chronic granulomatous herpes encephalitis: a rare entity posing a diagnostic challenge. *J Neurosurg Pediatr* 8: 402–6.

Agarwal M, Chawla S, Husain N, et al. (2004) Higher succinate than acetate levels differentiate cerebral degenerating cysticerci from anaerobic abscesses on in-vivo proton MR spectroscopy. *Neuroradiology* 46: 211–5.

Ali M, Safriel Y, Sohi J, et al. (2005) West Nile virus infection: MR imaging findings in the nervous system. *AJNR Am J Neuroradiol* 26: 289–97.

Amaral LL, Ferreira RM, da Rocha AJ, Ferreira NP (2005) Neurocysticercosis: evaluation with advanced magnetic resonance techniques and atypical forms. *Top Magn Reson Imaging* 16: 127–44.

Awasthi M, Parmar H, Patankar T, Castillo M (2001) Imaging findings in rabies encephalitis. *AJNR Am J Neuroradiol* 22: 677–80.

Barcelo C, Catalaa I, Loubes-Lacroix F, et al. (2010) Interest of MR perfusion and MR spectroscopy for the diagnostic of atypical cerebral toxoplasmosis. *J Neuroradiol* 37: 68–71.

Barinagarrementeria F, Cantú C (1998) Frequency of cerebral arteritis in subarachnoid cysticercosis: an angiographic study. *Stroke* 29: 123–5.

Barkovich AJ (2005) Infections of the nervous system. In: Barkovich AJ, ed. *Paediatric Neuroimaging, 4th edn.* Philadelphia: Lippincott Williams & Wilkins, pp. 801–5.

Baskin HJ, Hedlund G (2007) Neuroimaging of herpesvirus infections in children. *Pediatr Radiol* 37: 949–63.

Chandak NH, Kashyap RS, Kabra D, et al. (2009) Neurological complications of Chikungunya virus infection. *Neurol India* 57: 177–80.

da Rocha AJ, Maia AC Jr, Ferreira NP, do Amaral LL (2005) Granulomatous diseases of the central nervous system. *Top Magn Reson Imaging* 16: 155–87.

Demaerel P, Wilms G, Robberecht W, et al. (1992) MRI of herpes simplex encephalitis. *Neuroradiology* 34: 490–3.

Di Rocco A, Bottiglieri T, Werner P, et al. (2002) Abnormal cobalamin-dependent transmethylation in AIDS-associated myelopathy. *Neurology* 12: 58–60.

Dubberke ER, Tu B, Rivet DJ, et al. (2006) Acute meningoencephalitis caused by adenovirus serotype 26. *J Neurovirol* 12: 235–40.

Duckworth JL, Hawley JS, Riedy G, Landau ME (2005) Magnetic resonance restricted diffusion resolution correlates with clinical improvement and response to treatment in herpes simplex encephalitis. *Neurocrit Care* 3: 251–3.

Dung NM, Turtle L, Chong WK, et al. (2009) An evaluation of the usefulness of neuroimaging for the diagnosis of Japanese encephalitis. *J Neurol* 256: 2052–60.

Ferreira NP, Otta GM, do Amaral LL, da Rocha AJ (2005) Imaging aspects of pyogenic infections of the central nervous system. *Top Magn Reson Imaging* 16: 145–54.

Fink KR, Thapa MM, Ishak GE, Pruthi S (2010) Neuroimaging of pediatric central nervous system cytomegalovirus infection. *Radiographics* 30: 1779–96.

Galassi W, Phuttharak W, Hesselink JR, et al. (2005) Intracranial meningeal disease: comparison of contrast-enhanced MR imaging with fluid attenuated inversion recovery and fat-suppressed T1-weighted sequences. *AJNR Am J Neuroradiol* 26: 553–9.

Ganesan K, Diwan A, Shankar SK, et al. (2008) Chikungunya encephalomyeloradiculitis: report of 2 cases with neuroimaging and 1 case with autopsy findings. *AJNR Am J Neuroradiol* 29: 1636–7.

Garg A (2011) Vascular brain pathologies. *Neuroimaging Clin N Am* 21: 897–926.

Garg M, Gupta RK, Husain M, et al. (2004) Brain abscess, etiologic categorization with in vivo protron MR spectroscopy. *Radiology* 230: 519–27.

Ginsberg L (2004) Difficult and recurrent meningitis. *J Neurol Neurosurg Psychiatry* 75 (Suppl. 1): i16–i21.

Gupta RK, Kumar S (2011) Central nervous system tuberculosis. *Neuroimaging Clin N Am* 21: 795–814.

Gupta RK, Kathuria MK, Pradhan S (1999) Magnetization transfer MR imaging in CNS tuberculosis. *AJNR Am J Neuroradiol* 20: 867–75.

Gupta RK, Hasan KM, Mishra AM, et al. (2005) High fractional anisotropy in brain abscesses versus other cystic intracranial lesions. *AJNR Am J Neuroradiol* 26: 1107–14.

Gupta RK, Haris M, Husain N, et al. (2007) Relative cerebral blood volume is a measure of angiogenesis in brain tuberculoma. *J Comput Assist Tomogr* 31: 335–41.

Handique SK, Das RR, Barman K, et al. (2006) Temporal lobe involvement in Japanese encephalitis: problems in differential diagnosis. *AJNR Am J Neuroradiol* 27: 1027–31.

Handique SK, Das RR, Saharia B, et al. (2008) Coinfection of Japanese encephalitis with neurocysticercosis: an imaging study. *AJNR Am J Neuroradiol* 29: 170–5.

Haris M, Gupta RK, Husain M, et al. (2008) Assessment of therapeutic response on serial dynamic contrast enhanced MR imaging in brain tuberculomas. *Clin Radiol* 63: 562–74.

Heller C, Heinecke A, Junker R, et al. (2003) The Childhood Stroke Study Group. Cerebral venous thrombosis in children: a multifactorial origin. *Circulation* 108: 1362–7.

Holmes TM, Petrella JR, Provenzale JM (2004) Distinction between cerebral abscesses and high-grade neoplasms by dynamic susceptibility contrast perfusion MRI. *AJR Am J Roentgenol* 183: 1247–52.

Hughes DC, Raghavan A, Mordekar SR, et al. (2010) Role of imaging in the diagnosis of acute bacterial meningitis and its complications. *Postgrad Med J* 86: 478–85.

Kastrup O, Wanke I, Maschke M (2008) Neuroimaging of infections of the central nervous system. *Semin Neurol* 28: 511–22.

Khandelwal N, Gupta V, Singh P (2011) Central nervous system fungal infections in tropics. *Neuroimaging Clin N Am* 21: 859–66.

Kojan S, Al-Jumah M (2006) Infection related cerebral venous thrombosis. *J Pak Med Assoc* 56: 494–7.

Küker W, Nägele T, Schmidt F, et al. (2004) Diffusion-weighted MRI in herpes simplex encephalitis: a report of three cases. *Neuroradiology* 46: 122–5.

Kumar N, Ahlskog JE, Klein CJ, Port JD (2006) Imaging features of copper deficiency myelopathy: a study of 25 cases. *Neuroradiology* 48: 78–83.

Laothamatas J, Sungkarat W, Hemachudha T (2011) Neuroimaging in rabies. *Adv Virus Res* 79: 309–27.

Lee KY, Lee YJ, Kim TH, et al. (2014) Clinico-radiological spectrum in enterovirus 71 infection involving the central nervous system in children. *J Clin Neurosci* 21: 416–20. doi: 10.1016/j.jocn.2013.04.032.

Lim CC, Lee KE, Lee WL, et al. (2002) Nipah virus encephalitis: serial MR study of an emerging disease. *Radiology* 222: 219–26.

Lim CC, Lee WL, Leo YS, et al. (2003) Late clinical and magnetic resonance imaging follow up of Nipah virus infection. *J Neurol Neurosurg Psychiatry* 74: 131–3.

Liow K, Spanaki MV, Boyer RS, et al. (1999) Bilateral hippocampal encephalitis caused by enteroviral infection. *Pediatr Neurol* 21: 836–8.

Luthra G, Parihar A, Nath K, et al. (2007) Comparative evaluation of fungal, tubercular, and pyogenic abscesses with conventional and diffusion MR imaging and proton MR spectroscopy. *AJNR Am J Neuroradiol* 28: 1332–8.

Marjelund S, Jaaskelainen A, Tikkakoski T, et al. (2006) Gadolinium enhancement of cauda equina: a new MR imaging finding in the radiculitic form of tick-borne encephalitis. *AJNR Am J Neuroradiol* 27: 995–7.

Martins HS, da Silva TR, Scalabrini-Neto A, Velasco IT (2010) Cerebral vasculitis caused by *Aspergillus* simulating ischemic stroke in an immunocompetent patient. *J Emerg Med* 38: 597–600.

Morgado C, Ruivo N (2005) Imaging meningo-encephalic tuberculosis. *Eur J Radiol* 55: 188–92.

Mukherjee P, Berman JI, Chung SW, et al. (2008) Diffusion tensor MR imaging and fiber tractography: theoretic underpinnings. *AJNR Am J Neuroradiol* 29: 633–42.

Nagasawa H, Wada M, Kurita K, et al. (2006) A case of non-herpetic acute limbic encephalitis associated with a type-2 adenovirus infection. *Rinsho Shinkeigaku* 46: 322–7.

Petropoulou KA, Gordon SM, Prayson RA, Ruggierri PM (2005) West Nile virus meningoencephalitis: MR imaging findings. *AJNR Am J Neuroradiol* 26: 1986–95.

Phuong LK, Link M, Wijdicks E (2002) Management of intracranial infectious aneurysms: a series of 16 cases. *Neurosurgery* 51: 1145–51.

Post MJ, Berger JR, Duncan R, et al. (1993) Asymptomatic and neurologically symptomatic HIV-seropositive subjects: results of long-term MR imaging and clinical follow-up. *Radiology* 188: 727–33.

Prakash M, Kumar S, Gupta RK (2004) Diffusion-weighted MR imaging in Japanese encephalitis. *J Comput Assist Tomogr* 28: 756–61.

Pretell EJ, Martino C Jr, Garcia HH, et al. (2005) Differential diagnosis between cerebral tuberculosis and neurocysticercosis by magnetic resonance spectroscopy. *J Comput Assist Tomogr* 29: 112–4.

Provenzale JM, van Landingham KE, White LE (2010) Clinical and imaging findings suggesting human herpesvirus 6 encephalitis. *Pediatr Neurol* 42: 32–9.

Razek AA, Watcharakorn A, Castillo M (2011) Parasitic diseases of the central nervous system. *Neuroimaging Clin N Am* 21: 815–41.

Reiche W, Schuchardt V, Hagen T, et al. (2010) Differential diagnosis of intracranial ring enhancing cystic mass lesions—role of diffusion-weighted imaging (DWI) and diffusion-tensor imaging (DTI). *Clin Neurol Neurosurg* 112: 218–25.

Robin S, Ramful D, Le Seach F, et al. (2008) Neurologic manifestations of pediatric chikungunya infection. *J Child Neurol* 23: 1028–35.

Rumboldt Z (2008) Imaging of topographic viral CNS infections. *Neuroimaging Clin N Am* 18: 85–92.

Rumboldt Z, Thurnher MM, Gupta RK (2007) Central nervous system infections. *Semin Roentgenol* 42: 62–91.

Rushing EJ, Liappis A, Smirniotopoulos JD, et al. (2008) Immune reconstitution inflammatory syndrome of the brain: case illustrations of a challenging entity. *J Neuropathol Exp Neurol* 67: 819–27.

Saini J, Gupta AK, Jolapara MB, et al. (2010) Imaging findings in intracranial aspergillus infection in immunocompetent patients. *World Neurosurg* 74: 661–70.

Salzman KL (2004) Meningitis. In: Osborn AG, ed. *Diagnostic Imaging—Brain.* Salt Lake City: Amirsys, pp. 8–24.

Santy K, Nan P, Chantana Y, et al. (2011) The diagnosis of brain tuberculoma by (1)H-magnetic resonance spectroscopy. *Eur J Pediatr* 170: 379–87.

Shetty PG, Shroff MM, Sahani DV, et al. (1998) Evaluation of high-resolution CT and MR cisternography in the diagnosis of cerebrospinal fluid fistula. *AJNR Am J Neuroradiol* 19: 633–9.

Smirniotopoulos JG, Murphy FM, Rushing EJ, et al. (2007) Patterns of contrast enhancement in the brain and meninges. *RadioGraphics* 27: 525–51.

Smith AB, Rushing JR (2008) Central nervous system infections associated with human immunodeficiency virus infection: radiologic–pathologic correlation. *RadioGraphics* 28: 2033–58.

Tardieu M, Brunelle F, Raybaud C, et al. (2005) Cerebral MR imaging in uninfected children born to HIV-seropositive mothers and perinatally exposed to zidovudine. *AJNR Am J Neuroradiol* 26: 695–701.

Thurnher MM, Thurnher SA, Mühlbauer B, et al. (1997) Progressive multifocal leukoencephalopathy in AIDS: initial and follow-up CT and MRI. *Neuroradiology* 39: 611–8.

Thurnher MM, Post MJ, Jinkins JR (2000) MRI of infections and neoplasms of the spine and spinal cord in 55 patients with AIDS. *Neuroradiology* 42: 551–63.

Trivedi R, Saksena S, Gupta RK (2009) Magnetic resonance imaging in central nervous system tuberculosis. *Indian J Radiol Imaging* 19: 256–65.

Verboon-Maciolek MA, Groenendaal F, Cowan F, et al. (2006) White matter damage in neonatal enterovirus meningoencephalitis. *Neurology* 66: 1267–9.

Vossough A, Zimmerman RA, Bilaniuk LT, Schwartz EM (2008) Imaging findings of neonatal herpes simplex virus type 2 encephalitis. *Neuroradiology* 50: 355–66.

Wasay M, Channa R, Jumani M, et al. (2008) Encephalitis and myelitis associated with dengue viral infection clinical and neuroimaging features. *Clin Neurol Neurosurg* 110: 635–40.

Wong M, Connolly AM, Noetzel MJ (1999) Poliomyelitis-like syndrome associated with Epstein–Barr virus infection. *Pediatr Neurol* 20: 235–7.

Zagardo MT, Shanholtz CB, Zoarski GH, Rothman MI (1998) Rhombencephalitis caused by adenovirus: MR imaging appearance. *AJNR Am J Neuroradiol* 19: 1901–13.

Zeng H, Wen F, Gan Y, Huang W (2012) MRI and associated clinical characteristics of EV71-induced brainstem encephalitis in children with hand–foot–mouth disease. *Neuroradiology* 54: 623–30.

5
CONGENITAL INFECTIONS

James F Bale, Jr

Approximately 40 years ago investigators at Emory University, Atlanta, Georgia, and the United States Centers for Disease Control and Prevention coined the term TORCH, an acronym denoting *Toxoplasma gondii*, rubella, cytomegalovirus and herpesviruses, to promote the identification of congenital infections in newborn infants (Nahmias 1974). Though congenital herpes simplex virus infection occurs very rarely, and congenital rubella syndrome has largely disappeared in nations with compulsory rubella immunization, the pathogens signified by TORCH, with the addition of syphilis, parvovirus, varicella, and more recently recognized agents including lymphocytic choriomeningitis virus, remain major causes of deafness, blindness and permanent neurodevelopmental disabilities worldwide. This chapter provides current information regarding the TORCH agents and emphasizes the epidemiology, clinical manifestations, treatment and prevention of these important human infections.

Epidemiology

CONGENITAL TOXOPLASMOSIS

Congenital toxoplasmosis, caused by the intracellular parasite *Toxoplasma gondii*, currently represents the second most commonly recognized congenital infection after congenital cytomegalovirus (CMV) infection in most regions. Rates of congenital toxoplasmosis range from less than 0.1 per 1000 live births in many areas to approximately 1 per 1000 live births in highly endemic regions, whereas rates of congenital CMV infection are approximately 10-fold higher, particularly in many locations of the USA. The seroprevalence of toxoplasmosis among adults, a measure of acquired infection with *T. gondii*, is highest in France, intermediate in Latin America, sub-Saharan Africa and central Europe, and lowest in North America, southeast Asia and Oceania. A US population-based study detected very low rates of congenital toxoplasmosis (<0.02/1000 births) and observed that the mother's country of origin, educational level and number of pregnancies were linked to the risk of delivering an infant with congenital toxoplasmosis (Jara et al. 2001).

Toxoplasma gondii, a ubiquitous protozoan, infects birds and many mammals, especially felines, worldwide (Hill et al. 2005). Human infection results from ingesting meats that contain viable *T. gondii* tissue cysts, or foods, including leafy vegetables, that become contaminated with infectious oocysts. Theoretically, cases of congenital toxoplasmosis could be prevented by stringent processing of meats and avoidance of cats, cat excrement and under-cooked foods during a woman's pregnancy. Infectious cysts in meat can be inactivated by freezing meats at –20°C for more than 48 hours or by cooking at temperatures over 100°C for 10 minutes (El-Nawawi et al. 2008).

CONGENITAL RUBELLA SYNDROME

Prior to widespread immunization, rubella virus (the agent causing German measles) was the most common cause of congenital infection in humans. Epidemics of rubella occurred worldwide at 6–9 year intervals. Humans represent the only reservoir of rubella virus; thus, transmission results from contact with infected humans and their virus-contaminated respiratory secretions. During the 1962–5 pandemic, the last major US rubella outbreak, approximately 20 000 infants were affected by congenital rubella syndrome (CRS); there were more than 10 000 fetal deaths and 2000 neonatal deaths (Centers for Disease Control and Prevention 2005). Fortunately, CRS largely disappeared from the USA and other resource-rich nations by the late 1980s because of compulsory immunization programmes. A comprehensive epidemiology study of French-born infants with CRS confirmed the success of compulsory immunization for rubella virus by observing an incidence of 28 cases per 100 000 live births during the 1970s and 1980s and a 10-fold reduction by 2002 after an aggressive immunization programme. CRS remains a major health concern in resource-poor nations, with 112 000 cases in 2008. Infants with CRS still appear sporadically in the USA and other resource-rich nations as the result of immunization noncompliance or importation from countries without immunization programmes. Reinfection of seroimmune women can occasionally result in fetal infection and CRS, although this seems to be an exceptionally rare event (Bullens et al. 2000). Eliminating CRS worldwide remains a major goal of the World Health Organization.

CONGENITAL CYTOMEGALOVIRUS INFECTION

With the near-elimination of CRS from resource-rich nations, congenital CMV infection has emerged as the most commonly recognized congenital infection in many regions. Studies from many different locations indicate that 0.25%–1% of infants shed CMV in urine or saliva at birth, indicating congenital infection, and because 5%–10% of these infants have signs of infection at birth, approximately 4000 infants are born annually in the USA with symptomatic CMV infections, also known as congenital CMV disease (Istas et al. 1995). Detailed natural history studies indicate that the remaining infants, corresponding to 90%–95% of the infants with congenital CMV infection, lack symptoms of CMV at birth and have low risks of sequelae except for hearing loss, a complication discussed later in this chapter.

CMV latently infects 40%–100% of the human adult population, and such persons serve as an important reservoir of the virus. Infections periodically reactivate, leading to excretion of infectious virus in saliva, urine, breast milk and cervical secretions in women, and semen in men. Transmission requires direct contact with the infected body fluid; transfusion of CMV-infected blood products and transplantation of CMV-infected organs or tissues are also potential mechanisms of CMV transmission. Acquired CMV infections pose little or no risk of severe disease in immunocompetent hosts, but such infections can pose serious or potentially life-threatening risks for persons with immunocompromising conditions such as human immunodeficiency virus/autoimmune deficiency syndrome (HIV/AIDS) or post-transplant patients. In addition, up to 50% of toddlers shed CMV in their saliva and urine, indicating active infection (Murph and Bale 1988), and frequently transmit the virus to their playmates. Other persons, including parents and care providers, can acquire CMV from these infected individuals through exposure to virus-containing body fluids. Maternal risk factors for delivering a congenitally infected infant thus include close contact with young children, who are a major reservoir of CMV, as well as young maternal age and having multiple sexual partners (Murph et al. 1998).

CONGENITAL SYPHILIS

Each year as many as 12 million adults and 1 million pregnant women worldwide acquire syphilis, the consequence of infection with the ubiquitous spirochaete *Treponema pallidum* (Woods 2005). Infection results from direct contact with infected human secretions via oral, anal or vaginal intercourse; fomites do not participate in the transmission of *T. pallidum*. Transmission of the spirochaete to the fetus occurs in as many as 50% of the maternal infections, leading to fetal death, stillbirth and congenital infection (McClure and Goldenberg 2009). Rare in most resource-rich countries, congenital syphilis affects several hundred infants annually in the USA, especially in densely populated urban areas and the rural South. In the USA, rates of syphilis are highest in women 20–24 years of age and men 35–39 years of age; in 2008, the most recent year with available data, the Centers for Disease Control and Prevention received reports of 10.1/100 000 live births with congenital syphilis (Centers for Disease Control and Prevention 2010).

OTHER AGENTS

Several additional pathogens, including herpes simplex viruses (HSV), varicella-zoster virus (VZV), human parvovirus B19, lymphocytic choriomeningitis virus, *Trypanosoma cruzi*, Venezuelan equine encephalitis virus and, possibly, West Nile virus, pose potential threats to the fetus and the developing nervous system (Rasmussen et al. 2007).

The incidence of neonatal HSV infections averages 0.025–0.3 per 1000 live births, but only 5%–10% of these represent congenital infections (Kimberlin 2004). Women acquire HSV, either type 1 or type 2, through sexual or oral contact with the virus-containing secretions of infected persons. The rates of varicella infection, usually acquired through contact with the respiratory secretions of infected children, range from less than 1 to 3 per 1000 pregnancies, and very few (<2%) of these pregnancies result in infants with the congenital varicella syndrome.

Congenital infections with lymphocytic choriomeningitis virus (LCMV), a rodent-borne arenavirus, have been reported in infants from several regions (Bonthius et al. 2007b), but the precise incidence of congenital LCMV infection remains poorly defined. Humans presumably become infected with LCMV through contact with aerosols or fomites that contain infectious virus; occasional infected adults have an influenza-like illness with malaise, myalgias and low-grade fever. Current data regarding the incidence of congenital Chagas disease, caused by maternal infection with the parasite *T. cruzi*, although imprecise, may suggest that as many as 10 000 infants have congenital infections with this agent annually in the Americas. Despite considerable angst about the potential consequences of West Nile virus (WNV) infection during pregnancy, only a single case of congenital WNV infection has been reported to date (O'Leary et al. 2006).

Human parvovirus B19 infection, the cause of fifth disease, a mild childhood illness associated with low-grade fever and erythematous 'slapped cheek' rash, can be transmitted to the fetus during infections of seronegative women and lead to fetal anaemia and hydrops fetalis (de Jong et al. 2006). Outcomes of this infection can include spontaneous resolution in utero or, occasionally, fetal death. Approximately 50% of adults have serological evidence of prior infection with this small DNA virus; a seropositive woman of childbearing age is protected from the serious fetal consequences of this infection. Management of severe fetal infections includes intrauterine transfusions to correct fetal anaemia and induction of labour if the infant is near term.

Clinical manifestations

Early Manifestations
The pathogens causing human congenital infections typically produce systemic and neurological signs that can be identified in the neonatal period. The early features of these infections, commonly consisting of jaundice, hepatomegaly, splenomegaly, rash, intrauterine growth retardation, microcephaly, hydrocephalus, cataracts or chorioretinitis, underscore the importance of the TORCH acronym. When considering one agent, such as *T. gondii*, as the cause of an infant's condition, clinicians must remember that other pathogens, such as CMV and LCMV, can produce similar clinical manifestations. Although the TORCH acronym reminds clinicians of the features shared by these agents, some infections have unique features. CRS, for example, is the only disorder associated with congenital heart lesions (classically patent ductus arteriosus, but also atrial and ventricular septal defects) (Webster 1998), while congenital varicella syndrome is the only one producing a unique dermatomal pattern of skin scarring called a cicatrix (Sauerbrei and Wutzler 2007). Prominent osteopathy can suggest either congenital syphilis or CRS (Ghadouane et al. 1995). Isolated chorioretinal scarring suggests congenital infection with CMV, *T. gondii*, LCMV or HSV, whereas congenital cataracts suggest CRS, VZV or syphilis (Mets 2001). LCMV characteristically affects only the brain and eye in congenital infections, producing microcephaly, hydrocephalus and chorioretinitis (Bonthius et al. 2007b).

Though most of the agents described in this chapter infect or replicate in the liver or spleen, causing organ enlargement, jaundice, hepatitis, direct hyperbilirubinaemia and consumptive thrombocytopenia, the relative frequency of these signs varies considerably among pathogens. Of symptomatic infants with congenital CMV and *Toxoplasmosa* infection, for example, approximately 70% or more have jaundice and hepatosplenomegaly (Boppana et al. 1992). Approximately 50% of infants with congenital Chagas disease or congenital syphilis also have these abnormalities (Bittencourt 1976). By contrast, infants with CRS have low frequency of jaundice or hepatosplenomegaly (20%), and reticuloendothelial system involvement is distinctly unusual in infants with congenital infections with VZV and LCMV (Bonthius et al. 2007b).

Infants with congenital infections commonly have skin lesions, and these lesions often provide an important clue as to the offending pathogen. Purpuric or petechial rash occurs in 70% of infants with congenital CMV disease and in 20%–25% of those with toxoplasmosis, syphilis or CRS, whereas a vesicular rash is observed in 70% of congenitally or perinatally acquired HSV infection. The classic 'blueberry muffin' rash, a sign indicating extra-medullary haematopoesis, can be observed in CRS or CMV infection. Zig-zag skin lesions (cicatrix) conforming to a dermatomal distribution suggests congenital varicella syndrome (Sauerbrei and Wutzler 2007); rarely, bullous lesions can be observed in congenital infections with HSV or LCMV. Infants with congenital syphilis can exhibit maculopapular or bullous rashes of the palms, mucous patches or condyloma lata, raised wart-like lesions.

All of the agents described in this chapter can damage the developing nervous system. The neonatal neurological manifestations of congenital infections consist of microcephaly, macrocephaly, seizures, meningoencephalitis and abnormalities of muscle tone. Microcephaly commonly accompanies infections with CMV, rubella virus, HSV and VZV, whereas macrocephaly, often indicating hydrocephalus, commonly accompanies congenital toxoplasmosis. Infants with congenital LCMV infections can have either microcephaly or macrocephaly at birth; rapidly increasing head circumference with suture splaying can appear postnatally as a result of obstructive hydrocephalus in LCMV-infected infants who were initially microcephalic or normocephalic. Seizures, focal or generalized, can be an early manifestation of congenital infection with any of several agents. Meningoencephalitis can complicate infections with CMV, rubella, LCMV or HSV and produce somnolence, irritability and bulging fontanelles.

Ophthalmological abnormalities, including chorioretinitis, cataract, pigmentary retinopathy, optic atrophy and microphthalmia, commonly accompany congenital infection and sometimes provide useful clinical clues regarding the aetiological agent (Mets 2001). Chorioretinal scarring occurs in more than 90% of infants with congenital LCMV infection, 75% of infants with congenital toxoplasmosis, around 50% of infants with congenital varicella syndrome, and 10%–20% of infants with congenital CMV disease. Approximately 80% or more of the infants with CRS have cataracts, and some also have pigmentary retinopathy or microphthalmia. Cataracts can be observed in congenital infections with VZV, HSV and LCMV, but are very uncommon in infants with CMV or *T. gondii*. Cerebral visual impairment, reflecting damage to the occipital cortex or optic pathways, can complicate nearly all of the infections described in this chapter.

Sensorineural hearing loss, a prominent complication of CRS and congenital CMV disease, can occur with other congenital infections, including untreated congenital toxoplasmosis (Andrade et al. 2008). Nearly 90% of the 20 000 infants born during the 1962–1965 US rubella epidemic had sensorineural hearing loss. In many, deafness was the only manifestation of CRS. Sensorineural hearing loss occurs in 50% of infants with congenital CMV disease and approximately 8% of the congenitally infected infants who lack signs of CMV infection at birth (Grosse et al. 2008). Hearing loss in congenital CMV infections appears to be associated with disseminated infection and higher viral loads (Rivera et al. 2002). Sensorineural hearing loss in congenitally infected infants can be unilateral or bilateral and ranges from mild to profound, and can appear abruptly in otherwise healthy young children who had silent congenital infections with CMV. Deafness is a relatively infrequent complication of congenital infections with *T. pallidum*, *T. cruzi*, VZV, LCMV or HSV.

LATE MANIFESTATIONS

Certain sequelae of congenital infections may not appear for months or years after the intrauterine infection (Dudgeon 1975, Townsend et al. 1975, Takasu et al. 2005, Dunin-Wasowicz et al. 2007). Examples of these phenomena are immune-mediated diabetes mellitus and hypothyroidism that appears in adolescence or the early twenties in patients with a history of CRS (Takasu et al. 2005). Late-onset sensorineural hearing loss in children with congenital CMV infection can be progressive or fluctuating, even in children who had no signs of CMV infection during the neonatal period (Grosse et al. 2008). Infants with congenital syphilis can have a constellation of late findings that includes sabre shins, saddlenose deformity, mulberry molars, frontal bossing, rhagades, and the Hutchinson triad of sensorineural deafness, interstitial keratitis and Hutchinson teeth (peg-shaped upper incisors) (Woods 2005). Obstructive hydrocephalus can occur in young children who had congenital infections with LCMV. Infantile spasms can appear during the first year of life in infants with congenital CMV infection, congenital toxoplasmosis, CRS or perinatal HSV infection (Dunin-Wasowicz et al. 2007). Infants with CRS are at risk of post-rubella panencephalitis, a very rare but fatal neurodegenerative disorder that can appear several years after CRS (Townsend et al. 1975).

Laboratory findings

Laboratory abnormalities compatible with intrauterine infection include direct hyperbilirubinaemia, haemolytic anaemia, thrombocytopenia and elevations of the serum transaminases. Approximately 70% of infants with congenital CMV disease have mild to moderate elevations of serum transaminases (Boppana et al. 1992); infants with CMV infections can occasionally have severe hepatitis leading to cirrhosis and, uncommonly, liver failure. Self-limited hepatic dysfunction is frequent in congenital toxoplasmosis, CRS and congenital syphilis.

Thrombocytopenia, often in the range of 15 000–50 000/µL, can be seen in infections with CMV, *T. gondii* or rubella virus. Approximately 50% or more of the infants with congenital CMV disease have thrombocytopenia, and about one-third of those will have platelet counts lower than 50 000/µL (Boppana et al. 1992). Most infants with symptomatic CRS have thrombocytopenia (Dudgeon 1975); nearly 20% of such infants have platelet counts below 20 000/µL. Thrombocytopenia in congenital CMV disease and other congenital infections results from marrow dysfunction, consumption of platelets due to hypersplenism, and autoimmune destruction of mature platelets.

TABLE 5.1
Methods to detect selected pathogens associated with congenital infection

Agent	*Preferred diagnostic method*
Cytomegalovirus	Urine PCR or culture
Herpes simplex viruses	CSF, serum, vesicle fluid PCR
Lymphocytic choriomeningitis virus	Serum LCMV-specific IgM
Rubella virus	Serum rubella-specific IgM; RT-PCR
Toxoplasma gondii	*T. gondii*-specific IgM; PCR
Treponema pallidum	CSF, serum VDRL test
Varicella-zoster virus	VZV-specific IgM; CSF PCR
West Nile virus	CSF WNV-specific IgM

PCR, polymerase chain reaction; CSF, cerebrospinal fluid; LCMV, lymphocytic choriomeningitis virus; RT-PCR, reverse transcription PCR; VDRL, Venereal Disease Research Laboratory; VZV, varicella-zoster virus; WNV, West Nile virus.

Anaemia, secondary to marrow dysfunction or haemolysis, can be observed in infants with congenital syphilis, toxoplasmosis, CMV disease, Chagas disease or CRS. Infants with haemolytic anaemia can have increased reticulocyte counts and peripheral blood smears with abnormal erythrocyte morphology. Marrow aspirates, if obtained, may reveal an increased erythroid:myeloid ratio in haemolytic anaemia or decreased erythrocyte precursors in virus-induced marrow suppression. Examination of the cerebrospinal fluid (CSF) may reveal a lymphocytic pleocytosis or elevations of the protein content (Boppana et al. 1992).

Microbiological diagnosis
The diagnosis of congenital infections relies on serological, molecular or culture methods, depending upon the pathogen (Table 5.1). Serological methods remain the most useful strategy when evaluating infants for infections with *T. gondii* or LCMV. Because IgM and IgA do not cross the placenta, detection of *T. gondii*-specific IgM or IgA in the infant's serum strongly suggests congenital toxoplasmosis; neonatal blood spots have been used as a screening method for congenital toxoplasmosis, with a sensitivity approaching 90%. Analysis of paired sera from the mother and infant can be a useful strategy in infants with suspected congenital infections. Absence of *T. gondii*-specific IgG or IgM in the infant's serum and absence of *T. gondii*-specific IgG in the mother's serum, for example, virtually eliminate congenital toxoplasmosis. Congenital LCMV infection is supported by detection of LCMV-specific IgM in the infant's serum using enzyme-linked immunosorbent assays (Bonthius et al. 2007b).

While detection of CMV in an infant's saliva or urine by cell culture during the first 3 weeks of life remains the criterion standard for the diagnosis of congenital CMV disease, congenital infection can be established by detection of CMV-specific IgM in the neonate's serum, or CMV nucleic acids in urine or saliva using polymerase chain reaction (PCR) testing. In many clinical laboratories, molecular methods of virus detection such as PCR are gradually supplanting labour-intensive cell-culture methods. Because CMV is commonly

TABLE 5.2
Common neurological manifestations of congenital infections

Agent	Microcephaly	Hydrocephalus	Chorioretinitis	Cataract	Other
CMV	✓		✓		CD[a]
HSV	✓		✓	✓	CD
LCMV	✓	✓	✓		CD
Parvovirus B16					CD
Rubella	✓		✓	✓	
Syphilis			✓	✓	
T. gondii		✓	✓	✓	
VZV	✓			✓	CD
West Nile virus	✓		✓		

The header row "Clinical feature" spans Microcephaly, Hydrocephalus, Chorioretinitis, Cataract, and Other.

[a]CD = cortical dysplasia: this includes polymicrogyria, lissencephaly/pachygyria and schizencephaly, depending upon the agent. Passive ventriculomegaly can also be observed secondary to cortical atrophy or dysplasia. CMV, cytomegalovirus; HSV, herpes simplex virus (usually HSV-2); LCMV, lymphocytic choriomeningitis virus; VZV, varicella-zoster virus.

acquired by nursing infants, congenital infection cannot be confirmed by culture or PCR detection of CMV in urine samples obtained after 4 weeks of age. PCR detection of CMV in neonatal blood spots using Guthrie cards represents a potentially important breakthrough in the ability to retrospectively establish congenital CMV infection (Walter et al. 2008). Subsequent studies indicated that blood-spot PCR has much lower sensitivity than cell culture or PCR analysis of urine or saliva, indicating that it may not be an effective means to screen infants prospectively for congenital CMV infection (Boppana et al. 2010). A positive blood-spot PCR for CMV supports congenital infection, whereas a negative PCR must be viewed with caution. Virus culture or PCR can be used to establish the diagnosis of intrauterine or perinatally acquired HSV infections. The diagnosis of congenital varicella syndrome can be made by detection of VZV-specific DNA in tissues or fluids, detection of VZV-specific IgM in neonatal serum, or persistence of VZV-specific IgG beyond 7 months of age (Walter et al. 2008).

Neuroimaging features
Damage to the developing CNS represents the most serious consequence of congenital infections (Table 5.2), and several imaging modalities including ultrasonography, computed tomography and magnetic resonance imaging can be used to evaluate infants with suspected congenital infections. Ultrasonography remains a useful bedside technique to image the brains of unstable infants who cannot be transported to an imaging suite. It can provide valuable information regarding periventricular hyperechogenicities, intracranial calcification, cystic encephalomalacia, passive ventriculomegaly and periventricular leukomalacia, all potential CNS features of congenital infections.

Intracranial calcification has long been recognized as a hallmark of congenital infections, especially among infants infected with CMV, rubella or *T. gondii*. Approximately 50%

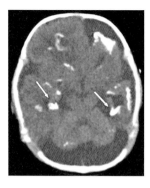

Fig. 5.1. Unenhanced head CT of a 6-day-old male infant with suspected congenital CMV infection shows bilateral periventricular calcifications (arrows) as well as cortical calcification of the left hemisphere and cerebellar hypoplasia.

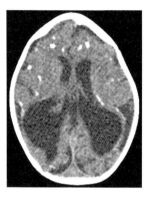

Fig. 5.2. Unenhanced head CT of a female infant with congenital toxoplasmosis shows passive ventriculomegaly, cortical dysplasia and calcification scattered throughout both cerebral hemispheres.

of infants with congenital CMV disease have intracranial calcification (Fig. 5.1), usually in a periventricular distribution, although this is also observed in infants with CRS, LCMV infection and congenital toxoplasmosis. In the latter disease, however, intracranial calcification tends to be scattered diffusely throughout the brain parenchyma (Fig. 5.2); some infants with CMV or LCMV infections can have a similar pattern of calcification (Bale et al. 1985). Calcification in infants with congenital HSV infections distinctively involve the thalamus and basal ganglia (Hutto et al. 1987). Infants with CRS have periventricular or parenchymal calcification, but because CRS largely disappeared in resource-rich nations prior to major advances in neuroimaging, the neuroimaging descriptions of CRS are rather limited.

Polymicrogyria, schizencephaly, pachygyria/lissencephaly, hydranencephaly and cleft cortical dysplasia can be observed in infants with congenital HSV, CMV, LCMV and VZV infections (Boppana et al. 1992, Iannetti et al. 1998, Bonthius et al. 2007b). CMV commonly causes polymicrogyria (Fig. 5.3) and can also produce lissencephaly and schizencephaly (Iannetti et al. 1998). Cerebellar hypoplasia can occur in infants with congenital CMV or LCMV infections (Boppana et al. 1992, Bonthius et al. 2007b). A single report indicates that passive ventriculomegaly, heterotopia and polymicrogyria can accompany congenital

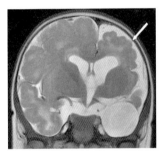

Fig. 5.3. T2-weighted, coronal MRI of a 7-month-old male infant with congenital CMV infection showing a dysplastic left hemisphere with cortical dysplasia (arrow).

human parvovirus B19 infection (Pistorius et al. 2008). As one might predict, congenitally infected infants with abnormal neuroimaging studies are more likely to have adverse neurodevelopmental outcomes (Noyola et al. 2001).

The neurodevelopmental consequences of congenital infection reflect several factors, including maternal immunity, the infectious agent, the cellular tropism of the infectious agent, and the timing of maternal infection. Because congenital infections must begin with maternal infection, maternal immune status is an important factor in determining the risk of infection and the spectrum of disease. The fetuses of women immune against rubella and CMV, as indicated by the presence of virus-specific IgG in mothers preconceptually, are protected from CRS and CMV infections in utero (Ferrante and Rowan-Kelly 1988).

The timing of maternal infection also influences the outcome of fetal infection and the spectrum of disease associated with congenital infection. Maternal rubella infection during the initial 8–12 weeks, for example, can be associated with cataracts and patent ductus arteriosus, and maternal infection during the initial 16 weeks can cause sensorineural hearing loss (Webster 1998). By contrast, infections after the 20th week, although associated with sensorineural hearing loss in some infants, are usually silent and unassociated with permanent neurodevelopmental disabilities. CMV-induced lissencephaly, schizencephaly, polymicrogyria and cortical dysplasia also imply that infections during critical periods of brain development (e.g. before the 20th week of gestation) produce more severe neurodevelopmental abnormalities. The outcome of LCMV infections is tightly linked to the timing of maternal infection, a conclusion supported by studies of LCMV infection of experimental animals (Bonthius et al. 2007a). Finally, congenital varicella syndrome rarely if ever happens when maternal infection occurs before the 5th week or after the 24th week of gestation.

For the most part, congenital infections begin with maternal and placental infections, and culminate in dissemination of the infectious pathogen to the fetus, replication in target organs, and damage to fetal tissues including the liver, spleen, eye, heart, cochlea and/or brain. Placental inflammation can cause placental insufficiency, leading to fetal death, stillbirth, intrauterine growth retardation and impaired brain growth. Although virus-induced necrosis is thought to cause intracranial dystrophic calcification, the pathogenesis of other neuropathological abnormalities, such as lissencephaly or schizencephaly, is not readily explained by direct viral replication in neural tissues. Studies of murine CMV infection suggest that virus-induced inflammatory responses participate in the pathogenesis of CMV-induced cerebellar hypoplasia (Koontz et al. 2008). The role that immune responses or genetic predilections may have in the pathogenesis of these birth defects has not been fully defined.

Prevention and treatment of congenital infections

Permanent neurodevelopmental disabilities, consisting of cerebral palsy, deafness, visual dysfunction, epilepsy and developmental delay/intellectual disability, commonly afflict children who survive congenital infection. To paraphrase Benjamin Franklin, an ounce of prevention is worth untold dollars of health-care costs for children with sequelae of congenital infections. Immunization of susceptible women prior to conception is the most effective means to eliminate the morbidity associated with many congenital infections. By September 2008, 65% of the world's countries had incorporated rubella vaccine into their national immunization schedule; eliminating CRS from all regions remains a major goal of the World Health Organization. Widespread utilization of VZV vaccine is likely to have comparable effects in eradicating the congenital varicella syndrome. Despite the lessons learned from the rubella vaccine campaign and the successful implementation of VZV immunization, progress in eliminating congenital CMV disease by vaccine has been painfully slow (Pass et al. 2009). Currently available public health strategies can diminish the health impacts of some congenital infections. The risk of congenital toxoplasmosis, for example, can be reduced by recommending that pregnant women avoid cleaning cat litter boxes and eating undercooked meats; avoiding contact with mice or hamsters and their excreta during pregnancy could also conceivably prevent some cases of congenital LCMV infection. Transmission of *T. cruzi*, the cause of Chagas disease, can be interrupted by screening blood products and controlling triatomine insects, the principal vectors of *T. cruzi* in Latin America (Rassi et al. 2009). Congenital syphilis can be prevented by identifying women infected with *T. pallidum* and treating them with penicillin.

Shunting of obstructive hydrocephalus and extended courses of anti-toxoplasma therapy with pyrimethamine and sulphadiazine improve considerably the neurodevelopmental prognosis for infants with congenital toxoplasmosis (McLeod et al. 2006). Resolution or improvement in intracranial calcification has been reported in treated children (Patel et al. 1996). Among infants with congenital toxoplasmosis treated with pyrimethamine/sulphadiazine, most have normal outcomes, and very few have sensorineural hearing loss or new eye lesions due to *T. gondii* recrudescence (McLeod et al. 2006). This contrasts with a greater than 50% morbidity associated with symptomatic congenital toxoplasmosis without treatment (McLeod et al. 2006). Longitudinal studies performed in infants with symptomatic congenital CMV infections before the availability of ganciclovir suggested that approximately 80% had permanent disability attributable to CMV infection (Pass et al. 1980) and at least 50% had sensorineural hearing loss. Ganciclovir treatment for 6 weeks results in improved hearing outcomes in congenital CMV, although its effect on other neurodevelopmental outcomes is uncertain (Kimberlin et al. 2003). The long-term morbidity associated with congenital syphilis can be prevented by perinatal penicillin therapy (Woods 2005,

McClure and Goldenberg 2009). Although the potential benefits of antiparasitic therapy in infants with congenital Chagas disease have not been established by randomized controlled clinical trials, consensus statements from the Southern Cone Initiative (Schofield and Dias 1999) and the World Health Organization (WHO 2013) currently recommend 30–60 days of antiparasitic therapy using benznidazole or nifurtimox. Although postnatal therapy with aciclovir seems appropriate in infants with congenital HSV or VZV infections, there are no data to suggest that aciclovir improves the outcome of such infants. No effective antiviral therapy currently exists for infants with CRS, emphasizing the value of preventing congenital infections.

REFERENCES

Andrade GM, Resende LM, Goulart EM, et al. (2008) Hearing loss in congenital toxoplasmosis detected by newborn screening. *Braz J Otorhinolaryngol* 74: 21–8.
Bale JF Jr, Bray PF, Bell WE (1985) Neuroradiographic abnormalities in congenital cytomegalovirus infection. *Pediatr Neurol* 1: 42–7.
Bittencourt AL (1976) Congenital Chagas disease. *Am J Dis Child* 130: 97–103.
Bonthius DJ, Nichols B, Harb H, et al. (2007a) Lymphocytic choriomeningitis virus infection of the developing brain: critical role of host age. *Ann Neurol* 62: 356–74.
Bonthius DJ, Wright R, Tseng B, et al. (2007b) Congenital lymphocytic choriomeningitis virus infection: spectrum of disease. *Ann Neurol* 62: 347–55.
Boppana SB, Pass RF, Britt WJ, et al. (1992) Symptomatic congenital cytomegalovirus infection: neonatal morbidity and mortality. *Pediatr Infect Dis J* 11: 93–9.
Boppana SB, Ross SA, Novak Z, et al. (2010) Dried blood spot real-time polymerase chain reaction assays to screen newborns for congenital cytomegalovirus infection. *JAMA* 303: 1375–82.
Bullens D, Smets K, Vanhaesebrouck P (2000) Congenital rubella syndrome after maternal reinfection. *Clin Pediatr (Phila)* 39: 113–6.
Centers for Disease Control and Prevention (2005) Elimination of rubella and congenital rubella syndrome – United States, 1969–2004. *MMWR Morb Mortal Wkly Rep* 54: 279–82.
Centers for Disease Control and Prevention (2010) Congenital syphilis – United States, 2003–2008. *MMWR Morb Mortal Wkly Rep* 59: 413–7.
de Jong EP, de Haan TR, Kroes AC, et al. (2006) Parvovirus B19 infection in pregnancy. *J Clin Virol* 36: 1–7.
Dudgeon JA (1975) Congenital rubella. *J Pediatr* 87: 1078–86.
Dunin-Wasowicz D, Kasprzyk-Obara J, Jurkiewicz E, et al. (2007) Infantile spasms and cytomegalovirus infection: antiviral and antiepileptic treatment. *Dev Med Child Neurol* 49: 684–92.
El-Nawawi FA, Tawfik MA, Shaapan RM (2008) Methods for inactivation of *Toxoplasma gondii* cysts in meat and tissues of experimentally infected sheep. *Foodborne Pathog Dis* 5: 687–90.
Ferrante A, Rowan-Kelly B (1988) The role of antibody in immunity against experimental naegleria meningoencephalitis ('amoebic meningitis'). *Immunology* 64: 241–4.
Ghadouane M, Benjelloun BS, Elharim-Roudies L, et al. (1995) Skeletal lesions in early congenital syphilis (a review of 86 cases). *Rev Rhum Engl Ed* 62: 433–7.
Grosse SD, Ross DS, Dollard SC (2008) Congenital cytomegalovirus (CMV) infection as a cause of permanent bilateral hearing loss: a quantitative assessment. *J Clin Virol* 41: 57–62.
Hill DE, Chirukandoth S, Dubey JP (2005) Biology and epidemiology of *Toxoplasma gondii* in man and animals. Anim Health Res Rev 6: 41–61.
Hutto C, Arvin A, Jacobs R, et al. (1987) Intrauterine herpes simplex virus infections. *J Pediatr* 110: 97–101.
Iannetti P, Nigro G, Spalice A, et al. (1998) Cytomegalovirus infection and schizencephaly: case reports. *Ann Neurol* 43: 123–7.
Istas AS, Demmler GJ, Dobbins JG, Stewart JA (1995) Surveillance for congenital cytomegalovirus disease: a report from the National Congenital Cytomegalovirus Disease Registry. *Clin Infect Dis* 20: 665–70.
Jara M, Hsu HW, Eaton RB, Demaria A Jr (2001) Epidemiology of congenital toxoplasmosis identified by population-based newborn screening in Massachusetts. *Pediatr Infect Dis J* 20: 1132–5.
Kimberlin DW (2004) Neonatal herpes simplex infection. *Clin Microbiol Rev* 17: 1–13.

Kimberlin DW, Lin CY, Sanchez PJ, et al. (2003) Effect of ganciclovir therapy on hearing in symptomatic congenital cytomegalovirus disease involving the central nervous system: a randomized, controlled trial. *J Pediatr* 143: 16–25.

Koontz T, Bralic M, Tomac J, et al. (2008) Altered development of the brain after focal herpesvirus infection of the central nervous system. *J Exp Med* 205: 423–35.

McClure EM, Goldenberg RL (2009) Infection and stillbirth. *Semin Fetal Neonatal Med* 14: 182–9.

McLeod R, Boyer K, Karrison T, et al. (2006) Outcome of treatment for congenital toxoplasmosis, 1981–2004: the National Collaborative Chicago-based, Congenital Toxoplasmosis Study. *Clin Infect Dis* 42: 1383–94.

Mets MB (2001) Eye manifestations of intrauterine infections. *Ophthalmol Clin North Am* 14: 521–31.

Murph JR, Bale JF Jr (1988) The natural history of acquired cytomegalovirus infection among children in group day care. *Am J Dis Child* 142: 843–6.

Murph JR, Souza IE, JD Dawson, et al. (1998) Epidemiology of congenital cytomegalovirus infection: maternal risk factors and molecular analysis of cytomegalovirus strains. *Am J Epidemiol* 147: 940–7.

Nahmias AJ (1974) The TORCH complex. *Hosp Pract* 9: 65–72.

Noyola DE, Demmler GJ, Nelson CT, et al. (2001) Early predictors of neurodevelopmental outcome in symptomatic congenital cytomegalovirus infection. *J Pediatr* 138: 325–31.

O'Leary DR, Kuhn S, Kniss KL, et al. (2006) Birth outcomes following West Nile Virus infection of pregnant women in the United States: 2003–2004. *Pediatrics* 117: e537–45.

Pass RF, Stagno S, Myers GJ, Alford CA (1980) Outcome of symptomatic congenital cytomegalovirus infection: results of long-term longitudinal follow-up. *Pediatrics* 66: 758–62.

Pass RF, Zhang C, Evans A, et al. (2009) Vaccine prevention of maternal cytomegalovirus infection. *N Engl J Med* 360: 1191–9.

Patel DV, Holfels EM, Vogel NP, et al. (1996) Resolution of intracranial calcifications in infants with treated congenital toxoplasmosis. *Radiology* 199: 433–40.

Pistorius LR, Smal J, de Haan TR, et al. (2008) Disturbance of cerebral neuronal migration following congenital parvovirus B19 infection. *Fetal Diagn Ther* 24: 491–4.

Rasmussen SA, Hayes EB, Jamieson DJ, O'Leary DR (2007) Emerging infections and pregnancy: assessing the impact on the embryo or fetus. *Am J Med Genet A* 143A: 2896–903.

Rassi A Jr, Dias JC, Marin-Neto JA, Rassi A (2009) Challenges and opportunities for primary, secondary, and tertiary prevention of Chagas' disease. *Heart* 95: 524–34.

Rivera LB, Boppana SB, Fowler KB, et al. (2002) Predictors of hearing loss in children with symptomatic congenital cytomegalovirus infection. *Pediatrics* 110: 762–7.

Sauerbrei A, Wutzler P (2007) Herpes simplex and varicella-zoster virus infections during pregnancy: current concepts of prevention, diagnosis and therapy. Part 2: Varicella-zoster virus infections. *Med Microbiol Immunol* 196: 95–102.

Schofield CJ, Dias JC (1999) The Southern Cone Initiative against Chagas disease. *Adv Parasitol* 42: 1–27.

Takasu N, Ikema T, Komiya I, Mimura G (2005) Forty-year observation of 280 Japanese patients with congenital rubella syndrome. *Diabetes Care* 28: 2331–2.

Townsend JJ, Baringer JR, Wolinsky JS, et al. (1975) Progressive rubella panencephalitis. Late onset after congenital rubella. *N Engl J Med* 292: 990–3.

Walter S, Atkinson C, Sharland M, et al. (2008) Congenital cytomegalovirus: association between dried blood spot viral load and hearing loss. *Arch Dis Child Fetal Neonatal Ed* 93: F280–5.

Webster WS (1998) Teratogen update: congenital rubella. *Teratology* 58: 13–23.

WHO (2013) Chagas disease (American trypanosomiasis). Fact sheet no. 340. Updated March 2013. Geneva: World Health Organization (online: http://www.who.int/mediacentre/factsheets/fs340/en/).

Woods CR (2005) Syphilis in children: congenital and acquired. *Semin Pediatr Infect Dis* 16: 245–57.

6
FEBRILE SEIZURES

Brian GR Neville

Febrile seizures are the most common seizure disorder, affecting about 2%–4% of children in Europe and North America, but with higher frequencies reported elsewhere, e.g. 8% in Japan.

High rates of childhood infection in resource-poor countries underline the need to recognize febrile seizures. In this chapter the difficulties of using definitions developed in different settings will be addressed, together with the risk factors, sequelae and management.

Historically it has been recognized that a benign convulsive disorder occurred with fever in young children, and the designation of febrile convulsions has been the common usage until very recently. Remarkably the school of Hippocrates recognized the major features that remain true today. The re-recognition of these essentially benign seizures occurred in the mid-19th century by separating them from neonatal and symptomatic seizures. To reinforce the benign nature of the disorder, the designation of febrile convulsions was used widely, including in epilepsy classifications. Epidemiological studies have not found any attributable risk of acquired impairments as a result of brief febrile seizures.

Definition

In 1980 the National Institute of Health Consensus Panel defined febrile seizures as "An event in infancy or early childhood, usually occurring between three months and five years of age, associated with fever but without evidence of intracranial infection or defined cause. Seizures with fever in children who have experienced a previous non-febrile seizure are excluded. Febrile seizures are to be distinguished from epilepsy which is characterised by recurrent non-febrile seizures" (Nelson and Ellenberg 1981).

The International League Against Epilepsy (ILAE) defined febrile seizures as "Seizures occurring in childhood after the age of 1 month, usually between 3 months and 6 years of age that are associated with a febrile illness, not caused by an infection of the central nervous system, without previous neonatal or unprovoked seizure and not meeting the criteria for other acute symptomatic seizures" (ILAE 1993).

Each aspect of these definitions can be questioned. The age range down to 3 months may seem rather low, and a degree of diagnostic care looking for symptomatic seizures including the first manifestations of Dravet syndrome (see below) is required. Many experts would extend the age range to the 7th birthday.

The level of fever is a matter for discussion but most clinicians rely on a history of a febrile illness, although some have suggested 38°C rectally or 38.5°C orally, as derived from the vaccine trial literature. However, precise temperatures may not be available, particularly in resource-poor countries.

A major issue is the exclusion of intracranial infection of defined cause. This would exclude meningitis, encephalitis or an associated toxic encephalopathy. However, *Shigella* infection seems relatively more epileptogenic than the levels of fever might suggest, and neurotoxin may be the cause. In malaria-endemic areas where infection is universal, seizures are common in *Plasmodium falciparum* and *P. vivax* malaria infections; however, the definition of brain involvement is not clear. It seems likely that many short seizures that occur with malaria-induced fever are genetically febrile seizures, but the cut-off point on the spectrum of clinical severity is arbitrary. One solution to this problem is to split seizures into subgroups as febrile seizures associated with shigella, malaria and herpes simplex virus-6 infection.

A much more practical issue is that a proportion of young children seen with fever and seizures will have an intracranial infection, and a fifth who have prolonged seizures with fever have potentially fatal meningitis or other infections (Chin et al. 2005). Thus the practical rules for managing these patients (even if they later prove to be outside the definition of febrile seizures) are critical. Unless the clinician can be absolutely sure that clinical examination excludes meningitis, they should be managed and investigated as if that were the diagnosis, i.e. with early lumbar puncture and treatment, or treatment and stabilization before a delayed lumbar puncture. In general, the younger and sicker the child, and those with prolonged seizures, fall into this group. However, having a previous febrile seizure or concurrent upper respiratory infection does not exclude meningitis. Status epilepticus due to febrile seizures rarely causes cerebrospinal fluid (CSF) pleocytosis, and the CSF glucose and protein levels remain normal (Frank et al. 2012). Presence of a cellular response in the CSF and/or hypoglycorrhachia (CSF glucose <0.4mmol/L) suggests meningitis.

Focal mesial temporal encephalitis, an uncommon entity with moderate fever, a cluster of seizures with partial features, reduced consciousness level and memory impairment may be confused with febrile seizures, but the evidence of parenchymal brain dysfunction and magnetic resonance imaging (MRI) findings differ from febrile seizures (Neville and Scott 2007).

Febrile seizures have been characterized as simple, i.e. lasting less than 15 minutes, and generalized. In fact most episodes are less than 5 minutes. Complex febrile seizures are prolonged, multiple within 24 hours, or focal. The issue of seizure semiology suggesting focality may depend on how carefully seizures are documented. In a recent study, 7 of 10 patients had early features ('aura') that pointed to a focal origin and this was often compatible with a temporal lobe source (Neville and Gindner 2009).

Stephenson has provided good evidence that a proportion of 'febrile seizures' are in fact vagally induced non-epileptic reflex asystolic attacks or what used to be called 'white breath-holding attacks' (Stephenson 1990). The evidence supporting this hypothesis compares the semiology of attacks induced by ocular compression and clinical seizures. It may be that within what we currently recognize as febrile seizures are a group with pain- and fever-induced reflex asystole, but there are no epidemiological studies to support this difference.

There are two issues about prolonged febrile seizures, i.e. those lasting 30 minutes or more and satisfying the criteria for convulsive status epilepticus. First, are they part of the same phenomenon as simple febrile seizures? Evidence from resource-rich countries suggests that the genetic background, i.e. a family history of febrile seizures, is very similar between those with short and long febrile seizures and that in any series of febrile seizures, about 35% will be complex with about 10% prolonged. In a population-based study of childhood convulsive status epilepticus, prolonged febrile seizures formed the single largest group (35%) (Chin et al. 2006). Second, do they cause damage, particularly hippocampal damage? This is discussed below.

It seems inappropriate to include in febrile seizures the group of children having a clear underlying acute CNS illness and thus a generally poor prognosis related to the underlying cause and its complications. Currently the suggested solution is to classify febrile seizures separately.

Epidemiology

Population-based studies in the USA and UK estimate the prevalence of febrile seizures to be 3%–4%. The prevalence in malaria-endemic areas will depend upon the definition used as discussed above. However, the rate of prolonged and often very prolonged seizures in a population-based study in rural Kenya was at least six times that in North London (Sandarangani et al. 2008), with a much higher mortality and morbidity. Several studies have shown a slight over-representation of boys. The subsequent prevalence of non-febrile epilepsy is about 2%–3%, with higher prevalence being predicted by young age of onset, previously abnormal development and a family history of epilepsy (Nelson and Ellenberg 1978, Verity and Golding 1985).

Risk factors

The risk factors for an initial febrile seizure compared to febrile controls include a higher temperature (Berg 1993, Rantala et al. 1995), an immediate family history (Berg et al. 1995) and, in some studies, a low plasma ferritin. Pertussis immunization is a risk factor for febrile seizures.

There is a 40% risk of recurrence of febrile seizures, associated with the following factors: young age of first febrile seizure (Verity et al. 1985, Berg et al. 1997); family history of febrile seizures (Van Esch et al. 1994, Rantala et al. 1995); low fever at time of seizure; and a short duration of fever before first febrile seizure (Berg et al. 1992). Half the recurrences occur within 6 months of the first seizure, three-quarters within 1 year, and 90% within 2 years (Vestergaard and Christensen 2009). Only 10% of children will have more than three febrile seizure recurrences.

Genetics

There is an excess of affected parents, and the risk to siblings is 10%–20% or higher if a parent is affected. Concordance for febrile seizures in monozygotic twins has been found to be significantly greater than in dizygotic twins (Eckhaus et al. 2013). Several linkage sites have been identified, either polygenic or dominant with incomplete penetrance have been suggested.

At least two genetically determined epilepsy syndromes are now recognized that present with what appear to be febrile seizures, but with a different natural history. Dravet syndrome (severe myoclonic epilepsy of infancy) usually begins with a prolonged hemiseizure with an often low-grade fever in the first months or year of life. The seizures may recur, and then from about the age of 1 year, myoclonic, atypical absences and partial seizures begin. Development, which had previously been normal, plateaus or regresses, with the gradual appearance of a motor disorder and significant behaviour problems (Dravet et al. 2002). About 80% have de novo mutations in the SCN1A subunit (Claes et al. 2001). Interestingly, of 14 children categorized as having pertussis vaccine encephalopathy, 12 had the Dravet phenotype and 11 had SCN1A mutations (Berkovic et al. 2006).

Generalized epilepsy, now renamed genetic epilepsy with febrile seizures plus (GEFS+) (Scheffer and Berkovic 1997) is autosomal dominant with 80% penetrance. There is quite a wide range of phenotypes within a family: some have just febrile seizures although they may occur around 5 years of age, others have more severe epilepsy syndromes including childhood absence, myoclonic astatic epilepsy or Dravet syndrome. The mutations identified included SCN1A and GABA2.

Presentation

The seizure usually occurs early in the illness, often before the presence of fever has been realized. Although tonic–clonic seizures are the most common, partial and atonic seizures also occur. Partial seizures may be followed by a Todd's paresis (post-ictal weakness). Seizure semiology, however, may be fragmentary and not conform to traditional seizure descriptions.

Immediate management and diagnostic evaluation

Most seizures are short, but about 10% are prolonged and the aim of initial medical contact is to stop them as soon as possible using intravenous antiepileptic drugs. If IV access is not available, the buccal or rectal route can be used, and a number of drugs can be given by intramuscular injection. Seizures that have lasted for 5 minutes or more should be treated urgently as potential convulsive status epilepticus. Children presenting with convulsions for 30 minutes or more may require cardiorespiratory stabilization. In an epidemiological study, around 50% of prolonged seizures in childhood including febrile seizures were intermittent, i.e. motor features stopped without recovery of consciousness, and there was evidence of ineffective treatment (Chin et al. 2008).

The management of febrile status epilepticus is similar to any convulsive status epilepticus and is discussed in Chapter 3.

The history should explore family history, previous risk factors for seizures including development, evidence of infectious illness in the child or close contacts, medication, and possible toxin exposure. An eyewitness description of the seizure is very important. It is also important to exclude any intracranial infection, particularly meningitis.

The physical examination looks for evidence of infection, consciousness level, meningeal signs, a bulging fontanelle and neurological deficit.

If a child has had many febrile seizures, thought should be given to chronic infection or increased susceptibility to infection.

Investigations apart from lumbar puncture have a very low yield, and practice statements of the American Academy of Pediatrics concluded that routine investigations including blood counts, chemistry and culture were not indicated (AAP 1999). Imaging is only justified if there is evidence of a neurological deficit. Likewise there is no indication for routine electroencephalography for either diagnostic or prognostic reasons (Yoong et al. 2009).

Lumbar puncture
Stopping a continuing seizure and ensuring cardiovascular and respiratory stability are first priorities, followed by the decision about lumbar puncture. If a child has recovered from the seizure, is over 18 months old and is well, without any indication of meningitis, lumbar puncture is very unlikely to be helpful.

Accepting that clinical exclusion of meningitis is the priority and that this may vary with the experience of the physician, indications for lumbar puncture include the following:

• prolonged seizures with fever
• reduced consciousness level and other evidence of incomplete recovery
• age under 18 months
• previous use of antibiotics for the child's illness.

A family history or prior personal history of febrile seizures should not influence this decision.

The differential diagnosis of febrile seizures includes the following:

• rigors
• syncope in the presence of pallor, atonic collapse or tonic extension
• afebrile seizures with minor infection. These children often have had febrile seizures and have a family history of febrile seizures (Lee and Ong 2004), and they have a much higher risk of long-term recurrence of afebrile seizures (7.8% compared with 1.6% for a single simple febrile seizure).

Management
The management of convulsive status epilepticus has been dealt with in Chapter 3, and the underlying infection may need treatment. The issue of antiepileptic prophylaxis has been through cycles. The essentially benign nature of febrile seizures suggested that they should not be treated. There was concern in the 1960s and 1970s about the risk of hippocampal damage, and studies demonstrated that phenobarbital appeared to lower the risk of recurrence

of seizures, but the behavioural side-effects of phenobarbital have restricted its use. A compelling problem of prophylaxis is that the vast majority of prolonged febrile seizures are the first such episode that the child has experienced (Nelson and Ellenberg 1978). The consensus view is that there is no case for routine prophylaxis, but that if a child is subject to repeated seizures, an antiepileptic drug can be used, probably sodium valproate or phenobarbital to reduce seizure recurrences. Intermittent prophylaxis using diazepam or clobazam at the onset of fever has been used for children during recurrence. However, a recent Cochrane analysis of 26 randomized clinical trials did not find any clinically important benefit of intermittent oral or rectal diazepam, phenobarbital or valproate for prophylaxis of febrile seizures (Offringa and Newton 2012). Also, while the use of antipyretics is comforting to the child, antipyretics do not prevent the recurrence of febrile seizures (Rosenbloom et al. 2013).

The long-term outcome of febrile seizures
Overall fewer than 5% of all children with febrile seizures develop later non-febrile seizures, although in population-based studies 15% of those with childhood-onset epilepsy have had earlier febrile seizures. The three risk factors for epilepsy are: early age of onset, slow development, and family history of epilepsy. Children with no risk factors had an afebrile seizure risk by the age of 7 years of 2%; those with one risk factor, 3%; and those with two or more risk factors, 13%. However, children with slow development are usually excluded from the definition of febrile seizures. A recent study found that the presence of prolonged ($\geq$10min) seizures, multiple seizures for 24 hours and the presence of epileptiform discharges were significantly associated with the development of subsequent epilepsy (Kim et al. 2013).

The relationship between prolonged febrile seizures and later temporal lobe epilepsy caused by mesial temporal sclerosis (MTS) has been discussed now for 50 years. The facts are as follows.

1 In surgical series of MTS patients, 30%–40% had a history of prolonged febrile seizures.
2 Population-based studies suggest this relationship to be rare, perhaps 1 in 150 000.
3 Animal studies of non-febrile status epilepticus produced similar mesial temporal damage. Febrile seizure animal models developed recently suggest that this can produce hippocampal damage, but that it may require a second insult to produce ongoing epilepsy.
4 Varying rates of dual pathology, i.e. a malformation as well as MTS, have been found.
5 Human studies have shown evidence of hippocampal swelling after prolonged febrile seizures that resolves by 6 months (Scott et al. 2003), but the completed sequence to MTS has not been documented. Although the rate of MTS with this background may be falling in Europe and North America, this does not mean that this sequence may not be more common in resource-poor countries, as appeared to be the case in the study from rural Kenya (Idro et al. 2008).

Population-based studies show that febrile seizures do not affect cognitive ability. The National Perinatal Collaborative Study and the British National Perinatal Collaborative Study found no differences in cognitive testing or school performance of children with febrile seizures from controls (Nelson and Ellenberg 1978, Verity et al. 1998). There are other studies that support this view.

In summary, febrile seizures are essentially benign and have a strong genetic basis. However, they are a common cause of convulsive status epilepticus, which constitutes a medical emergency. The major medical issue is to rapidly identify and treat those with seizures and fever caused by serious intracranial infection, particularly bacterial meningitis.

REFERENCES

AAP (1999) Practice parameter: long-term treatment of the child with simple febrile seizures. American Academy of Pediatrics. Committee on Quality Improvement, Subcommittee on Febrile Seizures. *Pediatrics* 103: 1307–9.

Berg AT (1993) Are febrile seizures provoked by a rapid rise in temperature? *Am J Dis Child* 147: 1101–3.

Berg AT, Shinnar S, Hauser WA, et al. (1992) A prospective study of recurrent febrile seizures. *N Engl J Med* 327: 1122–7.

Berg AT, Shinnar S, Shapiro ED, et al. (1995) Risk factors for a first febrile seizure. A matched case–control study. *Epilepsia* 36: 334–41.

Berg AT, Shinnar S, Hauser WA, et al. (1997) Predictors of recurrent febrile seizures: a prospective cohort study. *Arch Pediatr Adol Med* 151: 371–8.

Berkovic SF, Harkin L, McMahon JM, et al. (2006) De-novo mutations of the sodium channel gene SCN1A in alleged vaccine encephalopathy: a retrospective study. *Lancet Neurol* 5: 488–92.

Chin RF, Neville BG, Scott RC (2005) Meningitis is a common cause of convulsive status epilepticus with fever. *Arch Dis Child* 90: 66–9.

Chin RF, Neville BG, Scott RC (2006) Incidence, cause and short-term outcome of convulsive status epilepticus in childhood: prospective population-based study. *Lancet* 368: 222–9.

Chin RF, Neville BG, Peckham C, et al. (2008) Treatment of community-onset, childhood convulsive status epilepticus: a prospective, population-based study. *Lancet Neurol* 7: 696–703.

Claes L, Del-Favero J, Ceulemans B, et al. (2001) De novo mutations in the sodium-channel gene SCN1A cause severe myoclonic epilepsy of infancy. *Am J Hum Genet* 68: 1327–32.

Dravet C, Bureau M, Oguni H, et al. (2002) Severe myoclonic epilepsy in infancy (Dravet syndrome). In: Roger J, Bureau M, Dravet C, et al., eds. *Epileptic Syndromes in Infancy, Childhood and Adolescence, 3rd edn.* Eastleigh: John Libbey, pp. 81–103.

Eckhaus J, Lawrence KM, Helbig I, et al. (2013) Genetics of febrile seizure subtypes and syndromes: a twin study. *Epilepsy Res* 105: 103–9. doi: 10.1016/j.eplepsyres.2013.02.011.

Frank LM, Shinnar S, Hesdorffer DC, et al. (2012) Cerebrospinal fluid findings in children with fever-associated status epilepticus: results of the consequences of prolonged febrile seizures (FEBSTAT) study. *J Pediatr* 161: 1169–71. doi: 10.1016/j.jpeds.2012.08.008.

ILAE (1993) Guidelines for epidemiologic studies on epilepsy. Commission on Epidemiology and Prognosis, International League Against Epilepsy. *Epilepsia* 34: 592–6.

Idro R, Gwer S, Kahindi M, et al. (2008) The incidence, aetiology and outcome of acute seizures in children admitted to a rural Kenyan district hospital. *BMC Pediatr* 8: 5. doi: 10.1186/1471-2431-8-5.

Kim H, Byun SH, Kim JS, et al. (2013) Clinical and EEG risk factors for subsequent epilepsy in patients with complex febrile seizures. *Epilepsy Res* 105: 158–63. doi: 10.1016/j.eplepsyres.2013.02.006.

Lee W, Ong H (2004) Afebrile seizures associated with minor infections: comparison with febrile seizures and unprovoked seizures. *Pediatr Neurol* 31: 157–64.

Nelson KB, Ellenberg JH (1978) Prognosis in children with febrile seizures. *Pediatrics* 61: 720–727.

Nelson KB, Ellenberg JH (1981) Consensus statement on febrile seizures. In: *Febrile Seizures.* New York: Raven Press, pp. 301–6.

Neville BGR, Gindner D (2009) Febrile seizures – Semiology in humans and animal models: evidence of focality and heterogeneity. *Brain Dev* 32: 33–6.

Neville BGR, Scott RC (2007) Severe memory impairment in a child with bihippocampal injury after status epilepticus. *Dev Med Child Neurol* 49: 396–9.

Offringa M, Newton R (2012) Prophylactic drug management for febrile seizures in children. *Cochrane Database Syst Rev* 4: CD003031. doi: 10.1002/14651858.CD003031.pub2.

Rantala H, Uhari M, Hietala J (1995) Factors triggering the first febrile seizure. *Acta Paediatr* 84: 407–10.

Rosenbloom E, Finkelstein Y, Adams-Webber T, Kozer E (2013) Do antipyretics prevent the recurrence of febrile seizures in children? A systematic review of randomized controlled trials and meta-analysis. *Eur J Paediatr Neurol* 17: 585–8.

Sandarangani M, Seaton C, Scott AG, et al. (2008) Incidence and outcome of convulsive status epilepticus in Kenyan children: a cohort study. *Lancet Neurol* 2: 145–50.

Scheffer IE, Berkovic SF (1997) Generalized epilepsy with febrile seizures plus. A genetic disorder with heterogenous clinical phenotypes. *Brain* 120: 479–90.

Scott RC, King MD, Gadian DG, et al. (2003) Hippocampal abnormalities after prolonged febrile convulsion: a longitudinal MRI study. *Brain* 126: 2551–7.

Stephenson JBP (1990) *Fits and Faints. Clinics in Developmental Medicine No. 109.* London: Mac Keith Press.

Van Esch A, Steyerberg EW, Berger MY, et al. (1994) Family history and recurrence of febrile seizures. *Arch Dis Child* 70: 395–9.

Verity CM, Golding J (1985) Risk of epilepsy after febrile convulsions: a national cohort study. *BMJ* 303: 1373–6.

Verity CM, Butler NR, Golding J (1985) Febrile convulsions in a national cohort followed up from birth. I. Prevalence and recurrence in the first five years of life. *BMJ* 290: 1307–10.

Verity CM, Greenwood R, Golding J (1998) Long-term intellectual and behavioral outcomes of children with febrile convulsions. *N Engl J Med* 338: 1723–8.

Vestergaard M, Christensen J (2009) Register-based studies on febrile seizures in Denmark. *Brain Dev* 31: 372–7.

Yoong M, Chin RFM, Scott RC (2009) Management of convulsive status epilepticus in children. *Arch Dis Child Educ Pract Ed* 94: 1–9. doi: 10.1136/adc.2007.134049.

7
VIRAL ENCEPHALITIS AND MENINGITIS

Diane E Griffin

Viral infection of the CNS is an important cause of morbidity and mortality worldwide and in many regions disproportionately affects children (Griffin 2010, Wilson 2013). Infection and inflammation of the meninges is referred to as meningitis, of the brain is encephalitis, and of the spinal cord is myelitis. Many infections result in combinations of these syndromes such as meningoencephalitis or encephalomyelitis. In humans, the viruses most commonly identified as causes of viral encephalomyelitis are several herpesviruses (e.g. herpes simplex, cytomegalovirus, human herpesvirus 6) and RNA viruses in the picornavirus (e.g. polio, enterovirus 71), rhabdovirus (e.g. rabies), alphavirus (e.g. eastern equine, Venezuelan equine and western equine encephalitis), flavivirus (e.g. West Nile, Japanese encephalitis, Murray Valley and tick-borne encephalitis) and bunyavirus (e.g. LaCrosse, Toscana) families. Other virus families with members that can cause acute encephalitis are the paramyxoviruses (e.g. Nipah, Hendra) and arenaviruses (e.g. lymphocytic choriomeningitis, Junin) (Wilson 2013). However, this is certainly not a complete list, because for most cases of human viral encephalitis the aetiological agent is not identified, even when heroic attempts are made to do so.

The primary target cells for most encephalitic viruses are neurons, although a few viruses attack cerebrovascular endothelial cells to cause ischaemia and stroke or glial cells to cause demyelination, encephalopathy or dementia. Widespread infection of neurons may occur or viruses may display preferences for particular types of neurons in specific locations in the central nervous system (CNS). For instance, herpes simplex virus (HSV) type 1 often infects neurons in the hippocampus to cause behavioural changes, while poliovirus preferentially infects motor neurons in the brainstem and spinal cord to cause paralysis, and Japanese encephalitis virus infects basal ganglia neurons to cause symptoms similar to those of Parkinson disease.

Milder forms of disease involve infection of cells of the leptomeninges. Most infections begin with a flu-like prodrome that progresses to fever, stiff neck and headache when infection is confined to the meninges (meningitis) and altered mental status that may be accompanied by seizures and focal neurological signs when the brain parenchyma is involved (encephalitis).

Cerebrospinal fluid (CSF) should be examined to help differentiate between bacterial and viral infections and can provide information on the aetiology of the disease through culture, antigen detection or polymerase chain reaction (PCR) identification of the infectious organism. If a space-occupying lesion is suspected, computerized tomography (CT) of the brain should be performed before the lumbar puncture. Typically the pressure is somewhat elevated and a mild to moderate pleocytosis is present. Lymphocytes usually predominate, but early in infection neutrophils may be present. CSF red cell count may be increased in HSV encephalitis. Glucose is usually normal or slightly reduced, and the protein is usually modestly elevated.

Imaging techniques are useful to detect localized lesions, magnetic resonance imaging (MRI) being more sensitive than CT. Electroencephalography is useful for detecting seizure activity. A definitive aetiological diagnosis depends on culture or PCR identification of the organism or detection of virus-specific IgM antibody or a four-fold rise in IgG antiviral antibody.

Treatment with aciclovir for herpesvirus infection should be initiated pending outcome of the PCR test, as delay in treatment is associated with increased morbidity. Appropriate management of the airway, electrolytes, intracranial pressure, seizures and secondary infection is the mainstay for treatment of viral infections of the CNS.

Enterovirus and parechovirus infections

Enteroviruses and parechoviruses belong to the *Picornavirus* family of small plus-strand non-enveloped RNA viruses and are among the most common causes of virus infection of the CNS. The more than 100 different human enteroviruses have traditionally been subclassified based on biological characteristics into the polioviruses (*n*=3), coxsackie A viruses (*n*=23), coxsackie B viruses (*n*=6) and echoviruses (*n*=31). Newer enterovirus (EV) serotypes have been numbered. With sequence data now available, these viruses have been reclassified by VP1 capsid genotyping into five species: poliovirus, human enterovirus (HEV) A (coxsackie A viruses 2–8, 10, 12, 13, 16; EV71, EV76), HEV B (coxsackie A virus 9; coxsackie B viruses 1–6; echoviruses 1–7, 9, 11–21, 24–27, 29–33), HEV C (coxsackie A viruses 1, 11, 13, 17, 19–22, 24) and HEV D (EV68, EV70). This classification closely parallels the previous classification by serotyping (Oberste et al. 2003). Former echoviruses 22 and 23 are substantially different in sequence and biology from the rest of the enteroviruses and have been designated as a separate genus, the parechoviruses (*n*=6).

Within these groups, some viruses are frequently associated with neurological disease, while others rarely are. The viruses most commonly associated with symptomatic CNS infection are polioviruses 1, 2 and 3; HEV A virus EV71; HEV B coxsackie B viruses 3, 4 and 5; echoviruses 4, 6, 7, 9, 11, 18, 30 and EV75; and parechovirus type 3. The most severe disease and greatest likelihood of long-term sequelae result from infection with the polioviruses and EV71. In addition to virus type, age is an important determinant of disease severity. More severe disease with HEV B infection generally occurs in the youngest individuals. Perinatal infection can produce a sepsis-like syndrome that can be fatal (Abzug 2004), while in older infants and children infection of the CNS causes aseptic meningitis and occasional encephalitis with a benign outcome (Rorabaugh et al. 1993).

In temperate climates, infections occur primarily during the summer and autumn, while in tropical areas they appear throughout the year. Humans are the only reservoir for these viruses and infection is usually acquired by ingestion of contaminated food or water, but is occasionally spread by respiratory droplets or transplacentally. Initial virus replication is in the oropharynx and intestinal tract. Subsequently, virus infects lymphoid tissue and, in a small percentage of infections, spreads through the blood to multiple organs (e.g. muscle, skin, heart, lung, liver, brain) or by neuronal transport directly to the CNS (Racaniello 2006). CNS infection can lead to meningitis, focal or generalized encephalitis, myelitis or flaccid paralysis. Onset of disease is typically abrupt with the appearance of fever, constitutional symptoms, headache, photophobia and nuchal rigidity, but can be biphasic. Virus shedding from the gastrointestinal tract can be prolonged, and individuals with hypogammaglobulinaemia may develop persistent infection.

EPIDEMIOLOGICAL AND CLINICAL CHARACTERISTICS OF INFECTION

Poliomyelitis
Although it is an ancient disease, polio emerged as an epidemic problem first in the resource-rich countries of Europe and North America. Subsequent analysis of the epidemiology showed that infection was common and usually occurred early in childhood when maternal antibody protection waned, allowing virus entry into the CNS. Adults are more likely to experience paralysis: as infection was postponed to later ages with increased sanitation, paralysis became a more frequent complication. Nevertheless, as with the other enteroviruses, most infections are asymptomatic and only one in 100–200 will develop virus spread to the CNS and acute flaccid paralysis due to infection of lower motor neurons. Virus can continue to be shed from the gastrointestinal tract for weeks after infection, so poliovirus can circulate widely in the population without being recognized. Surveillance relies on identifying individuals with acute flaccid paralysis associated with poliovirus in the stool.

Virus that reaches the nervous system infects neurons, with a particular tropism for motor neurons. Therefore, flaccid paralysis is a common outcome of CNS infection. Disease begins with flu-like symptoms that progress to meningitis and paralysis. The course in children may be monophasic and rapid or biphasic. Paralysis is often preceded by myalgias and loss of superficial and deep tendon reflexes. The distribution is characteristically asymmetrical with proximal muscles more affected than distal muscles and legs more than arms. Paralysis of muscles of the diaphragm can result in respiratory failure. Bladder paralysis and intestinal atonia are common, and cranial nerve paresis (bulbar paralysis) can result in difficulties with speech, swallowing, breathing and eye movement. There may be recovery or progression to permanent paralysis, with the outcome generally apparent within the first 6 months.

Although wild-type polioviruses have been eliminated from most resource-rich countries, polio continues to resist eradication efforts, and disease emerges periodically due to both reintroduction of wild-type strains of poliovirus from areas with continuing endemic disease (Nigeria, Pakistan and Afghanistan) and circulation of vaccine-derived viruses that have regained virulence (Wringe et al. 2008). The oral poliovirus vaccine is composed of three strains of live poliovirus that have been attenuated (Sabin strains 1–3). These vaccine viruses are shed from the gastrointestinal tract and can spread to susceptible individuals when coverage with the oral poliovirus vaccine is inadequate. These circulating vaccine viruses can reacquire virulence through mutation or recombination with HEV C species enteroviruses and have raised substantial challenges for the poliovirus eradication effort (Minor 2009).

Other enteroviruses, primarily EV71 and EV75, can also target brain and spinal-cord motor neurons and cause outbreaks of acute flaccid paralysis similar to those caused by polioviruses.

Enterovirus 71

EV71 is closely related to coxsackievirus A16 and is one of several HEV A viruses that cause hand–foot–mouth disease in young children. However, EV71 has also gained the ability to invade the CNS and cause a spectrum of serious neurological diseases (Chang et al. 2007, Modlin 2007). EV71 was first isolated in California in 1969 from a child with encephalitis and was subsequently detected globally in association with cases of aseptic meningitis, encephalitis and acute flaccid paralysis. In addition to mimicking poliovirus infection, EV71 can also cause brainstem encephalitis that leads to cardiac dysfunction, pulmonary oedema and fatal respiratory failure. In 1997 outbreaks of hand–foot–mouth disease complicated by brainstem encephalitis occurred in Malaysia, and since then, there have been epidemics in multiple countries in Asia. The reasons for more severe neurological disease in the Asia–Pacific region are not clear, but may be related to genetic susceptibility or virus genotype. The epidemiology is reminiscent of the epidemics of polio in Europe and North America in the first half of the 20th century (Modlin 2007).

Symptomatic EV71 infection is most often associated with hand-foot-and-mouth disease or herpangina in children under 5 years of age and is characterized by rapid onset of fever and sore throat. Oral vesicles and ulcerations are common features that can be accompanied by vesicular lesions on the hands, feet or buttocks. The disease with neurological complications is biphasic with appearance of aseptic meningitis, encephalomyelitis, ataxia or acute flaccid paralysis 2–5 days after the onset of fever. Meningitis presents with headache, vomiting, fever and neck stiffness. Acute flaccid paralysis is usually unilateral involving an arm or leg. Survivors of flaccid paralysis are frequently left with residual weakness and atrophy, as well as lower intelligence test scores (Chang et al. 2007).

The most severe neurological complication is rhombencephalitis that can lead to rapid onset of respiratory distress, shock, apnoea and coma. Early neurological signs include myoclonus, vomiting, tremor, ataxia, abnormal respiration and oculomotor paresis. Within hours, pulmonary oedema, haemorrhage and cardiopulmonary failure occur in those with the most severe disease (Wilson 2013). CNS pathology shows neuronal infection with degeneration, inflammation and necrosis (Wong et al. 2008). If patients survive the acute period, they recover cardiopulmonary function over 3–5 days, but may be left with paresis, internuclear ophthalmoplegia and apnoea as sequelae.

Aseptic meningitis and encephalitis

Echoviruses, coxsackie B viruses and EV75 in the HEV B genogroup are more likely to cause neurological disease than the coxsackie A viruses (Yen et al. 2009). The most common neurological complication of infection with these enteroviruses is aseptic meningitis, occurring mostly in infants less than 6 months of age. In a minority of patients, there is evidence of encephalitis with seizures, increased intracranial pressure or coma.

Infants who acquire enterovirus infections in the first 2 weeks of life are more likely to have high levels of viraemia with infection of multiple organs and to develop severe neurological disease (Yen et al. 2007). Often there is a history of peripartum maternal illness. Signs of neonatal infection appear 3–7 days after birth, with fever, irritability, anorexia and lethargy. The course of disease can be fulminant with appearance of rash, hypoperfusion, jaundice and respiratory abnormalities that are difficult to distinguish from sepsis. Nosocomial transmission from an infected infant to others in nurseries for newborn infants can be a significant problem. When infection occurs beyond 2 weeks of age, the outcome from meningitis and encephalitis is usually good (Rorabaugh et al. 1993).

Parechovirus
Parechoviruses 1, 2, 4, 5 and 6 are associated primarily with gastroenteritis and respiratory symptoms in young children, rather than neurological disease. However, parechovirus 3 causes a neonatal sepsis-like illness, encephalitis and flaccid paralysis, similar to the diseases caused by the HEV B viruses (Benschop et al. 2006). In neonates, infection typically presents in the first week of life with a sepsis-like picture, irritability, rash and seizures. Ultrasound and MRI may show cyst formation, petechial haemorrhages and white-matter damage. Neurodevelopmental abnormalities are common sequelae (Verboon-Maciolek et al. 2008).

DIAGNOSIS
In patients with acute flaccid paralysis, MRI can show hyperintense lesions in the anterior horn regions of the cord on T2-weighted images and, with contrast, ventral root enhancement on T1-weighted images (Chen et al. 2001). In those with rhombencephalitis, T2-weighted images show high-intensity lesions in the brainstem, most commonly in the pontine tegmentum, followed by the medulla oblongata, midbrain and dentate nuclei. Virus can often be isolated from stool, throat and CSF specimens. For EV71, the highest yield is from throat swabs and vesicle fluid rather than CSF. More commonly, reverse transcription PCR is used to detect viral RNA using virus-specific or group-specific primers (Nix et al. 2006). Sequencing of the amplicons can then be used for species identification. Detection of IgM has generally not been useful for diagnosis (Fowlkes et al. 2008).

TREATMENT
As with all causes of encephalitis, supportive care and management of seizures, intracranial pressure, secondary infections and respiration is important. For EV71 brainstem encephalitis, early cardiopulmonary support improves outcome (Chang et al. 2004, Wang et al. 2006). Intracardiac haemodynamic monitoring can guide the use of inotropic agents to improve cardiac output and that of intravenous fluids to avoid volume overload.

Intravenous administration of immune globulin selected for high titre antibody against the virus causing the infection improves virus clearance in acutely infected neonates and in

TABLE 7.1
Arboviruses that frequently cause encephalitis in humans

Family and examples	Primary vector	Distribution
Alphavirus		
Eastern equine encephalitis	Mosquito	Eastern USA, Caribbean, South America
Western equine encephalitis	Mosquito	Western North America, South America
Venezuelan equine encephalitis	Mosquito	Central and South America
Flavivirus		
West Nile/Kunjin	Mosquito	Americas, Africa, Middle East, Europe/Australia
St Louis encephalitis	Mosquito	North and South America
Japanese encephalitis	Mosquito	Asia, India, Australia
Murray Valley encephalitis	Mosquito	Australia
Tick-borne encephalitis	Tick	Russia, eastern and central Europe
Bunyavirus		
California/La Crosse	Mosquito	North America
Toscana	Sandfly	Europe

immunocompromised patients with persistent infection. Antiviral treatment with pleconaril has also shown some promise for treatment of enterovirus infections in infants, but the generally benign course of most infections makes toxicity a potential issue (Abzug et al. 2003, Rotbart et al. 2001).

PREVENTION

Effective live attenuated virus and inactivated virus vaccines are in wide use to prevent polio. Immunity must be induced to all three poliovirus types for full protection from paralytic disease. The inactivated vaccine induces serum antibody that prevents virus spread to the CNS, but does not necessarily prevent infection of the gut. The live attenuated vaccine is essential for eradication efforts because it is delivered orally, infects and induces immunity in the intestinal tract, and protects against subsequent wild-type virus infection and thus interrupts silent spread of wild-type virus from person to person. These vaccines have resulted in a dramatic decrease in paralytic polio. Wild poliovirus type 2 is no longer circulating, and types 1 and 3 are targeted for eradication as well, but challenges remain.

Vaccines have not yet been licensed for any of the other human enteroviruses, but efforts to develop a vaccine for EV71 are underway.

Arbovirus encephalitis

Arthropod-borne viruses (arboviruses) are transmitted by insects, usually mosquitoes, ticks or blood-feeding flies. More than 100 arboviruses are known to infect humans. The viruses that cause neurological disease belong to several different virus genera, the most important of which are *Alphavirus*, *Flavivirus* and *Bunyavirus* (Table 7.1). The natural cycle for these enveloped RNA viruses involves transmission between an insect vector and vertebrate host. Humans are only accidentally infected and are unimportant for maintaining the viruses in nature. Human infection is often asymptomatic, but when disease occurs it can be manifested by mild-to-severe febrile illness, rash, arthritis, meningitis, encephalitis, myelitis, radiculitis or flaccid paralysis (Saad et al. 2005, Gould and Solomon 2008, Tyler 2009). The primary target cells in the CNS are neurons, and each virus causes a characteristic spectrum of illness depending on the neuronal populations infected. However, the same virus can produce diseases of differing severity depending on the viral inoculum and host factors such as age, genetic background and immunological status.

Alphaviruses are transmitted by mosquitoes. Eastern, western and Venezuelan equine encephalitis viruses (EEEV, WEEV, VEEV) are endemic in the Americas and can cause meningitis or encephalomyelitis. Disease is generally more severe in children than in adults. The rash- and arthritis-causing viruses (Sindbis virus in northern Europe and South Africa, Ross River virus in Australia, and chikungunya virus in Africa, India and southeast Asia) are also occasionally associated with meningoencephalopathy or myelitis in very young children (Robin et al. 2008).

Flaviviruses that are important causes of human encephalitis include the mosquito-borne West Nile virus (WNV) and its close Australian relative Kunjin virus, St Louis encephalitis virus (SLEV), Murray Valley encephalitis virus (MVEV), Japanese encephalitis virus (JEV, discussed in Chapter 9) and the tick-borne encephalitis virus (TBEV) (Turtle et al. 2012). These infections have a tendency to infect motor neurons and cause flaccid paralysis, in addition to meningoencephalitis. For WNV, SLEV and TBEV, disease is generally more severe in older adults than in children, while for JEV and MVEV the most severe disease is in children, potentially because older individuals in endemic areas have acquired infection previously during childhood.

Bunyaviruses are the most varied and numerous of the arboviruses and include the mosquito-transmitted California serogroup La Crosse virus in North America, which causes diseases primarily in children, and sandfly-transmitted Toscana virus in Europe with disease primarily in adults.

EPIDEMIOLOGICAL AND CLINICAL CHARACTERISTICS OF INFECTION

Eastern equine encephalitis
EEEV is enzootic in the Americas along the Atlantic and Gulf coasts, in the Great Lakes Region, in the Caribbean, and in Central and South America. Birds are the primary reservoir host, and many avian species are susceptible to infection. In North America the primary enzootic cycle is maintained in swamps with the ornithophilic mosquito *Culiseta melanura* as the vector. The amplifying species are wading birds, migratory passerine songbirds and starlings. North American strains of EEEV are the most virulent of the encephalitic alphaviruses and cause high mortality in all age groups (Reimann et al. 2008), while South American strains have not been associated with human disease. Fortunately, cases in North America are few (approximately 7–10 per year) because the mosquito that transmits the

virus between marsh birds does not usually feed on humans. When mosquitoes that feed on mammals become infected, people and horses are at risk.

Children under 10 years of age are most susceptible, with 1 in 8 infections in children resulting in encephalitis compared with 1 in 23 infections in adults. A prodromal illness consisting of fever, chills, malaise and myalgias begins days after the bite of an infected mosquito. In cases of encephalitis these prodromal symptoms are followed by the onset of headache, confusion, vomiting, restlessness and irritability leading to seizures, obtundation and coma (Deresiewicz et al. 1997). Meningismus is frequent, and focal signs including cranial nerve palsies and paralysis are common. Hyponatraemia due to inappropriate secretion of antidiuretic hormone is a common complication, and oedema of the face and extremities has been noted. The case-fatality rate is 30%–40%, with the highest rates in children (Deresiewicz et al. 1997). Death typically occurs within 2–10 days after onset of encephalitis.

Poor outcome is predicted by high CSF white cell count or severe hyponatraemia. Recovery is more likely in individuals who have a long (5–7 day) prodrome and do not develop coma. Sequelae including paralysis, seizures and intellectual disability are common, and 35%–80% of survivors, particularly children, have significant long-term neurological impairment (Deresiewicz et al. 1997).

Histopathology in fatal cases of eastern equine encephalitis demonstrates a diffuse meningoencephalitis with widespread neuronal destruction, perivascular cuffing with polymorphonuclear as well as mononuclear leukocytes, and vasculitis with vessel occlusion in the cortex, basal ganglia and brainstem. The spinal cord is frequently spared. Virus antigen is localized to neurons, and neuronal death is marked by cytoplasmic swelling and nuclear pyknosis (Garen et al. 1999). Gliosis is present in the regions of affected neurons (Garen et al. 1999).

Western equine encephalitis

WEEV is endemic in the western portions of the USA and Canada and in South America. In North America WEEV is maintained in an endemic cycle involving domestic and passerine birds and *Culex tarsalis*, a mosquito adapted to irrigated agricultural areas. WEEV caused seasonal epidemics of equine and human encephalitis in the USA from 1955 to 1984, but numbers of cases have declined steadily since then.

Signs and symptoms of WEEV encephalitis are similar to those of EEEV, but the case fatality rate of 3%–7% is lower (Longshore et al. 1956). There is a 3–5 day prodrome of fever and headache that may progress to restlessness, tremor, irritability, nuchal rigidity, photophobia, altered mental status and paralysis. Infants often present with rigidity, seizures and a bulging fontanelle. Perinatal infection due to transplacental transmission manifests within the first week of life as fever, failure to feed and seizures.

Clinically apparent disease is most common in the very young and those over 50 (Longshore et al. 1956). The estimated case to infection ratio is 1:58 in children under 5 years and 1:1150 in adults. In older children, males are two to three times more likely to develop disease than females (Longshore et al. 1956). Infants and young children are more likely to develop seizures, fatal encephalitis and significant sequelae (Earnest et al. 1971).

In infants under 1 year approximately 60% of survivors have brain damage, and in some the disease is progressive. Common problems are intellectual disability associated with quadriplegia, spasticity, recurring seizures, cortical atrophy, ventricular dilation and intracranial calcification (Noran and Baker 1949, Earnest et al. 1971, Somekh and Glode 1991).

Pathology of acute cases of western equine encephalitis shows leptomeningitis and perivascular cuffing with polymorphonuclear leukocyte infiltration in the earliest cases, and lymphocytes, plasma cells and macrophages at later times. Inflammation is accompanied by endothelial hyperplasia, petechial haemorrhages and glial nodules in areas of neuronal degeneration. Lesions are found primarily in the basal ganglia, brainstem, cerebellum, cerebral cortex and spinal cord. In addition, there are areas of focal necrosis and demyelination, particularly in the subcortical white matter and basal ganglia. Occasionally in infants and children there is pathological evidence of progressive disease consistent with persistent infection. Individuals surviving months to years after onset of encephalitis (often with progressive disease) may have cystic lesions, gliosis and demyelination with areas of active mononuclear inflammation (Noran and Baker 1949).

Venezuelan equine encephalitis
Enzootic Venezuelan equine encephalitis complex viruses are involved in perennially active transmission cycles in subtropical and tropical areas of the Americas. Enzootic isolates are primarily from *Culex (Melanoconion)* spp. mosquitoes that breed near aquatic plants and feed on a wide variety of rodents, birds and other vertebrates. Epizootic viruses cause significant disease in horses (Weaver et al. 2004), and isolates are primarily from *Aedes taeniorhynchus*, *Psorophora confinnis* and *Aedes sollicitans* mosquitoes, suggesting that the epizootic and enzootic transmission cycles differ (Weaver et al. 2004).

Clinically evident human infection can occur with enzootic, as well as epizootic, VEEV (Ehrenkranz and Ventura 1974, Weaver et al. 2004). Humans living in areas of enzootic transmission have a high prevalence of antibody associated mostly with undiagnosed mild febrile illnesses. During epizootic outbreaks, human attack rates vary widely and neurological symptoms tend to appear 4–10 days after onset of illness, with headache and vomiting as the most common initial symptoms followed by focal or generalized seizures, paresis, behavioural changes, and stupor or coma (Rivas et al. 1997). Laboratory studies often show lymphopenia.

All ages and both sexes are equally susceptible to infection; however, individuals under the age of 15 are more likely to develop fulminant disease with reticuloendothelial infection, lymphoid depletion and encephalitis. Fetal abnormalities, spontaneous abortion and stillbirth may occur with infection during pregnancy. Congenitally infected infants show severe neurological damage occasionally resulting in hydranencephaly (Wenger 1977). The incidence of encephalitis is generally less than 5% and the mortality less than 1% (Rivas et al. 1997). Essentially all deaths occur in children. Children who recover from encephalitis may be left with neurological deficits, particularly seizure disorders (Leon et al. 1975).

In fatal cases, pathology has shown myocarditis, focal centrilobular hepatic necrosis and inflammation, and generalized lymphoid depletion (Johnson et al. 1968). Lesions in the brain are found primarily in the olfactory cortex and basal ganglia and consist of perivascular cuffing and glial nodules. Congenitally infected infants have widespread necrosis, haemorrhage and hypoplasia (Wenger 1977).

West Nile virus

WNV is widespread throughout Africa, the Middle East and southern Europe. Kunjin, a related virus, is found in Australia. WNV is maintained in a natural cycle between *Culex* mosquitoes and birds. The virus was not recognized as an important cause of neurological disease until the mid-1990s, suggesting the recent emergence of a new, more virulent strain. In 1999 WNV was introduced into the Western hemisphere where appropriate mosquito vectors and avian hosts were available, resulting in rapid spread across North America (Petersen et al. 2013). Most infections are mild and not diagnosed. All ages are susceptible to infection, but disease is milder in children who tend to have fever, rash or aseptic meningitis (Suthar et al. 2013). The median age of individuals with neurological disease is 77 years, and most deaths occur in those over age 60 (Hayes et al. 2005).

There is a 1–2 week incubation period before onset of fever, headache, nausea and lymphadenopathy. Signs and symptoms of meningitis, encephalitis or myelitis develop in a subset of those infected (Bode et al. 2006). The fatality rate for those with neurological signs and symptoms is 5%–10%, but recovery is prolonged and often incomplete in survivors, with lingering fatigue, memory problems, weakness and tremor (Carson et al. 2006, Sejvar 2007).

St Louis encephalitis virus

SLEV is endemic in the Americas where it is maintained in enzootic cycles involving *Culex* mosquitoes and passerine birds. Most infections are asymptomatic, but there are periodic outbreaks of meningitis and encephalitis. SLEV shares with WNV and TBEV the capacity to cause more severe disease in adults than in children (Reimann et al. 2008) and has a case fatality rate of 10%. Disease in children is mild and characterized by abrupt onset of fever, headache, lethargy, vomiting and seizures, followed by gradual improvement (Wootton et al. 2004).

Murray Valley encephalitis virus

MVEV is endemic in northern Australia and is maintained in a natural cycle between *Culex* mosquitoes and water birds. Most infections are subclinical, with approximately 1:1000 resulting in clinically recognized encephalitis. However, encephalitis can be severe, with a fatality rate of 30% and a similar proportion being left with long-term neurological deficits (Burrow et al. 1998). Disease is more severe in children than in adults, with seizures and acute flaccid paralysis common complications (Speers et al. 2013).

Tick-borne encephalitis virus

TBEV is focally endemic in forested regions from Japan through northern China and Russia to Europe, and is second only to JEV as a cause of morbidity due to neurotropic flaviviruses

(Dumpis et al. 1999, Mansfield et al. 2009). Related viruses, louping-ill virus in Britain and Powassan virus in North America, also cause encephalitis in humans (Reimann et al. 2008), but are epidemiologically less important than TBEV (Gritsun et al. 2003). TBEV infects wild and domestic animals and is usually transmitted to humans by ixodid ticks. However, oral transmission from consumption of unpasteurized dairy products can also occur.

The incubation period is 7–14 days and the disease course is often biphasic. The initial phase lasts 1–7 days and consists of fever, headache, muscular pain and vomiting that corresponds with the viraemia. In patients who develop neurological disease, the first phase is followed 3–21 days later by symptoms ranging from mild meningitis to severe meningo-encephalomyelitis and flaccid paralysis (Mansfield et al. 2009). Several syndromes are described that involve combinations of fever, headache, meningismus, somnolence, muscle pain, paresis, delirium and tremors (Dumpis et al. 1999). Severity of illness tends to increase with the age of the patient, and fatality rates in adults are up to 40% depending on virus subtype. Disease is generally milder in children than in adults, and mortality is low. Most children develop meningitis, while approximately 30% show signs of meningoencephalitis such as confusion, tremor, ataxia, seizures or paresis (Lesnicar et al. 2003, Fritsch et al. 2008). In adults, neurological sequelae are common and chronic forms of disease with epilepsia partialis continua, progressive muscle atrophy and mental deterioration may occur. Neuro-imaging shows a predilection for the thalami, basal ganglia, cerebellum and anterior horns of the spinal cord (Horger et al. 2012). Although severe disease can occur in children, death is unusual and long-term neurological sequelae uncommon, but milder symptoms such as attention deficits are frequent (Lesnicar et al. 2003, Fritsch et al. 2008). Vaccination is protective and recommended for children who live in endemic regions. Maternal vaccination can prevent disease in young infants.

La Crosse virus
La Crosse virus is the most pathogenic member of the California encephalitis serogroup of bunyaviruses and is endemic in central USA where it is an important cause of paediatric encephalitis (Reimann et al. 2008). The virus infects small mammals and is transmitted by the tree-hole mosquito *Aedes triseriatus.*

The spectrum of illness caused by the California serogroup viruses ranges from mild febrile illness to aseptic meningitis and encephalitis. Neurological disease occurs primarily in children under 10 years of age. Initial symptoms are headache, fever and vomiting, with progression to disorientation and seizures (McJunkin et al. 2001). Focal signs may be present that lead to diagnostic confusion with herpes simplex encephalitis.

Peripheral white blood cell count may be elevated, causing confusion with bacterial meningitis. Brain biopsy shows mononuclear inflammation and the presence of virus. Complications can include hyponatraemia and status epilepticus. The case fatality rate is less than 1%, but in survivors sequelae can include paresis, behavioural problems and intellectual disability (McJunkin et al. 2001).

Toscana virus

Toscana virus is transmitted by sandflies and has emerged as a major cause of viral meningitis and encephalitis in southern Europe (Cusi et al. 2010). Disease typically presents with a 2–7 day prodrome consisting of fever, malaise and headache that may be accompanied by a rash. Meningitis is the most frequent neurological disease associated with infection, but about 5% develop encephalitis that can be severe (Cusi et al. 2010). There is epidemiological evidence to suggest that adults are more likely than children to develop neurological symptoms after infection (Terrosi et al. 2009). Infection has not been associated with mortality.

DIAGNOSIS

Diagnosis of disease caused by any arbovirus on clinical grounds alone is difficult except in outbreak situations, because of the paucity of specific findings on physical examination. CSF is almost always abnormal. Pressure and protein are increased, glucose is low to normal, red blood cells and xanthochromia are commonly present, and white cell counts range from 10/mL to 2000/mL. Polymorphonuclear leukocytes may be abundant early, with a shift to mononuclear cells over the first few days. Electroencephalographic abnormalities are relatively non-specific, usually showing slowing but occasionally showing lateralizing epileptiform discharges. CT may be normal or show only oedema, while MRI is more often abnormal with focal lesions commonly observed, particularly when T2-weighted fluid-attenuated inversion recovery imaging is used (Marjelund et al. 2004).

A residence and travel history can provide important clues to virus exposure. Virus can be isolated from CSF, blood or CNS tissue by inoculation into newborn mice or onto a variety of tissue-culture cells. However, that is rarely done and definitive diagnosis is usually made by detection of virus-specific IgM in serum or CSF by enzyme immunoassay, viral RNA by reverse transcription PCR (Lambert et al. 2003, Saksida et al. 2005), or seroconversion.

TREATMENT AND PREVENTION

There is no specific therapy for any of the arbovirus diseases. No successful specific antiviral therapy has been identified for CNS infection, although interferon, ribavirin and immune globulin have been given empirically (Solomon 2004). The mainstay of treatment remains vigorous supportive therapy including respiratory assistance, maintenance of electrolyte balance, control of seizures, and monitoring and control of increased intracranial pressure (Griffin 1991).

Community mosquito-control programmes and the use of insect repellents, insecticide-treated bednets, appropriate clothing and window screens for personal protection against insect bites are important for prevention of infection (Mansfield et al. 2009). Widespread aerial spraying of insecticides can decrease adult populations of mosquitoes, and treatment of water to control larvae can inhibit emergence.

Effective vaccines against JEV and tick-borne encephalitis are available and should be used by people living in or travelling to regions where exposure to these viruses is likely.

Vaccines against other arboviruses, particularly WNV and VEEV, as well as new-generation JEV and TBEV vaccines are in development (Charles et al. 1997, Gritsun et al. 2003, Reed et al. 2005, Halstead and Thomas 2010).

REFERENCES

Abzug MJ (2004) Presentation, diagnosis, and management of enterovirus infections in neonates. *Paediatr Drugs* 6: 1–10.
Abzug MJ, Cloud G, Bradley J, et al. (2003) Double blind placebo-controlled trial of pleconaril in infants with enterovirus meningitis. *Pediatr Infect Dis J* 22: 335–41.
Benschop KS, Schinkel J, Minnaar RP, et al. (2006) Human parechovirus infections in Dutch children and the association between serotype and disease severity. *Clin Infect Dis* 42: 204–10.
Bode AV, Sejvar JJ, Pape WJ, et al. (2006) West Nile virus disease: a descriptive study of 228 patients hospitalized in a 4-county region of Colorado in 2003. *Clin Infect Dis* 42: 1234–40.
Burrow JN, Whelan PI, Kilburn CJ, et al. (1998) Australian encephalitis in the Northern Territory: clinical and epidemiological features, 1987–1996. *Aust N Z J Med* 28: 590–6.
Carson PJ, Konewko P, Wold KS, et al. (2006) Long-term clinical and neuropsychological outcomes of West Nile virus infection. *Clin Infect Dis* 43: 723–30.
Chang LY, Hsia SH, Wu CT, et al. (2004) Outcome of enterovirus 71 infections with or without stage-based management: 1998 to 2002. *Pediatr Infect Dis J* 23: 327–32.
Chang LY, Huang LM, Gau SS, et al. (2007) Neurodevelopment and cognition in children after enterovirus 71 infection. *N Engl J Med* 356: 1226–34.
Charles PC, Brown KW, Davis NL, et al. (1997) Mucosal immunity induced by parenteral immunization with a live attenuated Venezuelan equine encephalitis virus vaccine candidate. *Virology* 228: 153–60.
Chen C, Chang Y, Huang C, et al. (2001) Acute flaccid paralysis in infants and young children with enterovirus 71 infection: MR imaging findings and clinical correlates. *AJNR Am J Neuroradiol* 22: 200–5.
Cusi MG, Savellini GG, Zanelli G (2010) Toscana virus epidemiology: from Italy to beyond. *Open Virol J* 4: 22–8.
Deresiewicz RL, Thaler SJ, Hsu L, Zamani AA (1997) Clinical and neuroradiographic manifestations of eastern equine encephalitis. *N Engl J Med* 336: 1867–74.
Dumpis U, Crook D, Oksi J (1999) Tick-borne encephalitis. *Clin Infect Dis* 28: 882–90.
Earnest MP, Goolishian HA, Calverley JR, et al. (1971) Neurologic, intellectual and psychologic sequelae following western encephalitis. A follow-up study of 35 cases. *Neurology* 21: 969–74.
Ehrenkranz NJ, Ventura AK (1974) Venezuelan equine encephalitis virus infection in man. *Annu Rev Med* 25: 9–14.
Fowlkes AL, Honarmand S, Glaser C, et al. (2008) Enterovirus-associated encephalitis in the California encephalitis project, 1998–2005. *J Infect Dis* 198: 1685–91.
Fritsch P, Gruber-Sedlmayr U, Pansi H, et al. (2008) Tick-borne encephalitis in Styrian children from 1981 to 2005: a retrospective study and a review of the literature. *Acta Paediatr* 97: 535–8.
Garen PD, Tsai TF, Powers JM (1999) Human eastern equine encephalitis: immunohistochemistry and ultrastructure. *Mod Pathol* 12: 646–52.
Gould EA, Solomon T (2008) Pathogenic flaviviruses. *Lancet* 371: 500–9.
Griffin DE (1991) Therapy of viral infections of the central nervous system. *Antiviral Res* 15: 1–10.
Griffin DE (2010) Emergence and re-emergence of viral diseases of the central nervous system. *Prog Neurobiol* 91: 95–101.
Gritsun TS, Lashkevich VA, Gould EA (2003) Tick-borne encephalitis. *Antiviral Res* 57: 129–46.
Halstead SB, Thomas SJ (2010) Japanese encephalitis: new options for active immunization. *Clin Infect Dis* 50: 1155–64.
Hayes EB, Komar N, Nasci RS, et al. (2005) Epidemiology and transmission dynamics of West Nile virus disease. *Emerg Infect Dis* 11: 1167–73.
Horger M, Beck R, Fenchel M, et al. (2012) Imaging findings in tick-borne encephalitis with differential diagnostic considerations. *AJR Am J Roentgenol* 199: 420–7. doi: 10.2214/AJR.11.7911.
Johnson KM, Shelokov A, Peralta PH, et al. (1968) Recovery of Venezuelan equine encephalomyelitis virus in Panama. A fatal case in man. *Am J Trop Med Hyg* 17: 432–40.

Lambert AJ, Martin DA, Lanciotti RS (2003) Detection of North American eastern and western equine encephalitis viruses by nucleic acid amplification assays. *J Clin Microbiol* 41: 379–85.

Leon CA, Jaramillo R, Martinez S, et al. (1975) Sequelae of Venezuelan equine encephalitis in humans: a four year follow-up. *Int J Epidem* 4: 131–40.

Lesnicar G, Poljak M, Seme K, Lesnicar J (2003) Pediatric tick-borne encephalitis in 371 cases from an endemic region in Slovenia, 1959 to 2000. *Pediatr Infect Dis J* 22: 612–7.

Longshore WA, Stevens IM, Hollister AC, et al. (1956) Epidemiologic observations on acute infectious encephalitis in California with special reference to the 1952 outbreak. *Am J Hyg* 63: 69–86.

Mansfield KL, Johnson N, Phipps LP, et al. (2009) Tick-borne encephalitis virus – a review of an emerging zoonosis. *J Gen Virol* 90: 1781–94.

Marjelund S, Tikkakoski T, Tuisku S, Räisänen S (2004) Magnetic resonance imaging findings and outcome in severe tick-borne encephalitis. Report of four cases and review of the literature. *Acta Radiol* 45: 88–94.

McJunkin JE, de los Reyes EC, Irazuzta JE, et al. (2001) La Crosse encephalitis in children. *N Engl J Med* 344: 801–7.

Minor P (2009) Vaccine-derived poliovirus (VDPV): impact on poliomyelitis eradication. *Vaccine* 27: 2649–52.

Modlin JF (2007) Enterovirus déjà vu. *N Engl J Med* 356: 1204–5.

Nix WA, Oberste MS, Pallansch MA (2006) Sensitive, seminested PCR amplification of VP1 sequences for direct identification of all enterovirus serotypes from original clinical specimens. *J Clin Microbiol* 44: 2698–704.

Noran HH, Baker AB (1949) Sequels of equine encephalomyelitis. *Arch Neurol Psych* 49: 398–413.

Oberste MS, Nix WA, Maher K, Pallansch MA (2003) Improved molecular identification of enteroviruses by RT-PCR and amplicon sequencing. *J Clin Virol* 26: 375–7.

Petersen LR, Brault AC, Nasci RS (2013) West Nile virus: review of the literature. *JAMA* 310: 308–15. doi: 10.1001/jama.2013.8042.

Racaniello VR (2006) One hundred years of poliovirus pathogenesis. *Virology* 344: 9–16.

Reed DS, Lind CM, Lackemeyer MG, et al. (2005) Genetically engineered, live, attenuated vaccines protect nonhuman primates against aerosol challenge with a virulent IE strain of Venezuelan equine encephalitis virus. *Vaccine* 23: 3139–47.

Reimann CA, Hayes EB, DiGuiseppi C, et al. (2008) Epidemiology of neuroinvasive arboviral disease in the United States, 1999–2007. *Am J Trop Med Hyg* 79: 974–9.

Rivas F, Diaz LA, Cardenas VM, et al. (1997) Epidemic Venezuelan equine encephalitis in La Guajira, Colombia, 1995. *J Infect Dis* 175: 828–32.

Robin S, Ramful D, Le SF, et al. (2008) Neurologic manifestations of pediatric chikungunya infection. *J Child Neurol* 23: 1028–35.

Rorabaugh ML, Berlin LE, Heldrich F, et al. (1993) Aseptic meningitis in infants younger than 2 years of age: acute illness and neurologic complications. *Pediatrics* 92: 206–11.

Rotbart H, Webster A (2001) Treatment of potentially life-threatening enterovirus infections with pleconaril. *Clin Infect Dis* 32: 228–35.

Saad M, Youssef S, Kirschke D, et al. (2005) Acute flaccid paralysis: the spectrum of a newly recognized complication of West Nile virus infection. *J Infect* 51: 120–7.

Saksida A, Duh D, Lotric-Furlan S, et al. (2005) The importance of tick-borne encephalitis virus RNA detection for early differential diagnosis of tick-borne encephalitis. *J Clin Virol* 33: 331–5.

Sejvar JJ (2007) The long-term outcomes of human West Nile virus infection. *Clin Infect Dis* 44: 1617–24.

Solomon T (2004) Flavivirus encephalitis. *N Engl J Med* 351: 370–8.

Somekh E, Glode MP (1991) Multiple intracranial calcifications after western equine encephalitis. *Pediatr Infect Dis J* 10: 408–9.

Speers DJ, Flexxman J, Blyth CC, et al. (2013) Clinical and radiological predictors of outcome for Murray Valley encephalitis. *Am J Trop Med Hyg* 88: 481–9.

Suthar MS, Diamond MS, Gale M Jr (2013) West Nile virus infection and immunity. *Nat Rev Microbiol* 11: 115–28. doi: 10.1038/nrmicro2950.

Terrosi C, Olivieri R, Bianco C, et al. (2009) Age-dependent seroprevalence of Toscana virus in central Italy and correlation with the clinical profile. *Clin Vaccine Immunol* 16: 1251–2.

Turtle L, Griffiths MJ, Solomon T (2012) Encephalitis caused by flaviviruses. *QJM* 105: 219–23. doi: 10.1093/qjmed/hcs013.

Tyler KL (2009) Emerging viral infections of the central nervous system. Part 1. *Arch Neurol* 66: 939–48.

Verboon-Maciolek M, Groenendaal F, Hahn C, et al. (2008) Human parechovirus causes encephalitis with white matter injury in neonates. *Ann Neurol* 64: 266–73.

Wang JN, Yao CT, Yeh CN, et al. (2006) Critical management in patients with severe enterovirus 71 infection. *Pediatr Int* 48: 250–6.

Weaver SC, Ferro C, Barrera R, et al. (1996) Venezuelan equine encephalomyelitis. *Annu Rev Entomol* 49: 141–74.

Wenger F (1977) Venezuelan equine encephalitis. *Teratology* 16: 359–62.

Wilson MR (2013) Emerging viral infections. *Curr Opin Neurol* 26: 301–6.

Wong KT, Munisamy B, Ong KC, et al. (2008) The distribution of inflammation and virus in human enterovirus 71 encephalomyelitis suggests possible viral spread by neural pathways. *J Neuropathol Exp Neurol* 67: 162–9.

Wootton SH, Kaplan SL, Perrotta DM, et al. (2004) St. Louis encephalitis in early infancy. *Pediatr Infect Dis J* 23: 951–4.

Wringe A, Fine PEM, Sutter RW, Kew OM (2008) Estimating the extent of vaccine-derived poliovirus infection. *PLoS ONE* 3: e3433. doi:10.1371/journal.pone.0003433.

Yen FB, Chang LY, Kao CL, et al. (2009) Coxsackieviruses infection in northern Taiwan – epidemiology and clinical characteristics. *J Microbiol Immunol Infect* 42: 38–46.

Yen M, Tsao K, Huang Y, et al. (2007) Viral load in blood is correlated with disease severity of neonatal coxsackievirus B3 infection: early diagnosis and predicting disease severity is possible in severe neonatal enterovirus infection. *Clin Infect Dis* 44: e78–81.

8
HERPES SIMPLEX VIRUS INFECTIONS

Richard J Whitley

Herpes simplex virus (HSV) infections of the central nervous system (CNS) are among the most devastating infections acquired by humans, in spite of efficacious antiviral therapy. Two distinct types of HSV infection of the CNS are recognized: (1) neonatal HSV encephalitis that occurs during the first month of life and is usually caused by HSV-2; and (2) herpes simplex encephalitis (HSE) that is recognized as the most common cause of sporadic fatal encephalitis and is almost uniformly caused by HSV-1. Intranuclear inclusion bodies consistent with HSV infection were demonstrated first in the brain of a neonate with encephalitis from which virus was isolated (Smith et al. 1941). The first adult patient with HSE providing similar proof of viral disease was described in 1944 (Zarafonetis et al. 1944). The most striking pathological findings in this patient's brain were in the left temporal lobe, in which perivascular cuffs of lymphocytes and numerous small haemorrhages were found. This temporal lobe localization subsequently has been determined to be characteristic of HSE in individuals older than 3 months.

Pathology

The histopathological findings of HSV infection of the CNS following either neonatal encephalitis or HSE are similar. These findings include ballooning of infected cells and the appearance of chromatin within the nuclei followed by degeneration of the cellular nuclei. Cells lose intact plasma membranes and form multinucleated giant cells. As host defenses are mounted, an influx of mononuclear cells can be detected in infected tissue. Macroscopically, HSE results in acute inflammation, congestion and/or haemorrhage, most prominently in the temporal lobes and usually asymmetrically in adults and more diffusely in newborn infants. The meninges are clouded or congested. After approximately 2 weeks, these changes proceed to frank necrosis and liquefaction of the involved brain tissue in the absence of antiviral therapy.

Microscopically, involvement extends beyond areas that appear grossly abnormal. At the earliest stage, the histological changes are not dramatic and may be non-specific, such as congestion of capillaries and other small vessels in the cortex and subcortical white matter, petechiae and areas of haemorrhagic necrosis and perivascular cuffing. Glial nodules are common findings after the second week (Boos and Kim 1984, Kapur et al. 1994). The microscopic appearance becomes dominated by evidence of necrosis and inflammation; the latter is characterized by a diffuse perivascular subarachnoid mononuclear cell infiltrate, gliosis and satellitosis–neuronophagia. In such cases, widespread areas of haemorrhagic necrosis, mirroring the area of infection, become most prominent. Oligodendrocytic involvement and gliosis are common findings, developing very late in the disease. Although found in only approximately 50% of patients, intranuclear Cowdry type A inclusions are characterized by an eosinophilic homogeneous appearance and surrounded by a clear, unstained zone beyond which lies a rim of marginated chromatin.

Pathogenesis

NEONATAL HERPES SIMPLEX INFECTION

The newborn infant usually acquires infection by contact with infected maternal genital secretions, accounting for 85% of cases. Approximately 5% of cases are acquired in utero, and the remainder postnatally. The most extensive evaluation of genital HSV infection in pregnant women reported that among 58 362 live births, there were 18 cases of neonatal HSV infection (one case per 3200 live births) (Brown et al. 2003). Of those 18 cases, 10 were caused by HSV-2 infection and eight by HSV-1. Of the 10 cases of neonatal HSV-2 infection, seven were born to mothers with first-episode HSV-2 and three to mothers with reactivation disease. Of the eight infants with neonatal HSV-1 infection, four were born to mothers with primary HSV-1 and four to mothers with reactivation HSV-1. The majority of disease in the newborn infant is, thus, the consequence of maternal first-episode genital disease.

Risk factors for transmission were evaluated for the 202 deliveries from which HSV was isolated (Brown et al. 2003). Only one out of 85 infants (1.2%) delivered by caesarean section developed neonatal HSV disease compared with nine out of 117 (7.7%) delivered vaginally (p=0.47; odds ratio [OR] 0.14 [0.02–1.26 adjusted]). The use of invasive monitors was associated with an increased frequency of neonatal disease (10.1% vs 1.6%, OR 3.5 [0.6–19 adjusted], p= 0.02). A maternal first episode of disease was more likely to result in transmission (30.8%) than recurrent infection (1.3%, OR 59.3 [6.7–525 adjusted], p<0.001). Similarly, the isolation of HSV from the cervix – the site most likely to be encountered by the fetus – was also associated with increased transmission (18.4% vs 0.7%, OR 15.4 [1.8–133 adjusted], p<0.001].

Involvement of the CNS results in either focal temporal lobe disease that is likely to be secondary to neuronal spread to the brain, or diffuse involvement, presumably secondary to viraemia associated with disseminated multiorgan disease.

HERPES SIMPLEX ENCEPHALITIS

The pathogenesis of HSE in older children (>3 months of age), adolescents and adults is only partially understood but is likely to be similar for all age groups. Both primary and recurrent HSV infections can cause disease of the CNS. Approximately one-third of cases of HSE are the consequence of primary infection, generally occurring in those younger than 18 years of age. The remaining two-thirds of cases occur in the presence of pre-existing antibodies, but only approximately 10% of patients have a history of recurrent herpes labialis. Patients with pre-existing antibodies are thought to have HSE as a consequence of reactivation of HSV (Nahmias et al. 1982). There is a mendelian predisposition in some children (Abel et al. 2010). Susceptibility to HSE has been related to mutations in Toll-like receptor response pathways that directly reduce the intrinsic resistance of neurons and other cells in the CNS to HSV infection (Lafaille et al. 2012).

The route of access of virus to the CNS in primary infection, especially in humans, is a subject of debate. Classic studies defined pathways for access of HSV to the brain in animals and included both the olfactory and trigeminal nerves among others. However, it is unclear which of these nerve tracts more commonly leads to HSV infection in the CNS of humans. The anatomical distribution of nerves from the olfactory tract into the limbic system, along with the recovery of virus from the temporal lobe (the site of apparent onset of HSE in the human brain), suggests that viral access to the CNS via this route is a tenable hypothesis. In patients with HSE, electron microscopic evidence has demonstrated herpesvirus particles along the olfactory tract in some individuals.

Reactivation of HSV, leading to focal HSE, is a similarly confusing problem from the standpoint of pathogenesis. Evidence of latent virus within infected brain tissue exists (Rock and Frasher 1983); however, virus reactivation at that site remains purely hypothetical. Reactivation of virus peripherally (namely, in the olfactory bulb or the trigeminal ganglion) with subsequent neuronal transmission to the CNS has been suggested (Griffith et al. 1967, Johnson et al. 1968, Davis and Johnson 1979, Stroop and Schaefer 1986). Nonetheless, a relevant observation is that with recurrent herpes labialis, whereby reactivation of virus from the trigeminal ganglia occurs, HSE is a very uncommon event.

Some patients (around 30%) develop autoantibodies against N-methyl-D-aspartate receptor antibodies, which may have potential pathogenic disease-modifying effects, and may benefit from immunotherapy (Pruss et al. 2012). Association with psychiatric symptoms and tumours has been uniquely seen with autoimmune encephalitis, whereas acute onset with fever and absence of basal ganglia involvement in magnetic resonance imaging (MRI) support a diagnosis of HSE (Oyanguren et al. 2013).

Clinical presentation of herpes simplex virus infections of the brain

NEONATAL HERPES SIMPLEX VIRUS INFECTION

The most extensive evaluation of the natural history and presentation of infants with neonatal HSV infection was reported by Kimberlin et al. (2001a). Infants were classified according to the extent of disease. Those with disease limited to the skin were identified as having skin, eye and mouth infection. Those with CNS disease with or without involvement of the skin were defined as having encephalitis. Those with multi-organ involvement, including those with CNS disease, were labelled as having disseminated infection. This review will focus on those infants with CNS disease.

Infants with encephalitis and disseminated disease that involves the CNS present clinically at approximately 17 days and 12 days, respectively, for therapy (Kimberlin et al. 2001b, Berger and Houff 2008). The mean duration of disease is between 5.7 and 7.4 days. For infants with encephalitis, a smaller number had skin lesions (63%) that were present on average for 6.1 days at the time of presentation; 49% were lethargic, 44% had fever, 16% had conjunctivitis, and 57% had seizures at presentation. For those infants with disseminated disease and CNS disease, 58% had skin vesicles that were present for an average of 3.7 days; 47% were lethargic, 56% had fever, 17% had conjunctivitis, 22% had seizures, 34% had disseminated intravascular coagulopathy, and 37% had pneumonia.

The outcome correlated with the virus type and disease classification. For those infants with encephalitis, the neurological outcome was significantly better with HSV-1 than with HSV-2 infection. For example, 25% of those having HSV-1 infection were left with severe impairment, compared with 55% for HSV-2 infection. The outcome reversed, however, for infants with disseminated disease. In this circumstance, 70% of those with HSV-1 infection were either dead or were left with severe neurological impairment compared with 50% with HSV-2 infection. In addition to poor cognitve outcome, survivors have speech impairment, attention deficit and poor social skills (Engman et al. 2008).

The neurodiagnostic and laboratory evaluation of these children is similar to that for HSE (see below).

HERPES SIMPLEX ENCEPHALITIS

HSE is estimated to occur in approximately 1 in 250 000 to 1 in 500 000 individuals per year (Longson 1984, Skoldenberg 1984). In the USA, HSE is thought to account for as many as 10%–20% of all encephalitic viral infections of the CNS before the occurrence of West Nile virus encephalitis (Corey and Spear 1986). In the UK, HSV was estimated to cause serious neurological disease in 1 in 64 000 young children and 1 in 230 000 older children (Ward et al. 2012). A recent study of 581 patients in Spain determined the incidence of viruses causing aseptic meningitis, meningoencephalitis and encephalitis (de Ory et al. 2013). Among those with meningitis, 57.1% were characterized; echovirus was the most frequent (76.8%), followed by varicella-zoster virus (10.3%) and HSV (3.1%; HSV-1: 1.6%; HSV-2: 1.0%, HSV non-typed: 0.5%). For meningoencephalitis, 40.7% of cases were characterized, of which 43.2% were caused by HSV-1. For encephalitis, 27.6% of cases were characterized; 71% were caused by HSV-1. HSE occurs throughout the year and in patients of all ages, with approximately one-third of cases occurring in patients younger than 20 years but older than 3 months, and approximately one-half in patients older than 50 years (Whitley et al. 1982). Caucasians account for 95% of patients with diseases confirmed by either biopsy or polymerase chain reaction (PCR). Both sexes are affected equally.

In the absence of therapy or with the administration of an ineffective antiviral medication, the mortality is in excess of 70%; only approximately 2.5% of all patients with confirmed disease (9.1% of survivors) return to normal function after recovering from their illness (Whitley et al. 1977, 1981; Longson 1979; Longson et al. 1980). With antiviral therapy, good outcome has been reported in some centres (Hsieh et al. 2007).

Most patients with HSE confirmed by biopsy presented with a focal encephalopathic process, including (1) altered cognitive function and decreasing levels of consciousness with focal neurological findings; (2) cerebrospinal fluid (CSF) pleocytosis and proteinosis; (3) the absence of bacterial and fungal pathogens in the CSF; and (4) focal electroencephalographic

(EEG), computed tomographic (CT), and/or technetium brain scan findings (Whitley et al. 1982). Magnetic resonance imaging (MRI) is a more sensitive diagnostic tool and has, for the most part, replaced CT (Sener 2001, 2002; Schlesinger et al. 1995).

Patients with HSE present with fever and changes in personality, irrespective of age. The frequency of headache and CSF pleocytosis is higher in patients with confirmed HSE than in patients with diseases that mimic HSE. Seizures, whether focal or generalized, occur in only approximately two-thirds of all patients with confirmed disease. Thus, the clinical findings of HSE are non-specific and do not allow for empiric diagnosis of disease predicated solely on clinical presentation. Although clinical evidence of a localized temporal lobe lesion is often thought to indicate HSE, a variety of other diseases can mimic this condition such as other bacterial, fungal, *Mycoplasma*, tubercular and cryptococcal infections; viral infections (Epstein–Barr virus, cytomegalovirus, togavirus, echovirus, mumps); tumours, subdural haematomas and adrenal leukodystrophy (Whitley et al. 1989).

Unless contraindicated because of increased intracranial pressure, CSF examination is essential both to assess biochemical parameters and to perform an HSV PCR. In patients with HSE, CSF findings are non-diagnostic, being similar in patients with confirmed disease and in those with diseases that mimic HSE (Whitley et al. 1989). Both the CSF white blood cell count (lymphocytic predominance) and CSF protein become elevated as the disease progresses. The average CSF white blood cell count is 100 cells/L; the protein averages approximately 100mg/dL. The presence of red blood cells in CSF is not diagnostic for HSE. Approximately 5%–10% of patients have a normal CSF formula on first evaluation.

Non-invasive neurodiagnostic studies support a presumptive diagnosis of HSE. These studies have included EEG, CT and MRI. Focal changes of the EEG are characterized by spike and slow-wave activity and periodic lateralized epileptiform discharges, which arise from the temporal lobe (Radermecker 1956, Miller and Coey 1959, Upton and Grumpert 1970, Smith et al. 1975, Chien et al. 1977). Early in the disease, the abnormal electrical activity usually involves one temporal lobe and then spreads to the contralateral temporal lobe as the disease evolves, usually during a period of 7–10 days. The sensitivity of the EEG is approximately 84%, but the specificity is only 32.5%. CT initially shows low-density areas with mass effect localized to the temporal lobe, which can progress to radiolucent and/or haemorrhagic lesions (Enzmann et al. 1978, Zimmerman et al. 1980, Baskin and Hedlund 2007). Bitemporal disease occurs commonly in the absence of therapy, particularly late in the course of the disease. When these neurodiagnostic tests are used in combination, the sensitivity is enhanced; however, the specificity remains inadequate. None of these neurodiagnostic tests is uniformly satisfactory for diagnosing HSE. MRI detects evidence of HSE before CT demonstration (Schlesinger et al. 1995).

Laboratory considerations for diagnosis

Serological assessments are rarely, if ever, used for diagnostic purposes in newborn infants. However, in older children and adults, several strategies utilizing antibody production have been employed (Cesario et al. 1969). Because most encephalitic patients are HSV-seropositive at presentation, seroconversion is usually not helpful as fever alone can reactivate labial herpes, resulting in antibody elevations. A four-fold rise in serum antibody was neither sensitive nor specific enough to be useful. A four-fold or greater rise in CSF antibody will occur significantly more often within a month after onset of disease in patients with biopsy-proven HSE as opposed to those with other diagnoses: 85% versus 29%, respectively. By 10 days after clinical presentation, however, only 50% of brain-biopsy-positive patients had a four-fold rise in CSF antibody. Thus, this test is useful only for retrospective diagnosis. The use of a serum to CSF antibody ratio of 20 or less did not improve sensitivity during the first 10 days of disease.

Polymerase Chain Reaction Detection of Viral DNA
PCR detection of HSV DNA in the CSF has become the diagnostic method of choice for both neonatal HSV infection and HSE (Rowley et al. 1990; Aurelius et al. 1991, 1993; Puchhammer-Stockl et al. 1993; Sakrauski et al. 1994; Shoji et al. 1994; Lakeman and Whitley 1995; DeBiasi and Tyler 1999). The sensitivity and specificity are 94% and 98%, respectively. These CSF specimens were obtained from patients with biopsy-confirmed and biopsy-negative disease. Notably, the specificity would have been higher except that some tissue specimens were fixed in formalin, which killed infectious virus, before attempts at isolation in cell culture were made. HSV DNA persists in 80% of tested specimens for 1 week or more despite antiviral therapy (Lakeman and Whitley 1995).

Real-time PCR has been applied to evaluation of CSF specimens from patients with HSE. Virus load in the CSF appears to correlate directly with clinical outcome. In an initial study, the quantity of virus (copies of viral DNA/mL) correlated statistically with decreased level of consciousness, the presence of a lesion detected by either CT or MRI, and a poor neurological outcome (Domingues et al. 1997, 1998a,b).

Therapy

Neonatal Herpes Simplex Virus Infection
The most extensive recently published treatment data have come from the NIAID Collaborative Antiviral Study Group (Whitley et al. 1991a,b; Kimberlin et al. 2001a,b). Aciclovir therapy at dosages of 10, 15 or 20mg/kg every 8 hours for 14 versus 21 days of treatment was assessed. For infants with either encephalitis or disseminated disease, a significant reduction in mortality occurred with high-dose therapy. For infants with disseminated disease, mortality was decreased from 61% for those receiving 10mg/kg every 8 hours to 31% for those receiving high-dose aciclovir. Predictors of mortality included disease severity (pneumonia, disseminated intravascular coagulopathy, seizures and hepatitis), virus type (HSV-1) and preterm birth.

Although survival was improved, there were no significant differences according to the disease classification in morbidity, as defined at 12 months. For infants with disseminated multi-organ disease, 83% of survivors developed normally after high-dose aciclovir compared with 60% of those receiving standard-dose aciclovir. For patients with encephalitis, 31% of survivors developed normally compared with 29% receiving standard therapy. These data indicate the efficacy of aciclovir in the management of neonatal HSV infection; however, the persistent morbidity and nagging mortality indicate a further need for both preventive and therapeutic interventions.

Ideally, the prevention of neonatal HSV infection is preferred to the treatment of established disease. However, no vaccine or therapeutic intervention for the pregnant woman has yet proved efficacious. An inactivated subunit vaccine was evaluated (Stanberry et al. 2002) and the results indicated that women who were seronegative for both HSV-1 and HSV-2 derived nearly 70% efficacy for the prevention of both infection and disease. However, both among individuals who were seropositive for HSV-1 and among men who were seronegative for HSV-1 and HSV-2, no effect of vaccination was demonstrated.

An alternative approach to the prevention of neonatal disease has been the administration of aciclovir to women during the third trimester of gestation, particularly the last 4 weeks. Over the past decade, three published clinical trials have addressed the efficacy of aciclovir. Recently, a double-blind, randomized placebo-controlled trial of aciclovir in late pregnancy documented a reduction in HSV shedding but not in the incidence of caesarean delivery (Watts et al. 2003). Lesion occurred at delivery in 11 out of 78 women (14%) who received placebo versus four out of 84 who received aciclovir (5%, p =0.08). Women who received placebo were culture-positive in 7% and PCR-positive in 34% of cases within 48 hours of delivery. For the comparative aciclovir group, no woman was culture-positive and 2% were PCR-positive (p=0.03 and p<0.01, respectively). Caesarean delivery for HSV occurred in eight of the placebo recipients (10%) and three of the aciclovir-treated women (4%), p=0.17. Aciclovir thus significantly decreased the virus shedding and evidence of viral infection using PCR, but did not impact on the frequency of caesarean delivery.

A similar randomized controlled study was performed with valaciclovir (500mg/d) (Andrews et al. 2006). Valaciclovir had no impact on viral shedding, the detection of lesions or caesarean delivery. Neonatal renal function was evaluated extensively; there was no evidence of elevated creatinine or blood urea nitrogen, or of decreased urine output or glomerular filtration rate.

Clearly, there is a lack of population-based data on the impact of aciclovir during the last 4 weeks of gestation on the maternal–fetal transmission of HSV. However, because of the high frequency of caesarean delivery in women with a known history of genital herpes, the American College of Obstetrics and Gynecology has suggested that antiviral therapy should be considered in women who have recurrent genital herpes, as well as in women who experience first-episode genital herpes in the last trimester of gestation.

HERPES SIMPLEX ENCEPHALITIS

The first antiviral drug proven efficacious for therapy of HSE was vidarabine (Whitley et al. 1977, 1981); however, it has been replaced by aciclovir in the physician's armamentarium. During these studies, the variables of age, duration of disease and level of consciousness at the onset of therapy proved to be major determinants of clinical outcome. Patients under 30 years of age and with a more normal level of consciousness (lethargic as opposed to comatose) were more likely to return to normal function than were older patients, especially those who were semicomatose or comatose. Notably, 90% of individuals under 30 years of age were children and adolescents. From these data, older patients (>30 years of age), whether comatose or semicomatose, had mortality rates that approached 70% – a figure very similar to that encountered in the placebo recipients of the previously cited studies. If therapy is to be effective, it must be instituted before the onset of haemorrhagic necrosis of a dominant temporal lobe and of significant deterioration of consciousness. Aciclovir is superior to vidarabine for the treatment of HSE (Whitley et al. 1986).

The mortality is 55% at 6 and 18 months after the onset of treatment for vidarabine recipients versus 19% and 28%, respectively, for the aciclovir-treated group. Late deaths were not a consequence of either persistent or reactivated HSV infection but occurred in patients who were severely impaired as a consequence of their disease. The mortality rate is somewhat lower in children and adolescents but not statistically different from that in older individuals. As noted above, previous studies indicated that age and level of consciousness influenced long-term outcome. A more objective reflection of level of consciousness is the Glasgow coma score (GCS). Scores that approached normal predicted enhanced survival. When GCS and age were assessed simultaneously, a GCS of 6 or less predicted a poor therapeutic outcome, irrespective of the agent administered or of the age of the patient (Whitley et al. 1986).

Regarding morbidity, with aciclovir therapy, 38% of patients returned to normal or had minor impairment, 9% of patients had moderate sequelae, and 53% of patients were left with severe impairment or died. Relapse of HSE has been reported, although not well documented, in a few patients after receiving vidarabine (Davis and McLaren 1983, Wang et al. 1994) and aciclovir (Van Landingham et al. 1988, Wang et al. 1994). Many patients were not afebrile at the conclusion of treatment, suggesting that a longer duration of therapy to a minimum of 14–21 days may be desirable. These findings indicate that the current therapy of choice for the management of HSE is aciclovir. Aciclovir is administered at a dosage of 10mg/kg every 8 hours (30mg/kg/d) for a period of only 14–21 days. High-dose aciclovir therapy (60mg/kg/d) has been recommended by some and found to be safe in children being treated for HSE when compared with standard low dose (Kendrick et al. 2014). Although the use of adjunctive steroid therapy with aciclovir has been shown to be associated with an improved outcome in experimental and clinical situations (Ciro et al. 2013), current evidence is not yet sufficient to recommend this as a standard practice.

Recent research shows emerging HSV drug resistance in both immunocompromised and immunocompetent persons when HSV infections involve 'immune-privileged sites' (Andrei and Snoeck 2013). Thus, drug-resistance typing and combination therapy is advisable in cases of aciclovir-unresponsive HSE.

Conclusion

Consistent advances in both treatment and diagnosis of HSV infections of the CNS have been achieved over the past 25 years. However, for both neonatal HSV infections and HSE, improvement in therapeutic strategies is imperative. Unfortunately, antiviral medications with high lipophilicity and mechanisms of action different from aciclovir, allowing for the opportunity for combination therapy, are not in the immediate future. Hopefully the current vaccine studies may offer an opportunity for prevention rather than therapy after the fact.

REFERENCES

Abel L, Plancoulaine S, Jouanguy E, et al. (2010) Age-dependent Mendelian predisposition to herpes simplex virus type 1 encephalitis in childhood. *J Pediatr* 157: 623–9.

Andrei G, Snoeck R (2013) Herpes simplex virus drug-resistance: new mutations and insights. *Curr Opin Infect Dis* 26: 551–60.

Andrews WW, Kimberlin DF, Whitley R, et al. (2006) Valacyclovir therapy to reduce recurrent genital herpes in pregnant women. *Am J Obstet Gynecol* 194: 774–81.

Aurelius E, Johansson B, Skoldenberg B, et al. (1991) Rapid diagnosis of herpes simplex encephalitis by nested polymerase chain reaction assay of cerebrospinal fluid. *Lancet* 337: 189–92.

Aurelius E, Johansson B, Skoldenberg B, Forsgren M (1993) Encephalitis in immunocompetent patients due to herpes simplex virus type 1 or 2 as determined by type-specific polymerase chain reaction and antibody assays of cerebrospinal fluid. *J Med Virol* 39: 179–86.

Baskin HJ, Hedlund G (2007) Neuroimaging of herpesvirus infections in children. *Pediatr Radiol* 37: 949–63.

Berger JR, Houff S (2008) Neurological complications of herpes simplex virus type 2 infection. *Arch Neurol* 65: 596–600.

Boos J, Kim JH (1984) Biopsy histopathology in herpes simplex encephalitis and in encephalitis of undefined etiology. *Yale J Bio Med* 57: 751–5.

Brown ZA, Wald A, Morrow RM, et al. (2003) Effect of serologic status and cesarean delivery on transmission rates of herpes simplex virus from mother to infant. *JAMA* 289: 203–9.

Cesario TC, Poland JD, Wulff H, et al. (1969) Six years experiences with herpes simplex virus in a children's home. *Am J Epidemiol* 90: 416–22.

Chien LT, Boehm RM, Robinson H, et al. (1977) Characteristic early electroencephalographic changes in herpes simplex encephalitis. *Arch Neurol* 34: 361–4.

Ciro Ramos-Estebanez, Lizarraga KJ, Merenda A (2013) A systematic review on the role of adjunctive corticosteroids in herpes simplex virus encephalitis: is timing critical for safety and efficacy? *Antivir Ther*. doi: 10.3851/IMP2683. [Epub ahead of print.]

Corey L, Spear P (1986) Infections with herpes simplex viruses. *N Engl J Med* 314: 686–91.

Davis LE, Johnson RT (1979) An explanation for the localization of herpes simplex encephalitis. *Ann Neurol* 5: 2–5.

Davis LE, McLaren LE (1983) Relapsing herpes simplex encephalitis following antiviral therapy. *Ann Neurol* 13: 192–5.

DeBiasi RL, Tyler KL (1999) Polymerase chain reaction in the diagnosis and management of central nervous system infections. *Arch Neurol* 56: 1215–9.

de Ory F, Avellón A, Echevarría JE, et al. (2013) Viral infections of the central nervous system in Spain: a prospective study. *J Med Virol* 85: 554–62.

Domingues RB, Lakeman FD, Pannuti CS, et al. (1997) Advantage of polymerase chain reaction in the diagnosis of herpes simplex encephalitis: presentation of 5 atypical cases. *Scand J Infect Dis* 29: 229–31.

Domingues RB, Fink MC, Tsanaclis SM, et al. (1998a) Diagnosis of herpes simplex encephalitis by magnetic resonance imaging and polymerase chain reaction assay of cerebrospinal fluid. *J Neurol Sci* 157: 148–53.

Domingues RB, Lakeman FD, Mayo MS, Whitley RJ (1998b) Application of competitive PCR to cerebrospinal fluid samples from patients with herpes simplex encephalitis. *J Clin Microbiol* 36: 2229–34.

Engman ML, Adolfsson I, Lewensohn-Fuchs I, et al. (2008) Neuropsychologic outcomes in children with neonatal herpes encephalitis. *Pediatr Neurol* 38: 398–405.

Enzmann DR, Ransom B, Norman D (1978) Computed tomography of herpes simplex encephalitis. *Radiology* 129: 419–25.

Griffith JR, Kibrick S, Dodge PR, Richardson EP (1967) Experimental herpes simplex encephalitis: electroencephalographic, clinical, virologic, and pathologic observations in the rabbit. *Electroencephalogr Clin Neurophysiol* 23: 263–7.

Hsieh WB, Chiu NC, Hu KC, et al. (2007) Outcome of herpes simplex encephalitis in children. *J Microbiol Immunol Infect* 40: 34–8.

Johnson RT, Olson LC, Buescher EL (1968) Herpes simplex virus infections of the nervous system. Problems in laboratory diagnosis. *Arch Neurol* 18: 260–4.

Kapur N, Barker S, Burrows EH, et al. (1994) Herpes simplex encephalitis: long term magnetic resonance imaging and neuropsychological profile. *J Neurol Neurosurg Psychiatry* 57: 1334–42.

Kendrick JG, Ensom MH, Steer A, et al. (2014) Standard-dose versus high-dose acyclovir in children treated empirically for encephalitis: a retrospective cohort study of its use and safety. *Paediatr Drugs.* [Epub ahead of print.]

Kimberlin DW, Lin CY, Jacobs RF, et al. (2001a) Natural history of neonatal herpes simplex virus infections in the acyclovir era. *Pediatrics* 108: 223–9.

Kimberlin DW, Lin CY, Jacobs RF, et al. (2001b) Safety and efficacy of high-dose intravenous acyclovir in the management of neonatal herpes simplex virus infections. *Pediatrics* 108: 230–8.

Lafaille FG, Pessach IM, Zhang SY, et al. (2012) Impaired intrinsic immunity to HSV-1 in human iPSC-derived TLR3-deficient CNS cells. *Nature* 491: 769–73.

Lakeman FD, Whitley RJ (1995) Diagnosis of herpes simplex encephalitis: application of polymerase chain reaction to cerebrospinal fluid from brain biopsied patients and correlation with disease. National Institute of Allergy and Infectious Diseases Collaborative Antiviral Study Group. *J Infect Dis* 172: 857–63.

Longson M (1979) Le defi des encephalitis herpetiques. *Ann Microbiol (Paris)* 130: 5.

Longson M (1984) The general nature of viral encephalitis in the United Kingdom. In: Ellis LS, ed. *Viral Diseases of the Central Nervous System.* London: Baillière Tindall, pp. 19–31.

Longson MM, Bailey AS, Klapper P (1980) Herpes encephalitis. In: Waterson AP, ed. *Recent Advances in Clinical Virology.* New York: Churchill Livingston, pp. 147–57.

Miller JHD, Coey A (1959) The EEG in necrotizing encephalitis. *Electroencephalogr Clin Neurophysiol* 2: 582–5.

Nahmias AJ, Whitley RJ, Visintine AN, et al. (1982) Herpes simplex encephalitis: laboratory evaluations and their diagnostic significance. *J Infect Dis* 145: 829–36.

Oyanguren B, Sánchez V, González FJ, et al. (2013) Limbic encephalitis: a clinical–radiological comparison between herpetic and autoimmune etiologies. *Eur J Neurol* 20: 1566–70.

Pruss H, Finke C, Holtje M, et al. (2012) N-methyl-D-aspartate receptor antibodies in herpes simplex encephalitis. *Ann Neurol* 72: 902–11.

Puchhammer-Stockl E, Heinz FX, Kundi M, et al. (1993) Evaluation of the polymerase chain reaction for diagnosis of herpes simplex virus encephalitis. *J Clin Microbiol* 31: 146–8.

Radermecker J (1956) Systematique des electrocencephalographic des encephalitis it encephalopathies. *Electroencephalography* Suppl 5: 1–243.

Rock DL, Frasher NW (1983) Detection of HSV-1 genome in central nervous system of latently infected mice. *Nature* 302: 523–31.

Rowley A, Lakeman F, Whitley R, Wolinsky S (1990) Rapid detection of herpes simplex virus DNA in cerebrospinal fluid of patients with herpes simplex encephalitis. *Lancet* 335: 440–1.

Sakrauski A, Weber B, Kessler HH, et al. (1994) Comparison of two hybridization assays for the rapid detection of PCR amplified HSV genome sequences from cerebrospinal fluid. *J Virol Meth* 50: 175–84.

Schlesinger Y, Tebas P, Gaudreault-Keener M, et al. (1995) Herpes simplex type 2 meningitis in the absence of genital lesions: improved recognition using the polymerase chain reaction. *Clin Infect Dis* 20: 842–8.

Sener RN (2001) Herpes simplex encephalitis: diffusion MR imaging findings. *Comput Med Imaging Graph* 25: 391–7.

Sener RN (2002) Diffusion MRI in Rasmussen's encephalitis, herpes simplex encephalitis, and bacterial meningoencephalitis. *Comput Med Imaging Graph* 26: 327–32.

Shoji H, Koga M, Kusuhara T, et al. (1994) Differentiation of herpes simplex virus 1 and 2 in cerebrospinal fluid of patients with HSV encephalitis and meningitis by stringet hybridization of PCR-amplified DNAs. *J Neurol* 241: 526–30.

Skoldenberg B, Forsgren M, Alestig K, et al. (1984) Acyclovir versus vidarabine in herpes simplex encephalitis: a randomized multicentre study in consecutive Swedish patients. *Lancet* 2: 707–11.

Smith JB, Westmoreland BF, Reagan TJ, Sandok BA (1975) A distinctive clinical EEG profile in herpes simplex encephalitis. *Mayo Clin Proc* 50: 469–74.

Smith MG, Lennette EH, Reames HR (1941) Isolation of the virus of herpes simplex and the demonstration of intranuclear inclusions in a case of acute encephalitis. *Am J Pathol* 17: 55–68.

Stanberry LR, Spruance SL, Cunningham AL, et al. (2002) Glycoprotein-D-adjuvant vaccine to prevent genital herpes. *N Engl J Med* 347: 1652–61.

Stroop WG, Schaefer DC (1986) Production of encephalitis restricted to the temporal lobes by experimental reactivation of herpes simplex virus. *J Infect Dis* 153: 721–31.

Upton A, Grumpert J (1970) Electroencephalography in diagnosis of herpes simplex encephalitis. *Lancet* 1: 650–2.

Van Landingham KE, Marsteller HB, Ross GW, Hayden FG (1988) Relapse of herpes simplex encephalitis after conventional acyclovir therapy. *JAMA* 259: 1051–3.

Wang HS, Kuo MF, Huang SC, Chou ML (1994) Choreoathetosis as an initial sign of relapsing of herpes simplex encephalitis. *Pediatr Neurol* 11: 341–5.

Ward KN, Ohrling A, Bryant NJ, et al. (2012) Herpes simplex serious neurological disease in young children: incidence and long-term outcome. *Arch Dis Child* 97: 162–5.

Watts DH, Brown ZA, Money D, et al. (2003) A double-blind, randomized, placebo-controlled trial of acyclovir in late pregnancy for the reduction of herpes simplex virus shedding and cesarean delivery. *Am J Obstet Gynecol* 188: 836–43.

Whitley RJ, Soong S-J, Dolin R, et al. (1977) Adenine arabinoside therapy of biopsy-proved herpes simplex encephalitis: National Institute of Allergy and Infectious Diseases Collaborative Antiviral Study. *N Engl J Med* 297: 289–94.

Whitley RJ, Soong S-J, Hirsch MS, et al. (1981) Herpes simplex encephalitis: vidarabine therapy and diagnostic problems. *N Engl J Med* 304: 313–8.

Whitley RJ, Soong S-J, Linneman C Jr, et al. (1982) Herpes simplex encephalitis: clinical assessment. *JAMA* 247: 317–20.

Whitley RJ, Alford CA Jr, Hirsch MS, et al. (1986) Vidarabine versus acyclovir therapy in herpes simplex encephalitis. *N Engl J Med* 314: 144–9.

Whitley RJ, Cobbs CG, Alford CA Jr, et al. (1989) Diseases that mimic herpes simplex encephalitis: diagnosis, presentation and outcome. *JAMA* 262: 234–9.

Whitley RJ, Arvin A, Prober C, et al. (1991a) A controlled trial comparing vidarabine with acyclovir in neonatal herpes simplex virus infection. *N Engl J Med* 324: 444–9.

Whitley RJ, Arvin A, Prober C, et al. (1991b) Predictors of morbidity and mortality in neonates with herpes simplex virus infections. *N Engl J Med* 324: 450–4.

Zarafonetis CJD, Smodel MC, Adams JW, Haymaker V (1944) Fatal herpes simplex encephalitis in man. *Am J Pathol* 20: 429–45.

Zimmerman RD, Russell EJ, Leeds NE, Kaufman D (1980) CT in the early diagnosis of herpes simplex encephalitis. *AJR Am J Roentgenol* 134: 61–6.

9
JAPANESE ENCEPHALITIS

Rashmi Kumar and Rupa R Singh

Japanese encephalitis, referred to as a "plague of the Orient", is the most common cause of epidemic acute viral encephalitis in the world (Monath 1988). According to the World Health Organization (WHO), approximately 3 billion people live in Japanese-encephalitis-endemic regions (WHO 2007, PATH 2009). An estimated 67 900 cases of Japanese encephalitis occur annually (CDC 2013); about 10–15 000 deaths are reported to the WHO each year but this may be an underestimate due to inadequate surveillance systems and lack of viral diagnostic facilities in affected regions (Tsai 2000). In endemic areas, the annual incidence ranges from 10 to 100 per 100 000 population (Tirounourougane et al. 2002). The disease carries a high case-fatality rate of 20%–30%, with a risk of neurological or psychiatric sequelae in survivors (Campbell et al. 2011) posing a heavy economic burden on the poor rural families who are primarily affected.

History

The Japanese encephalitis virus (JEV) was first isolated from autopsied monkey brain in Japan in 1935, though descriptive accounts of the disease date back to the late 1800s (Solomon 2003). Nowadays, Japanese encephalitis is rare in Japan owing to JEV vaccination, the use of agricultural pesticides and controlled pig farming (WHO 2007). The first case from India was recorded in 1954 and from Nepal in 1978 (Halstead 2004). Recently, the virus has been introduced into northern mainland Australia (Hanna et al. 1999).

The virus

The Japanese encephalitis virus is a small, single-stranded, positive-sense RNA virus belonging to the genus *Flavivirus*, family *Flaviviridae* of the arboviruses. Closely related flaviviruses include the West Nile, St Louis encephalitis and Murray Valley encephalitis viruses. The Japanese encephalitis virion consists of the RNA strand wrapped in a nucleocapsid and surrounded by a glycoprotein-containing envelope. There are three structural proteins – core (C), premembrane (PrM) and envelope (E) – and seven nonstructural proteins (NS1, NS2A, NS2B, NS3, NS4A, NS4B, NS5). The E protein is the largest structural protein with nearly 500 amino acids. It is considered important for viral entry into host cells and is the main target for humoral immune response (Solomon 2003).

To date, the PrM and E protein-encoding genes have usually been used for the phylogenetic analysis of JEV. Five genotypes of JEV are known at present; of these, types I, II and III are the most prevalent. Different genotypes of JEV (associated with different virulence

126

patterns) thrive in a particular climatic condition: genotypes IV (the oldest) and V are isolated in the tropical endemic region of Indonesia–Malaysia, whereas genotypes I and III are found in the temperate epidemic regions (Ghosh and Basu 2009).

Transmission and life cycle

Japanese encephalitis is primarily transmitted between vertebrate animals by an insect vector – the mosquito. The main vertebrate host and reservoir of infection all over Asia is the pig (Medappa 1980). The animal has a prolonged viraemic stage, which makes it an effective reservoir of the infection, but it does not exhibit symptoms except for abortion. Besides the pig, birds of the family *Ardeidae* (pond heron, water egrets, etc.) are also capable of transmitting the infection. Human beings and horses suffer from illness but act as 'deadend' hosts because they are incapable of transmitting the infection further, the period of viraemia being too short (ARMCANZ 1998). Cattle do not transmit the infection either, although they may help to support a large population of mosquitoes (Medappa 1980). The main vector all over Asia is the *Culex tritaeiorrhynchus*, rice-field breeding mosquito. Therefore, Japanese encephalitis tends to occur in rural rice-growing populations that rear pigs. However, other mosquito vectors are also known. In India, isolates from other species of *Culex* (*whitmorei, vishnui, epidesmus, bitaeniorrhynchus*) and even some anophelines indicate that other mosquitos may play a role as complementary vectors (Medappa 1980).

Epidemiology

The disease primarily occurs in outbreaks and epidemics that coincide with periods of peak mosquito activity. However, some baseline incidence must be present that makes the occurrence of outbreaks possible. It has now been reported that JEV lineages can be divided into four endemic cycles, comprising southern Asia, eastern coastal Asia and western Asia. Central and southernmost Asia are the source of JEV (genotype 1) diversity from which the viruses disperse and evolve throughout Asia (Gao et al. 2013). The ratio of apparent to non-apparent infection is estimated as 1:300 to 1:1000. There is a scattered pattern of occurrence: only one or two cases per village, with some villages completely spared (Medappa 1980). Children between 5 and 15 years of age bear the brunt of the disease. Adults living in endemic areas have generally acquired antibodies to JEV, and adult infection most often occurs in areas where the disease is newly introduced (Halstead 2004). A study of laboratory-proven cases of the disease in children hospitalized during the 2005 epidemic in Uttar Pradesh revealed that almost all cases were confined to rural areas, children below 2 years of age were not affected, and boys accounted for almost three-quarters of the cases (Kumar et al. 2006).

Pathogenesis

The E protein has been shown to have a major role in determination of virulence phenotype. Even single amino-acid substitutions are sufficient to cause loss of neuro-invasiveness. Changes in the putative receptor-binding site and hinge regions E52 and E270–279 have been shown to result in loss of virulence. After entering the body through a mosquito bite, the virus resides and multiplies within host leukocytes (probably T lymphocytes), which act as carriers to the central nervous system (CNS). JEV virions bind to the endothelial surface of the CNS vessels and are internalized by endocytosis (Mathur et al. 1989); however, it is still not clear whether macrophages and B lymphocytes can also harbour JEV. In other flaviviral infections, such as West Nile virus, macrophages could serve as a reservoir, spreading the virus from the peripheral areas to the CNS (Rios et al. 2006). Damage in flaviviral encephalitis appears to result from both direct virally mediated damage and host inflammatory response. Uncontrolled overactivation of microglia occurs (Ghoshal et al. 2007), which releases proinflammatory cytokines such as interleukin 6 (IL-6), tumour necrosis factor alpha (TNFα), monocyte chemotactic protein 1 (MCP1) and RANTES (regulated upon activation, normal T cell expressed and secreted), promoting massive leukocyte migration and infiltration into the brain (Chen et al. 2004). The production of interferon-c-inducible protein 10 (IP-10) by activated astrocytes also contributes to the infiltration of natural killer cells and monocytes, among others (Bhowmick et al. 2007). Recently, attention has focused on the role of apoptosis in the pathogenesis of arboviral encephalitis. Apoptosis has been shown in vitro in different cell lines for various arboviruses. T lymphocytes and immunoglobulin M (IgM) play a major role in the recovery and clearance of the virus after infection (Liao et al. 1997).

Pathology

The brain bears the brunt of the disease, although changes also occur in the lungs, myocardium and reticuloendothelial system. The brain shows swelling, and intense congestion of the grey matter with confluent areas of haemorrhage. The thalamus and hippocampus are particularly involved (Sips et al. 2012). A characteristic but not pathognomonic finding is focal, punched-out areas of necrosis observed exclusively in the grey matter. Microscopically there is meningeal and perivascular mononuclear infiltration. The cerebral cortex shows diffuse microglial infiltration with circumvascular necrolytic zones in the grey matter that show total loss of neurons. White matter is fairly well preserved (Shankar et al. 1983).

Clinical features

Infection with JEV can be asymptomatic, or present with an acute undifferentiated febrile illness, an aseptic meningitis-like illness or an encephalitis-like illness (Solomon 2003). The last of these has been the most studied. The course of the illness can be divided into a prodromal stage, an acute encephalitic stage and a convalescent stage. After an incubation period of 5–15 days the disease starts abruptly with high-grade fever. Headache, vomiting and diarrhoea may occur. Typically, this is followed in a matter of hours to a few days by seizures, usually generalized tonic spasms, following which the child lapses into coma. In severe cases, hyperventilation, signs of raised intracranial pressure, shock and death may occur in quick succession. Gastric haemorrhage is a common acute or terminal manifestation in seriously ill children. About a third of children succumb during the acute stage of the infection, a third recover quickly within the next few days, and the remaining third have a prolonged convalescence. During this period, pronounced extrapyramidal signs and focal deficits may become apparent. Focal deficits may be in the form of hemiplegia, monoplegia or even triplegia without corresponding lesions seen on imaging. Severe dystonia and abnormal movements may occur, the latter gradually improving over a period of weeks to a few months (Kumar et al. 2006). Two clinical signs – hyperventilation and extrapyramidal features – were significantly and independently associated with a diagnosis of Japanese encephalitis (Kumar et al. 1994) and help differentiate it from other viral encephalitides. It is now well recognized that Japanese encephalitis can involve spinal-cord anterior horn cells and occasionally present with polio-like lower motor neuron weakness (Kumar et al. 1991, Solomon et al. 1998).

CSF examination may be normal or may show mild to moderate pleocytosis with elevated protein but normal sugar. The CSF was normal in half the children described from Lucknow seen during the 2005 epidemic. In the remainder there was mild pleocytosis with a maximum cell count of 300/mm^3 and only 12.3% of patients having counts beyond 100/mm^3 (Kumar et al. 2006).

Neuroimaging in Japanese encephalitis reveals changes in the basal ganglia, thalamus and brainstem. A study comparing cranial computerized tomography (CCT) with magnetic resonance imaging (MRI) found that 21 of 38 patients showed abnormalities on CCT compared to all on MRI (Kumar et al. 1997).

Electrophysiological studies revealed abnormalities on electroencephalogram in 80%, mostly in the form of non-specific theta or delta slowing, with alpha coma and epileptiform discharges in a small proportion each. Motor evoked potentials were abnormal in 70% and correlated with weakness and 3-month outcome. Electromyograms and somatosensory evoked potentials also revealed abnormalities in a few patients (Kalita and Misra 2002).

Laboratory diagnosis

Viral isolation by intracerebral inoculation in infant mice followed by identification and haemagglutination inhibition test in paired sera were commonly used for diagnosis until the 1990s. Other serological tests included the neutralization test, agar gel diffusion test, single radial haemolysis and complement fixation test. There is considerable cross-reactivity between flaviviruses, because of which these tests should be performed in parallel with other circulating flaviviruses (Medappa 1980). However, the mainstay for diagnosis now is the IgM-capture, enzyme-linked immunosorbent assay (ELISA) test in cerebrospinal fluid (CSF) or serum. Sensitivity as well as specificity of the test is higher in CSF, making it the preferred sample. After about 10 days from onset of illness, detection of IgM in CSF or serum reaches about 95%. A negative test especially in serum very early in the illness should therefore be repeated after an interval of 10 days if the diagnostic suspicion is strong (WHO 2007, CDC 2012). Three kits are available commercially – the Excyton kit developed by the National Institute of Mental Health and Neurosciences (NIMHANS), India; the Inbios kit (USA); and a combination kit for dengue and Japanese encephalitis marketed by Panbio, Australia. A comparative study of these kits revealed that the sensitivity of all three was comparable but the Panbio kit had the highest specificity. Specificity of the Excyton kit was higher if dengue was excluded or only encephalitis cases were tested (Jacobson et al. 2007). Another kit has been developed by the National Institute of Virology, Pune, India.

More recently, polymerase chain reaction techniques are being used in the diagnosis of

Japanese encephalitis. The test is likely to be positive in the early stages of the infection when serology may be noncontributory. However, it is not very sensitive as viral genome may be undetectable in clinically ill Japanese encephalitis patients. Therefore a negative result should not be used to rule out Japanese encephalitis (WHO 2007).

Treatment

To date, treatment of Japanese encephalitis is essentially supportive. Anticonvulsants, antipyretics, intravenous fluids, measures to lower intracranial pressure, and nursing care of the comatose patient should be provided. Intravenous antibiotics are usually given to seriously ill patients and in cases where doubt exists about bacterial meningitis. Critically ill patients are managed in intensive care settings and may require respiratory and haemodynamic support. Randomized controlled trials with antivirals, α-interferon (Solomon et al. 2003) and ribavirin (Kumar et al. 2009a) did not yield benefit. Minocycline, a tetracycline drug with neuroprotective properties, has recently been shown to be effective against the virus in an animal model (Mishra and Basu 2006).

Sequelae

Clinical sequelae are seen in the majority of survivors. A study on 55 laboratory-proven childhood cases showed major sequelae such as intellectual disability and motor deficits in 45.5%. Academic difficulties, subtle neurological signs or behavioural abnormalities were found in another 25%, and only 29% were completely normal (Kumar et al. 1993).

Prevention

The WHO has developed a Japanese encephalitis laboratory network that provides training workshops, technical support, proficiency testing and confirmatory testing for 18 countries (CDC 2013). The case definition, laboratory criteria for confirmation and recommendations for surveillance by the WHO are shown in Tables 9.1–9.3. Measures for prevention of the infection include better water management in rural areas, control of mosquitoes, control of pig populations in proximity to humans, and vaccination. Of these, vaccination remains the most effective short-term strategy, the remaining measures being related to poverty, lack of development and lifestyle. It must be borne in mind that vaccination of humans does not interrupt Japanese encephalitis transmission in nature. The reservoir of infection remains, and individuals who are not vaccinated remain susceptible to the disease.

The earliest vaccine to be marketed against JEV was the inactivated mouse-brain-derived vaccine originally produced by BIKEN, Japan, and marketed in the USA as JE-VAX®. Since the vaccine is derived from neural tissue, a risk of neurological events (acute disseminated encephalomyelitis) does exist. An apparently new pattern of adverse reactions has been reported since 1989, mostly among travellers vaccinated in Australia, Europe and North America. These include urticaria, angio-oedema, respiratory distress and collapse due to hypotension. Rates for these reactions have varied from 0.7/1000 to 104/1000. These safety concerns led to suspension of vaccine production in most countries including Japan, USA and India.

TABLE 9.1
World Health Organization case definition and classification[a]

Clinical case definition

Clinically, a case of acute encephalitis syndrome (AES) is defined as a person of any age, at any time of year with acute onset of fever and at least one of: (1) change in mental status (including symptoms such as confusion, disorientation, coma, or inability to talk); (2) new onset of seizures (excluding simple febrile seizures). Other early clinical findings may include irritability, somnolence or abnormal behaviour greater than that seen with usual febrile illness.

Case classification

AES (suspected Japanese encephalitis) case: a case that meets the clinical case definition of AES. AES cases should be classified in one of the following four ways.

1   Laboratory-confirmed Japanese encephalitis. An AES case that has been laboratory confirmed as Japanese encephalitis.

2   Probable Japanese encephalitis. An AES case that occurs in close geographical and temporal relationship to a laboratory-confirmed case of Japanese encephalitis, in the context of an outbreak.

3   AES – other agent. An AES case in which diagnostic testing is performed and an aetiological agent other than Japanese encephalitis virus is identified.

4   AES – unknown. An AES case in which no diagnostic testing is performed or in which testing was performed but no aetiological agent was identified or in which test results were indeterminate.

[a]PATH (2006).

Another commonly used JEV vaccine is the live attenuated vaccine (SA 14-14-2 strain) produced in China by Chengdu Biologicals in partnership with global health organization PATH. This vaccine has been used in the public sector in China since 1998, Nepal since 1999 and India since 2006. Efficacy in a Nepalese study was 99.3% in the same year, 98.5% after 1 year and 96.2% after 5 years. Another Indian study found vaccine efficacy to be 94.5% after 6 months (Kumar et al. 2009b). The safety profile has been good, with only 5%–10% of recipients developing transient fever, and no more than 1%–3% showing local reactions, rash or irritability. It has recently been approved by WHO (PATH 2013).

The cell-culture-derived, inactivated JEV vaccine based on the Beijing P-3 strain is another vaccine in wide use in China. Primary immunization of infants with this formalin-inactivated vaccine results in about 76%–95% protection, but immunity wanes relatively rapidly, leading to requirement of booster doses (Solomon 2010).

The IC51 vaccine (marketed as Ixiaro® by Intercell/Novartis) is a new-generation formalin-inactivated vaccine prepared from the SA 14-14-2 strain grown in Vero cells. Adverse events brought to medical attention were 12.7% versus 12.2% in the vaccine and placebo groups respectively. Serious adverse events occurred in 0.5% for IC51 versus 0.9% for placebo. No serious allergic or neurological events were reported (FDA 2013). However, going by the experience with the mouse brain, killed vaccine, rare events may not be detectable by the numbers treated so far with IC51. This JEV vaccine received US Food and

TABLE 9.2
World Health Organization laboratory criteria for confirmation[a]

Clinical signs of Japanese encephalitis are indistinguishable from other causes of AES. Laboratory confirmation is therefore essential for accurate diagnosis of Japanese encephalitis. Detection of IgM antibody by capture enzyme-linked immunosorbent assay (ELISA) in cerebrospinal fluid (CSF) or serum reaches ≥95% sensitivity 10 days after onset of first symptoms.

The recommended method for laboratory confirmation of a Japanese encephalitis virus (JEV) infection is:

1 The presence of JEV-specific IgM antibody in a single sample of CSF or serum as detected by an IgM-capture ELISA specifically for JEV. However, further confirmatory tests (e.g. looking for cross-reactivity with other flaviviruses circulating in the geographical area) should be carried out when (a) there is an ongoing dengue or other flavivirus outbreak, (b) when vaccination coverage is very high, or (c) in cases or areas with no epidemiological or entomological data supportive of JEV transmission; *or*

2 Detection of JEV antigens in brain tissue by immunohistochemistry or immunofluorescence assay; *or*

3 Detection of JEV genome in CSF, serum, plasma, blood or brain tissue by reverse transcriptase polymerase chain reaction or an equally sensitive and specific nucleic acid amplification test; or

4 Isolation of JEV in CSF, serum, plasma, blood or brain tissue; *or*

5 Detection of a four-fold or greater rise in JEV-specific antibody as measured by haemagglutination inhibition test or plaque reduction neutralization assay in serum collected during the acute and convalescent phase of illness. The two specimens for IgG should be collected at least 14 days apart. These should be performed in parallel with other flaviviruses.

It may be noted that detection of virus genome or virus isolation in serum, plasma or blood is very specific for Japanese encephalitis diagnosis; however it is not sensitive as virus levels are usually undetectable in clinically ill Japanese encephalitis patients. Therefore a negative result by these tests should not be used to rule out Japanese encephalitis in a suspected case. Similarly, virus genome or virus in CSF is usually found only in fatal cases and is therefore not a very sensitive method and should not be used to rule out a diagnosis of Japanese encephalitis.

[a]PATH (2006).

Drug Administration (FDA) approval for use in adults 17 years of age or older in 2009 (FDA 2013) and has also been approved in Europe and Australia. Provisionally, the US Advisory Committee on Immunization Practices advises JEV vaccine for travellers if they plan to stay in an endemic area for at least a month or to visit rural areas. However, with availability of the new-generation vaccine these recommendations may be revised. This vaccine produced with Austrian collaboration is available in India as Jeev® (Biological E Ltd).

Another Vero-cell-derived purified inactivated JEV vaccine, Jenvac®, has received manu-facturing and marketing approval from the Drug Controller General of India. The virus strain (821564 XZ) used in this vaccine was isolated in Kolar, Karnataka, during the early 1980s and characterized by the National Institute of Virology at Pune. It is expected to meet the need for quick augmentation of immunity during an epidemic (Dhar 2013).

Other candidate JEV vaccines being developed include the live attenuated YFV-

TABLE 9.3
World Health Organization recommendations for Japanese encephalitis surveillance[a]

Japanese encephalitis surveillance should be conducted year round. When feasible, surveillance should be performed within the context of integrated disease surveillance and linked with similar surveillance activities such as those for acute flaccid paralysis or meningitis. Two types of surveillance are recommended:

1 In all Asian countries:

Comprehensive syndromic surveillance for acute encephalitis syndrome with aggregate reporting is recommended. In sentinel hospitals, surveillance should be case based with specimens collected for laboratory confirmation. The number of sentinel hospitals should be gradually increased if feasible.

2 In Asian countries where a high level of Japanese encephalitis control has been achieved:

Surveillance should be case based throughout the country and include laboratory confirmation of all suspect cases.

[a]PATH (2006).

17D/JEV vaccine (Acambis). A chimeric yellow fever/Japanese encephalitis virus was constructed by insertion of the premembrane and envelope (prME) genes of an attenuated human vaccine strain (SA 14-14-2) of JEV between core and nonstructural genes of a YFV-17D infectious clone. Phase 2 trials have shown a seroconversion rate of 94% following a single shot. Recruitment for phase 3 studies is ongoing in Thailand (Monath et al. 2003).

REFERENCES

ARMCANZ (1998) Australian Veterinary Emergency Plan AUSVETPLAN 1998. Disease Strategy: Japanese Encephalitis. Agriculture and Resources Management Council of Australia and New Zealand (online: http://www.animalhealthaustralia.com.au/wp-content/uploads/2011/04/jedfinal.pdf).

Bhowmick S, Duseja R, Das S, et al. (2007) Induction of IP-10 (CXCL10) in astrocytes following Japanese encephalitis. *Neurosci Lett* 414: 45–50.

Campbell GL, Hills SL, Fischer M, et al. (2011) Estimated global incidence of Japanese encephalitis: a systematic review. *Bull World Health Organ* 89: 766E–774E.

CDC (2012) Japanese encephalitis. Diagnostic testing (online: http://www.cdc.gov/japaneseencephalitis/healthCareProviders/healthCareProviders-Diagnostic.html).

CDC (2013) Japanese encephalitis surveillance and immunization – Asia and the Western Pacific, 2012. *MMWR Morb Mortal Wkly Rep* 62: 658–62.

Chen CJ, Chen JH, Chen SY, et al. (2004) Upregulation of RANTES gene expression in neuroglia by Japanese encephalitis virus infection. *J Virol* 78: 12107–19.

Dhar A (2013) India launches vaccine to prevent Japanese encephalitis. *The Hindu*, October 4, 2013 (online: http://www.thehindu.com/news/national/india-launches-vaccine-to-prevent-japanese-encephalitis/article5201813.ece).

FDA (2013) Intercell AG IXIARO – highlights of prescribing information (online: http://www.fda.gov/downloads/BiologicsBloodVaccines/Vaccines/ApprovedProducts/UCM142569.pdf).

Gao X, Liu H, Wang H, et al. (2013) Southernmost Asia is the source of Japanese encephalitis virus (genotype 1) diversity from which the viruses disperse and evolve throughout Asia. *PLoS Negl Trop Dis* 7: e2459. doi: 10.1371/journal.pntd.0002459.

Ghosh D, Basu A (2009) Japanese encephalitis: a pathological and clinical perspective. *PLOS Negl Trop Dis J* 3: e437. doi:10.1371/journal.pntd.0000437.

Ghoshal A, Das S, Ghosh S, et al. (2007) Proinflammatory mediators released by activated microglia induces neuronal death in Japanese encephalitis. *Glia* 55: 483–96.

Halstead SB (2004) Arboviral encephalitis outside North America. In: Behrman RE, Kleigman RM, Jenson HB, eds. *Nelson Textbook of Pediatrics, 17th edn.* New Delhi: Elsevier, pp. 1089–91.

Hanna J, Ritchie S, Phillips D, et al. (1999) Japanese encephalitis in north Queensland, Australia, 1998. *Med J Aust* 170: 533–6.

Jacobson JA, Hills SL, Winkler JL, et al. (2007) Evaluation of three immunoglobulin M antibody capture enzyme-linked immunosorbent assays for diagnosis of Japanese encephalitis. *Am J Trop Med Hyg* 77: 164–8.

Kalita J, Misra UK (2002) Neurophysiological changes in Japanese encephalitis. *Neurol India* 50: 262–6.

Kumar R, Agarwal SP, Wakhlu I, Mishra KL (1991) Japanese encephalitis—an encephalomyelitis. *Indian Pediatr* 28: 1525–8.

Kumar R, Mathur A, Singh KB, et al. (1993) Clinical sequelae of Japanese encephalitis in children. *Indian J Med Res* 97: 9–13.

Kumar R, Senthilselvan A, Mathur A, et al. (1994) Clinical predictors of Japanese encephalitis. *Neuro-epidemiology* 13: 97–102.

Kumar R, Tripathi P, Singh S, Banerji G (2006) Clinical features in children hospitalized during the 2005 epidemic of Japanese encephalitis in Uttar Pradesh, India. *Clinical Infect Dis* 43: 123–31.

Kumar R, Tripathi P, Barawal M, et al. (2009a) Randomised controlled trial of oral ribavirin in children with Japanese encephalitis in Uttar Pradesh, India. *Clin Infect Dis* 48: 400–6.

Kumar R, Tripathi P, Rizvi A (2009b) Effectiveness of one dose of live-attenuated SA 14-14-2 vaccine against Japanese encephalitis. *N Engl J Med* 360: 1465–6 (letter).

Kumar S, Misra UK, Kalita J, et al. (1997) MRI in Japanese encephalitis. *Am J Med Sci* 39: 180–4.

Liao CL, Lin YL, Wang JJ, et al. (1997) Effect of enforced expression of human bcl-2 on Japanese encephalitis virus-induced apoptosis in cultured cells. *J Virol* 71: 5963–71.

Mathur A, Kulshreshtha R, Chaturvedi UC (1989) Evidence for latency of Japanese encephalitis virus in T lymphocytes. *J Gen Virol* 70: 461–5.

Medappa N (1980) Japanese encephalitis in India. *ICMR Bulletin* 10: 29–38.

Mishra MK, Basu A (2006) Minocycline neuroprotects, reduces microglial activation, inhibits caspase 3 reduction and viral replication following Japanese encephalitis. *J Neurochem* 105: 1582–95.

Monath TP (1988) Japanese encephalitis – a plague of the orient. *N Engl J Med* 319: 641–3.

Monath TP, Guirakhoo F, Nichols R, et al. (2003) Chimeric live, attenuated vaccine against Japanese encephalitis (ChimeriVax-JE): phase 2 clinical trials for safety and immunogenicity, effect of vaccine dose and schedule, and memory response to challenge with inactivated Japanese encephalitis antigen. *J Infect Dis* 188: 1213–30 (online: http://jid.oxfordjournals.org/content/188/8/1213.long).

PATH (2006) Japanese encephalitis surveillance standards (online: http://www.path.org/files/WHO_surveillance_standards_JE.pdf).

PATH (2009) Japanese encephalitis morbidity, mortality and disability. Reduction and control by 2015 (online: http://www.path.org/vaccineresources/files/JE_Reduction_and_Control_by_2015.pdf).

PATH (2013) SA 14-14-2 Live Japanese encephalitis (JE) vaccine (online: http://www.path.org/publications/files/SA14142-fact-sheet-1013.pdf).

Rios M, Zhang MJ, Grinev A, et al. (2006) Monocytes macrophages are a potential target in human infection with West Nile virus through blood transfusion. *Transfusion* 46: 659–67.

Shankar SK, Vasudev Rao T, Mruthyunjayanna BP, et al. (1983) Autopsy study of brain during the epidemic of Japanese encephalitis in Karnataka. *Indian J Med Res* 78: 431–40.

Sips GJ, Wilschut J, Smit JM (2012) Neuroinvasive flavivirus infections. *Rev Med Virol* 22: 69–87.

Solomon T (2003) Recent advances in Japanese encephalitis. *J Neurovirol* 9: 274–83.

Solomon T (2010) Japanese encephalitis vaccine. In: Zuckerman JN, Jong EC, eds. *Travelers' Vaccines, 2nd edn.* Shelton, CT: People's Medical Publishing, pp. 229–76 (online: http://www.liv.ac.uk/media/livacuk/infectionandglobalhealth/docs/vaccines-against.pdf).

Solomon T, Kneen R, Dung NM, et al. (1998) Poliomyelitis-like illness due to Japanese encephalitis virus. *Lancet* 351: 1094–7.

Solomon T, Dung NM, Wills B, et al. (2003) Interferon alfa-2a in Japanese encephalitis: a randomized double-blind placebo-controlled trial. *Lancet* 361: 821–6.

Tirounourougane SV, Raghava P, Srinivasan S (2002) Japanese viral encephalitis. *Postgrad Med J* 78: 205–15.

Tsai TF (2000) New initiatives for the control of Japanese encephalitis by vaccination: minutes of a WHO/CVI meeting, Bangkok, Thailand, 13–15 October 1998. *Vaccine* 18 Suppl 2: 1–25.

WHO (2007) *World Health Organization Manual for the Laboratory Diagnosis of Japanese Encephalitis Virus Infection.* Geneva: World Health Organization (online: http://www.who.int/immunization/monitoring_surveillance/burden/laboratory/Manual_lab_diagnosis_JE.pdf).

10
RABIES

Chandra Kanta and Rashmi Kumar

Rabies, a form of fatal, acute viral encephalomyelitis, is a zoonotic disease that is transmitted to humans from animals through infected saliva. The disease is endemic in 87 countries but about 95% of human deaths occur in Asia and Africa. Globally, more than 55 000 people die of rabies each year and more than 15 million people require post-exposure immunization (WHO 2010). Rabies-free countries and territories include both resource-rich (e.g. Japan, New Zealand) and resource-poor island countries (e.g. Barbados, Fiji, Maldives, Seychelles), and parts of northern and southern mainland Europe (e.g. Greece, Portugal, Sweden, Norway) and Latin America (e.g. Uruguay and Chile) (CDC 2013). A rabies-free area is defined as one in which no case of indigenously acquired rabies has occurred in man or any animal species for 2 years (WHO 1998).

Epidemiology

All warm-blooded mammals including humans are susceptible to rabies virus infection, but only a few species are important as reservoirs for the disease. Rabies is described in the following forms.

1 *Urban rabies.* Dogs continue to be the main carrier of rabies in Africa and Asia and are responsible for most of the human rabies deaths worldwide.
2 *Wildlife rabies.* In resource-rich countries rabies continues mainly in wild animals such as the jackal, fox, hyena, raccoon, skunk, coyote and mongoose.
3 *Bat rabies.* In the past few years, bat rabies has emerged as a public health problem in the Americas (Brazil, Venezuela, Mexico, USA, Trinidad and Tobago) and Europe (Germany, Denmark, Holland). The virus can be transmitted through these bats by either bite or aerosol. Bats provide a constant source of infection for wild animals and humans, and help the virus persist in nature (CDC 2011).

Over the last 100 years, the epidemiology of rabies in the developed world has changed dramatically. With use of modern-day prophylaxis, human fatalities have declined to one or two per year, occurring in people who fail to seek medical assistance. Before 1960 the majority of animal rabies cases occurred in domestic animals, whereas now more than 90% of all animal cases in the USA are in wildlife – mainly wild carnivores and bats (CDC 2011).

In resource-poor countries, most human deaths follow a bite from an infected dog. Dog rabies is responsible for more than 14 million courses of post-exposure treatment and this poses a great economic burden. In Asia, the average cost of rabies immunization after a suspicious animal bite is US$49. The estimated annual cost of rabies is US$583.5 million, most of which is borne by Asian and African countries, where it is responsible for 1.74 million disability-adjusted life-years lost annually (WHO 2004).

India is a high-incidence country and all states are endemic for rabies except for Lakshadweep, Andaman and Nicobar Islands (Sehgal and Bhatia 1985). Rabies is not a notifiable disease there, but 30 000 deaths are estimated to occur annually due to this infection. About 1–1.5 million individuals receive post-exposure vaccination annually. Dog bites are responsible for 99% of cases. There are an estimated 2.5 million dogs in the country, mostly unvaccinated.

The virus

Rabies virus is an RNA virus belonging to the family *Rhabdoviridae* of the genus Lyssavirus. The rhabdoviruses have a distinct 'bullet' shape and are approximately 180nm long and 75nm wide. The rabies genome encodes five proteins: nucleoprotein (N), phosphoprotein (P), matrix protein (M), glycoprotein (G) and polymerase (L). The glycoprotein forms approximately 400 trimeric spikes, which are tightly arranged on the surface of the virus. It is the only antigen capable of inducing the formation of neutralizing antibodies (WHO 1973). The presence of neutralizing antibodies in the blood of humans or animals is considered an index of protection against the rabies virus (Campbell et al. 1968).

Rabies virus is excreted in the saliva of all affected animals. The virus recovered from naturally occurring cases of rabies is called the 'street virus'. This is infectious for all mammals with a variable incubation period of 20–60 days in dogs. Serial brain-to-brain passage of the virus in rabbits modifies the virus such that its incubation period is progressively reduced until it becomes constant at 4–6 days. Virus isolated at this stage is called the 'fixed virus'. It does not form Negri bodies, does not multiply in extraneural tissues, and is used in vaccine production (WHO 1973).

MODES OF TRANSMISSION

The rabies virus may be transmitted (1) through animal bites, most commonly dog bites but also from other animals such as monkeys, cats, horses, sheep, goats, etc.; (2) licks on abraded skin; (3) aerosol infection in caves infested with infected bats, or among laboratory personnel; (4) rarely, person-to-person transmission following human bite and corneal and organ transplantation (Park 2011).

SOURCE OF INFECTION

The source of infection is the saliva of rabid animals. The saliva becomes infectious up to 5–6 days before onset of illness and remains so until death. However, even in rabid animals, not all saliva is infectious. The amount of virus in saliva is variable, and only about half the bites by proven rabid animals cause rabies (Park 2011).

CARRIER STATE

Serological surveys have shown that a small proportion of unvaccinated animals have antirabies antibodies. There are also reports of dogs living for years with rabies virus being repeatedly isolable from their saliva (Park 2011).

Pathogenesis

The fusion of the rabies virus envelope to the host cell membrane (adsorption) initiates the infectious process. After adsorption, the virus penetrates the host cell and enters the cytoplasm by pinocytosis, aggregating in large endosomes (cytoplasmic vesicles). The uptake of virus into peripheral nerves is important for progressive infection to occur. Rabies virus is then transported to the central nervous system (CNS) via retrograde axoplasmic flow through sensory and motor nerves, and rapidly disseminates within the CNS. The limbic system is involved early, and the classic behavioural changes associated with rabies develop during this period of cerebral infection. Active cerebral infection is followed by passive centrifugal spread of virus to peripheral nerves, which may lead to the invasion of highly innervated sites including salivary glands (CDC 2013b).

Pathology

Rabies infection typically produces encephalitis and myelitis. Perivascular infiltration with lymphocytes, neutrophils and plasma cells can occur throughout the CNS. Cytoplasmic eosinophilic inclusion bodies (Negri bodies) in neuronal cells, especially in pyramidal cells of the hippocampus and Purkinje cells of the cerebellum, are identified (CDC 2013b).

Incubation period

The incubation period can vary from as little as 4 days to several years but is commonly between 3 and 8 weeks. In no other communicable disease is the incubation period so variable and dependent on so many factors. It depends on site and severity of bite, number of wounds, amount of virus injected and species of the biting animal, protection afforded by clothing, and treatment undertaken. In general, it is shorter in severe bites on the upper limbs, head and neck, and in bites by wild animals (Park 2011).

Clinical features

Rabies in Dogs

Again the incubation period is variable – from as short as 10 days to more than 1 year. Once symptoms of the disease develop, rabies is rapidly fatal. In dogs the disease may manifest in two forms:

• *Furious rabies.* This is the typical 'mad dog' illness. There is a change in the behaviour of the animal, which becomes very aggressive, biting people and other animals without provocation, and biting at unusual objects like sticks, straw and mud. The animal may run amok, i.e. run away from home and wander aimlessly, biting people who pass by. There may be a change in the voice because of paralysis of laryngeal muscles, excessive salivation, and finally a paralytic stage just before death.

• *Paralytic rabies.* In this type of illness, the irritable phase is lacking. The disease is predominantly paralytic. When paralysis spreads to all parts of body, the animal becomes depressed, rapidly enters a coma and dies (Eng and Fishbein 1990).

RABIES IN HUMANS

Between 30% and 60% of victims are children under the age of 15 years who often play with animals and are less likely to report bites or scratches (WHO 2011). The first symptoms of rabies are flu-like, including fever, headache, sore throat and fatigue. About 80% of patients complain of pain or tingling at the site of the bite – the only prodromal symptom to be considered specific. This phase is followed by widespread excitation of the nervous system, involving sensory, motor, sympathetic and mental functions. The patient is intolerant to noise, bright light or draught of air (aerophobia). Attempts to swallow liquid induce spasm of pharyngeal muscles (hydrophobia). Examination may reveal increased reflexes and muscle spasms, along with dilated pupils, perspiration, lacrimation and salivation (sympathetic). Mental changes include fear of death, anger, irritability and depression. The patient may pass into a stage of coma or paralysis, or convulse. Without intensive care, death occurs within 7–10 days (WHO 2011). Paralytic rabies accounts for about 30% of the total number of human cases. It has a less dramatic and usually longer course than the furious form. The muscles gradually become paralysed, starting at the site of the bite or scratch. Later, coma develops, and eventually death occurs. The paralytic form of rabies is often misdiagnosed, contributing to the under-reporting of the disease (WHO 2013).

The differential diagnosis of rabies includes viral encephalitis, tetanus, poliomyelitis, Guillain–Barré syndrome, poisonings and drugs.

Table 10.1 gives the clinical case definition, case classification, and classification of exposure to rabies according to the World Health Organization (WHO 2011).

Laboratory diagnosis

IN ANIMALS

The direct fluorescent antibody test is the most frequently used diagnostic test for rabies. It can be performed in the brain tissue from suspect dead animals or even in corneal impressions or skin biopsies of live animals. Results are available within a few hours. Fluorescent-labelled anti-rabies antibody directed against the nucleoprotein antigen of the virus is incubated with rabies-suspect brain tissue and binds to rabies antigen. Unbound antibody is washed away, and areas where antigen is present can be visualized using a fluorescence microscope. If rabies virus is absent there will be no staining. The test is as accurate as virus isolation by animal inoculation. A negative result indicates that the bitten person need not be treated (CDC 2013a).

Histological findings of biopsy or autopsy tissues include (1) mononuclear infiltration, (2) perivascular cuffing of lymphocytes or polymorphonuclear cells, (3) lymphocytic foci, (4) Babès nodules consisting of glial cells, (5) Negri bodies, round or oval inclusions within the cytoplasm of neurons, most frequently located in the pyramidal cells of Ammon's horn,

TABLE 10.1
World Health Organization clinical case definition and classification of rabies and rabies exposure[a]

Clinical case definition

A person presenting with acute neurological syndrome (encephalitis) dominated by forms of hyperactivity (furious rabies) or paralytic syndromes (paralytic rabies) progressing towards coma and death, usually by respiratory failure within 7–10 days after the first symptom if no intensive care is instituted.

Case classification

1 Suspected: a case compatible with the clinical case definition
2 Probable: a suspected case plus history of contact with a suspected rabid animal
3 Confirmed: a suspected case that is laboratory confirmed

Classification of rabies exposure

1 Possible exposure: a person who had close contact (usually a bite or scratch) with a rabies-susceptible animal in (or originating from) a rabies-infected area
2 Probable exposure: a person who had close contact (usually a bite or scratch) with an animal displaying clinical signs consistent with rabies at the time of exposure, or within 10 days following exposure in a rabies-infected area
3 Exposed: a person who had close contact (usually a bite or scratch) with a laboratory-confirmed rabid animal

[a]WHO (2011).

the Purkinje cells of the cerebellum, the cells of the medulla and various other ganglia. The presence of Negri bodies is variable and may be found in about 50% of clinically rabid animals.

Intracerebral mouse inoculation is still a useful test. A 10% emulsion of suspected brain tissue is prepared in normal saline and centrifuged at 2000rpm for 5–10 minutes; 0.03mL of the supernatant is inoculated intracerebrally in at least four suckling mice using a tuberculin syringe. If infected, they show signs of rabies within 6–8 days. The infection can be further identified by the fluorescent antibody test or histopathology for Negri bodies.

IN HUMANS (Table 10.2)
Several tests are necessary to diagnose rabies ante mortem (before death) in humans, and no single test is sufficient. Tests are performed on samples of saliva, serum, spinal fluid, and skin biopsies of hair follicles at the nape of the neck. Saliva can be tested by virus isolation or reverse transcription followed by amplification. Serum and spinal fluid are tested for antibodies to rabies virus, which form by the 8th day. Skin biopsy specimens are examined for rabies antigen in the cutaneous nerves at the base of hair follicles. Immunohistochemical procedures are more sensitive than histological staining methods (WHO 2011).

Prevention of human rabies
Appropriate wound management, modern cell-culture vaccines and rabies immunoglobulins

TABLE 10.2
World Health Organization laboratory criteria for rabies[a]

One or more of the following:

• Detection of rabies viral antigen by FAT or ELISA in clinical specimen collected post mortem

• Detection by FAT on skin biopsy (ante mortem)

• FAT positive after inoculation of brain tissue, saliva or CSF in cell culture, or after intracerebral inoculation in mice

• Detectable rabies-neutralizing antibody titre in CSF or serum of an unvaccinated person

• Detection of viral nucleic acid by PCR on tissue collected post mortem or intra vitam in a clinical specimen (brain tissue or skin, cornea, urine or saliva)

[a]WHO (2011). FAT, fluorescent antibody test; ELISA, enzyme-linked immunosorbent assay; CSF, cerebrospinal fluid; PCR, polymerase chain reaction.

as soon as possible after suspect contact with an animal are almost 100% effective in preventing human rabies (Quiambao et al. 2005).

A significant contact with any warm-blooded animal should be treated as a medical emergency and post-exposure prophylaxis (PEP) initiated as soon as possible. Infancy, pregnancy and lactation are never contraindications for PEP. The animals include dog, cat, bat, cow, buffalo, sheep, goat, pig, donkey, horse, camel, fox, jackal, monkey, mongoose, bear and others. Post-exposure prophylaxis is not required if the biting animal is a small rodent or rabbit (Childs et al. 1997). Prophylaxis may be deferred if the biting animal is a pet, more than a year old, and has received proper vaccination against rabies. Whenever possible, the suspect animal should be tested for the virus. Post-exposure prophylaxis may be stopped if the animal is a dog or cat and remains healthy after 10 days (WHO 2010).

WOUND MANAGEMENT (Table 10.3)

Proper wound treatment is very effective in reducing rabies transmission (Wilde 2007). The first step in post-exposure care is thorough cleansing of the wound with soap and flushing under running water for 10 minutes, followed by irrigation with a virucidal agent such as 70% alcohol or povidone iodine as soon as possible after the bite. Antimicrobial therapy and tetanus vaccination should be given if indicated. Primary suturing of the wound should be avoided. Rabies immunoglobulin (RIG) must be infiltrated in the wound prior to suturing when suturing is unavoidable (Wilde 2007, Allan 2009).

RABIES IMMUNOGLOBULIN

RIG functions by neutralizing the rabies virus both locally and systemically during the first week after exposure. RIG is not indicated after 7 days and in individuals who have received pre- or post-exposure prophylaxis in the past.

Two types of RIGs are available: human (HRIG) and equine (ERIG). HRIG is preferred over ERIG because it has fewer side-effects, although it is more expensive and has limited availability (Helmick et al. 1982). Adverse effects of ERIG include anaphylactoid reaction

TABLE 10.3
World Health Organization categories of rabies exposure and management[a]

Category	Type of contact with a suspect or confirmed rabid domestic or wild animal, or animal unavailable for testing	Recommended treatment
I	Touching or feeding of animals, licks on intact skin	None if reliable case history is available
II	Nibbling of uncovered skin, minor scratches or abrasions without bleeding	Immediate vaccination and local treatment of the wound
III	Single or multiple transdermal bites or scratches, contamination of mucous membrane with saliva (i.e. licks), licks on broken skin or exposure to bats	Immediate vaccination and administration of rabies immunoglobulin; local treatment of the wound

[a]Adapted from WHO (2013).

and serum sickness-like reaction (Wilde et al. 1989). Skin testing before ERIG administration is not recommended (Cupo et al. 2001). With the use of purified ERIG, the adverse effects have been low (6%–8%).

ERIG (40 IU/kg) or HRIG (20 IU/kg) should be infiltrated around and into the wound(s), even if the lesion has begun to heal. If the volume of the calculated dose of ERIG/HRIG is insufficient, then it can be diluted with normal saline to permit thorough infiltration. Any remaining volume is injected intramuscularly at a site distant from vaccine administration. A recent study found monoclonal antibody cocktail against rabies virus instead of RIG to be safe and effective (Tesoro Cruz et al. 2008).

ANTIRABIES VACCINES
These are recommended for Category II and III exposures (Table 10.3).

Non-neural vaccines

• *Avian embryo vaccines.* Purified duck embryo vaccine (PDEV) was widely used before the cell-culture vaccines became available. This has less neuroparalytic effect but carries the risk of anaphylaxis and is poorly immunogenic compared to cell-culture vaccines (Shayam et al. 2006).

• *Primary cell-culture vaccines.* Cell-culture vaccines were first developed in 1964. Very few adverse effects have been reported with modern cell-culture vaccines.

1st generation vaccines:

— *Human diploid cell vaccine (HDCV)* is prepared from the Pitman Moore strain of rabies virus grown on MRC-5 human diploid cell-culture line. Then it is concentrated by ultrafiltration, and inactivated by BPL13. It may be administered by intramuscular or intra-dermal route. It is a potent and safe vaccine (Wiktor et al. 1978).

2nd generation vaccines:

— *Purified chick embryo cell vaccine (PCECV)* is prepared from fixed rabies virus strain FLURYLEP grown in primary cultures of chicken fibroblasts. It is cheaper and as effective as HDCV (Sehgal et al. 1995).
— *Purified Vero cell rabies vaccine (PVRV)* is prepared from the Wistar strain of virus grown in continuous Vero cell line. This is a potent vaccine but may contain potentially oncogenic substances. Such cell lines must be monitored for residual DNA (Wang et al. 2000).
— *Rabies vaccine adsorbed (RVA)* contains the Kissling strain of challenge virus standard rabies virus adapted to fetal rhesus lung diploid cell culture, BPL inactivated and concentrated by adsorption to aluminium phosphate. It is a liquid vaccine approved only for intramuscular use (Burgoyne et al. 1985).
— *Primary hamster kidney cell vaccine (PHKV)* is prepared with primary kidney cells of Syrian hamsters and used in China and Russia (Shayam et al. 2006).

Reported adverse effects of cell-culture vaccines include local pain, erythema, swelling, itching, headache, malaise, myalgia, local lymphadenopathy, allergic reactions, gastrointestinal symptoms and type III hypersensitivity reactions (Shayam et al. 2006).

Future vaccines
Recently, recombinant vaccine has been tried in humans and found to be safe and effective (Faber et al. 2009). DNA vaccines developed so far have shown good efficacy in animals but not in humans (Lodmell 1999).

VACCINATION SCHEDULE FOR NON-NEURAL VACCINES

Intramuscular schedule

• *Essen protocol.* Five doses of non-neural vaccine are given on days 0, 3, 7, 14 and 28. A booster dose on day 90 may be offered to immunocompromised or debilitated patients (WHO 2011). Vaccine should be given intramuscularly in the deltoid or anterolateral thigh but not in the gluteal region. The dose is 1mL IM at all ages for HDCV, PCECV and PDEV, and 0.5mL for PVRV.

• *Zagreb schedule.* Two IM doses on day 0, one IM dose each on days 7 and 21. An early antibody response is expected with this schedule (Park 2011).

Recently, the Centers for Disease Control and Prevention, USA, have revised the recommendations for the number of doses required for post-exposure prophylaxis in immunocompetent persons. Previously, the Advisory Committee on Immunization Practices recommended a five-dose rabies vaccination regimen with HDCV or PCECV. The new recommendations reduce the number of vaccine doses to four because the fifth dose did not further improve outcomes. The first dose of the four-dose course should be administered as soon as possible after exposure (day 0). Additional doses should then be administered on days 3, 7 and 14 (CDC 2013b).

Intradermal vaccination schedule
This is a cost-effective alternative to intramuscular vaccination, as the dose required is only 0.1mL. The WHO therefore recommends the use of cell-culture vaccines, except RVA, by this route. Intradermal route should not be used in immunocompromised patients or in those on chloroquine therapy.

• *Thai Red Cross regimen* (two-site intradermal regimen). Two intradermal doses of PVRV or PCECV in the deltoid on days 0, 3 and 7, and one dose on days 30 and 90.

• *Oxford regimen* (eight-site intradermal regimen). On day 0, eight intradermal doses of HDCV or PCECV (upper arms, lateral lower abdominal quadrants, thighs and suprascapular regions); day 7, four doses (each thighs and upper arm); days 30 and 90, one dose into upper arm.

  In both regimens less than two vials of vaccine is used per person (Lodmell 1999, WHO 2010, Park 2011).

POST-EXPOSURE TREATMENT OF PREVIOUSLY VACCINATED PERSONS
Passive immunization with RIG is not required when the person has received previous pre- or post-exposure prophylaxis. Antibody titre against rabies should be done. If it is above 0.5 IU/mL and the bite is not severe, only two doses of HDCV are needed, on days 0 and 3. In case of severe bite or in persons with unknown antibody titre, three doses of HDCV should be administered, on days 0, 3 and 7 (Park 2011).

PRE-EXPOSURE PROPHYLAXIS
Pre-exposure prophylaxis for rabies is recommended for travellers to endemic countries and for selected populations who are at risk of repeated exposure such as veterinarians, animal handlers, laboratory staff working with rabies virus and wildlife officers. Pre-exposure prophylaxis recommended by WHO consists of three doses of cell-culture vaccine given on days 0, 7 and 28. A booster dose is required every 2 years. Whenever feasible, 1 month after primary immunization a serum sample should be sent to test for virus-neutralizing antibodies. A booster dose needs to be administered if titres are less than 0.5 IU/mL (WHO 2010, Park 2011).

Prevention of rabies in animals

Animal rabies is prevented by vaccinating susceptible species. Primary immunization of dogs should be started at the age of 3–4 months followed by booster doses. Two types of vaccine are commonly used: BPL-inactivated neural vaccine and chick embryo vaccine. The dosage for BPL vaccine is 5mL for dogs and 3mL for cats. A booster dose is required after 6 months, and subsequently every year. The dosage for chick embryo vaccine is 3mL, and a booster needs to be administered after every 3 years (Park 2011).

Oral vaccination of wildlife with vaccine-containing bait offers hope of controlling the disease in susceptible wild animal populations. No suitable oral bait is available for use in dogs.

Public health measures to control rabies

Public health education regarding responsible pet ownership, routine veterinary care, avoiding contact with wildlife and professional continuing education are essential components of rabies prevention. Registration and licensing of domestic dogs, cats and ferrets should be done. Possible exposure to suspect animals should be reported. Mass vaccinations of dogs are financially justified by the future savings on discontinuing post-exposure preventive treatment for people. Stray and ownerless dogs need to be eliminated from public places.

REFERENCES

Allan K (2009) Grill approach to management of suspected rabies exposures, what primary care physicians need to know. *Can Fam Physician* 55: 247–51.
Burgoyne GH, Kajiya KD, Brown DW, Mitchell JR (1985) Rhesus diploid rabies vaccine (adsorbed): a new rabies vaccine using FRhL-2 cells. *J Infect Dis* 152: 204–10.
Campbell JB, Kaplan MM, Koprowski H, et al. (1968) Present trends and the future in rabies research. *Bull World Health Organ* 38: 373–81.
CDC (2013a) Protocol for postmortem diagnosis of rabies in animals by direct fluorescent antibody testing (online: http://www.cdc.gov/rabies/pdf/rabiesdfaspv2.pdf).
CDC (2013b) Rabies (online: http://www.cdc.gov/rabies/).
Childs JE, Colby L, Krebs JW, et al. (1997) Surveillance and spatiotemporal association of rabies in rodents and lagomorphs in the United States, 1985–1994. *J Wildl Dis* 33: 20–7.
Cupo P, Azevedo-Marques MM, Sarti W, Hering SE (2001) Proposal of abolition of the skin test before equine rabies immune globulin application. *Rev Med Trop Sao Paulo* 43: 51–3.
Eng TR, Fishbein DB (1990) Epidemiologic factors, clinical findings, and vaccination status of rabies in cats and dogs in the United States in 1988. National Study Group on Rabies. *J Am Vet Med Assoc* 197: 201–9.
Faber M, Li J, Kean RB, et al. (2009) Effective pre-exposure and post-exposure prophylaxis of rabies with a highly attenuated recombinant rabies virus. *Proc Natl Acad Sci U S A* 106: 11300–5.
Helmick CG, Johnstone C, Sumner J, et al. (1982) A clinical study of Mereux human rabies immune globulin. *J Biol Stand* 10: 357–67.
Lodmell DL (1999) Rabies DNA vaccines for protection and therapeutic treatment. *Expert Opin Investig Drugs* 8: 115–22.
Park K (2011) The epidemiology of communicable diseases – rabies. In: Park K, ed. *Park's Textbook of Preventive and Social Medicine, 21st edn.* Jabalpur: Banarsidas Bhanot, p. 205.
Quiambao BP, Dimaano EM, Ambas C, et al. (2005) Reducing the cost of post-exposure rabies prophylaxis: efficacy of 0.1 ml PCEC rabies vaccine administered intradermally using the Thai Red Cross post-exposure regimen in patients severely exposed to laboratory-confirmed rabid animals. *Vaccine* 23: 1709–14.
Sehgal H, Bhatia R (1985) *Rabies: Current Status and Proposed Control Programme in India.* Delhi: National Institute of Communicable Diseases.

Sehgal S, Bhattacharya D, Bhardwaj M (1995) Ten-year longitudinal study of efficacy and safety of purified chick embryo cell vaccine for pre- and post-exposure prophylaxis of rabies in Indian population. *J Commun Dis* 27: 36–43.

Shayam C, Duggal AK, Kamble U, Agarwal AK (2006) Post-exposure prophylaxis for rabies. *JIACM* 7: 39–46.

Tesoro Cruz E, Feria Romero IA, López Mendoza J, et al. (2008) First administration to humans of a monoclonal antibody cocktail against rabies virus: safety, tolerability, and neutralizing activity. *Vaccine* 26: 5922–7.

Wang XJ, Lang J, Tao XR, et al. (2000) Immunogenicity and safety of purified Vero-cell rabies vaccine in severely rabies exposed patients in China. *Southeast Asian J Trop Med Public Health* 31: 287–94.

WHO (1973) WHO Expert Committee on Rabies: sixth report. WHO Technical Report Series 523. Geneva: World Health Organization (online: http://whqlibdoc.who.int/trs/WHO_TRS_523.pdf).

WHO (1998) The World Health Report 1998. Life in the 21st century: a vision for all. Geneva: World Health Organization (online: http://www.who.int/whr/1998/en/).

WHO (2004) WHO Expert Consultation on Rabies: first report. WHO Technical Report Series 931. Geneva: World Health Organization (online: http://whqlibdoc.who.int/trs/WHO_TRS_931_eng.pdf).

WHO (2010) Rabies vaccines: WHO position paper. *Wkly Epidemiol Rec* 85: 309–20 (online: http://www.who.int/wer/2010/wer8532.pdf).

WHO (2011) Rabies. Excerpt from WHO recommended standards and strategies for surveillance, prevention and control of communicable diseases. Geneva: World Health Organization (online: http://www.who.int/rabies/epidemiology/rabiessurveillance.pdf).

WHO (2013) Rabies. Fact sheet no. 99. Updated July 2013. Geneva: World Health Organization (online: http://www.who.int/mediacentre/factsheets/fs099/en/).

Wiktor TJ, Plotkin SA, Koprowski H (1978) Development and clinical trials of the new human rabies vaccine of tissue culture (human diploid cell) origin. *Dev Biol Stand* 40: 3–9.

Wilde H (2007) Failures of post-exposure rabies prophylaxis. *Vaccine* 25: 7605–9.

Wilde H, Chomchey P, Punyaratabandhu P, et al. (1989) Purified equine rabies immune globulin: a safe and affordable alternative to human rabies immune globulin. *Bull World Health Organ* 67: 731–6.

11
HIV INFECTIONS

Jo M Wilmshurst, Brian S Eley and Bruce J Brew

The neurological complications of human immunodeficiency virus type 1 (HIV-1) acquired immunodeficiency disease (AIDS) contribute significantly to the morbidity of HIV infection in the paediatric age group (Belman et al. 1988). However, the majority of published data relate to HIV encephalopathy, with less focus on other complications such as cerebrovascular disease, epilepsy and peripheral neuropathy (Cooper et al. 1998). These conditions may display a more complex phenotype than in adult disease as a consequence of the effects on the immature brain.

HIV-2 is found primarily in West Africa and is associated with neurological complications, but to a lesser extent. This chapter will focus on the neurological complications of HIV-1, as the common variant, and will cover recent insights into the neurological pathogenesis of childhood HIV-1 and the implications for therapy, and highlight areas for future research that may offer novel treatment possibilities.

Epidemiology

It is estimated that 3.4 million children worldwide were living with HIV-1/AIDS at the end of 2010, of whom 90% lived in sub-Saharan Africa and 456 000 were receiving antiretroviral therapy (ART, formerly referred to as highly active antiretroviral therapy or HAART). The burden of HIV-1 on child health services in high-prevalence countries is considerable, with as many as 60% of the children admitted to general paediatric wards in some parts of South Africa being infected with HIV (Weakly et al. 2009, WHO 2011).

Neurological involvement has been reported in 50%–60% of infected children, and central nervous system (CNS) involvement may be the initial manifestation of AIDS in up to 18% of children (Belman et al. 1988). Sixty per cent of children with HIV-1 have behavioural difficulties and neurological problems including cerebrovascular insults, peripheral neuropathy and epilepsy (Govender et al. 2011).

Pathogenesis

The CNS is especially vulnerable to HIV-1 infection in the early stages of development. HIV encephalopathy (HIVE) occurs following CNS invasion. The clinical presentation and progression of disease in the developing brain is distinct from that in adults (Schwartz and Major 2006). Macrophages, microglia and astrocytes are targeted, resulting in neuronal loss and dysfunction, and impaired brain growth (Fig. 11.1) (Cooper et al. 1998). Deficits are

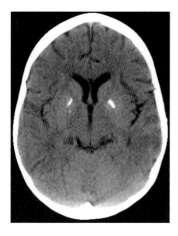

Fig. 11.1. CT of an 8-year-old male with HIV demonstrating the typical cerebral atrophy and basal ganglia calcification.

seen in motor, language, cognitive and social skills (Foster et al. 2006). Many antiretroviral agents penetrate the CNS poorly (Sonza and Crowe 2001).

Clinical manifestations

HIV ENCEPHALOPATHY
In the revised Centers for Disease Control and Prevention (CDC) classification system for HIV-1 infection in children less than 13 years of age, HIVE is a condition listed in Category C (CDC 1994). In the World Health Organization (WHO) classification system, HIVE is listed as a Stage 4 condition (i.e. severe HIV) (WHO 2007). HIVE is reported to occur in 13%–23% of infected children, which is lower than before the advent of ART (Blanche et al. 1997, Tardieu et al. 2000, Chiriboga et al. 2005).

Presentation may differ according to the age and mode of HIV-1 infection. Infants and young children manifest with the most severe neurological disease complications (Englund et al. 1996), and older children manifest with less global and more specific areas of dysfunction (Englund et al. 1996, Blanche et al. 1997, Mckinney et al. 1998, Koekkoek et al. 2008). Children with early onset of HIVE (before 1 year of age) have smaller head circumference, lower birthweight and more severe neurological disease, which suggests a different pathophysiology compared to the encephalopathy that occurs in older children (Tardieu et al. 2000). Children with vertically acquired infection have more severe CNS manifestations than those infected via blood or blood products, even in the neonatal period (Mintz 1994). Further, HIV-1-infected children who are naive to ART (Englund et al. 1996) or on monotherapy (McKinney et al. 1998) are at greater risk of developing CNS manifestations than children on combination ART (Tardieu and Boutet 2002). However, children with HIV-1 infection exposed to zidovudine in utero and for 6 weeks after birth did not differ in the incidence of encephalopathy or level of cognition, compared to children who were not treated (Tardieu et al. 2000). Many children infected with HIV-1 are born into poor socio-economic circumstances and suffer multiple health risks, which complicate the clinical scenario and inevitably lead to greater impact on neurobehavioural function (Ramey and Ramey 1998).

HIVE is defined as either progressive (subacute or plateau) or static (Brouwers et al. 1994). Subacute progressive encephalopathy is the most severe subtype, characterized by progressive global regression. In the plateau course of progressive encephalopathy, the acquisition of new skills slows or stops, but previously acquired milestones remain. Children with the subacute and plateau subtypes have a significant decline in standardized scores on serial neurodevelopmental screens. Children with static encephalopathy acquire new skills and abilities more slowly than normal, and their standardized test scores are below average. Since HIVE appears less prevalent since the introduction of ART, most new cases are in very young children (Blanche et al. 1997, Cooper et al. 1998, Tardieu et al. 2000), particularly those naive to ART (Englund et al. 1996), and among older children in advanced stages of HIV-1 disease (Mitchell 2001).

HIV-RELATED COMPROMISE

HIV-related compromise is associated with cognitive functioning that is within normal limits, but significant declines in psychometric test scores or deficits in one or more selective neurobehavioural functions occur (Wolters and Brouwers 1998). ART does not reduce the incidence of this complication, and neurobehavioural complications arise.

BEHAVIOURAL ISSUES

Attention deficits occur in patients with HIV-1, but there is debate as to whether this is related directly to the disease or to secondary sequelae (Watkins et al. 2000). Disruptions in the dopaminergic pathways are hypothesized. Prevalence rates of 28.6% for attention-deficit–hyperactivity disorder (ADHD), 24.3% for anxiety disorders and 25% for depression are reported (Melvin et al. 2007). However, most studies are small and there are few controlled trials (Scharko 2006). Children with HIVE have more severe impairments in everyday behaviour, such as activities of daily living and socialization, compared to children without encephalopathy. Hyperactivity does not appear to be specifically linked with HIV (Mellins et al. 2003). Since medication with methylphenidate is not contraindicated in children with HIV, intervention is feasible. Additional challenges faced by clinicians, who may have managed children with vertically acquired infection for many years, are the repercussions of disclosure, orphan status, and the implications for future life choices. Red Cross War Memorial Children's Hospital is a tertiary referral hospital in the Western Cape of South Africa and the main referral centre for complex HIV-infected children in the region. A cohort of vertically infected adolescents at this centre demonstrate complex behavioural phenotypes, with retained intelligence quotients, but have progressive deterioration in areas of executive functioning (Dr Rene Nassen, child psychiatrist, unpublished data). Fifty-five per cent of children aged 9–16 years with vertically transmitted HIV-1 met the criteria for a psychiatric disorder in one study (Mellins et al. 2006). They had combinations of anxiety disorders (40%), attention-deficit disorder (21%), conduct disorders (13%) and oppositional defiant disorders (11%). Treatment of children with ART may improve neurobehavioural functioning (Letendre 2011) and reverse cortical atrophy (DeCarli et al. 1991).

ART for these children must include at least one agent with good CNS penetration, such as zidovudine or nevirapine (Letendre 2011).

SPECIFIC NEUROLOGICAL COMPLICATIONS

The specific neurological complications of HIV-1 can be divided into primary disorders, i.e. those directly related to HIV-1 brain infection (e.g. HIVE), and secondary disorders, i.e. those due to CNS opportunistic infections, malignancies and cerebrovascular disease.

The opportunistic infections – cryptococcal meningitis, progressive multifocal leukoencephalopathy, toxoplasma encephalitis, and possibly cytomegalovirus (CMV) encephalitis – occur less frequently in children than in adults, since reactivation of prior infections is less likely in childhood. However, bacterial meningitis in unvaccinated children is more prevalent in HIV-infected children than in HIV-infected adults (Madhi et al. 2001, Molyneux et al. 2003). *Streptoccus pneumoniae* and *Haemophilus influenzae* type b are the most common bacteria implicated (Madhi et al. 2001, Molyneux et al. 2003). Tuberculous meningitis (TBM) is common in HIV-infected children who live in settings where the prevalence of tuberculosis is high. This coinfection of HIV and tuberculosis complicates the management of both diseases; for example, rifampicin reduces the concentration of protease inhibitors and non-nucleoside reverse transcriptase inhibitors (Ren et al. 2008). Specific recommendations are available (CDC 2013). Intervention with ART may also result in reconstitution of antimycobacterial immune responses, which lower the subsequent risk of developing tuberculosis in HIV-infected patients (Kampmann et al. 2006). The typical neuroimaging findings in TBM, hydrocephalus and basal enhancement, may be less marked in patients with HIV, warranting a lower threshold for diagnostic consideration in these patients (Van der Weert et al. 2006).

In centres other than in resource-poor settings, the most common opportunistic infecting organism may be CMV, which causes subacute or chronic encephalitis/ventriculitis, acute ascending radiculomyelitis, or acute or subacute neuropathy (Kozlowski et al. 1990). Herpes simplex virus (HSV) and varicella-zoster virus (VZV) are additional causes of acute or subacute encephalitis (Annunziato and Gershon 1998). Progressive multifocal leukoencephalopathy, caused by a human polyomavirus, the John Cunningham virus (JCV), has rarely been reported in HIV-infected children (Wilmshurst et al. 2006). MRI of the brain often has typical findings (Fig. 11.2), and JCV DNA can be detected in the CSF in a reasonable number of patients. Meningitis caused by *Candida* species, *Aspergillus fumigatus* or fungal abscesses is common in some settings (Kozlowski et al. 1990). Cryptococcal meningitis is less common in the paediatric population than in adults. *Toxoplasma* encephalitis is rare in children (Simmonds and Gonzalo 1998). Mass lesions in children are most likely to be caused by tuberculoma (Fig. 11.3) or lymphoma. Unusual pathogens should also be considered including atypical mycobacteria, *Treponema pallidum*, *Bartonella* species, *Listeria monocytogenes* and *Nocardia asteroides* complex.

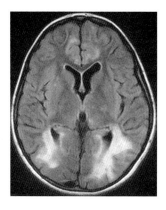

Fig. 11.2. MRI (axial fluid attenuated inversion recovery sequence) of an 11-year-old female with progressive multifocal leukoencephalopathy demonstrating symmetrical white-matter hyperintensity most marked over the posterior regions.

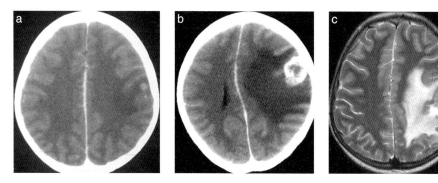

Fig. 11.3. (a) CT with contrast from an 11-year-old female with focal seizures demonstrating a tuberculous granuloma in the left hemisphere. (b) Follow-up imaging 6 months later despite additional treatment for active tuberculosis demonstrated progression in the lesion. (c) MRI axial T2-weighted image showed a low-signal lesion with surrounding oedema consistent with the diagnosis of a progressive tuberculous granuloma. The child was confirmed HIV positive despite having no other markers of the disease and subsequently responded well to the combination of highly active antiretroviral therapy and continued antituberculosis medication.

Primary CNS lymphoma is the most common CNS mass lesion in paediatric AIDS and is the second most common cause of focal neuropathy after stroke (Little 2006). Tumours tend to be high-grade, multifocal B-cell tumours. Affected children present with subacute onset of change in cognitive status or behaviour, reflected by the predilection for the deep grey matter, as well as headaches, seizures and new focal neuropathy. Lesions enhance with contrast, and are associated with mass effect and oedema. Outcome is poor (Little 2006). Confirmation of the diagnosis may be challenging, and empiric treatments for tuberculosis and toxoplasmosis are logical interventions in case of doubt (Little 2006). If laboratory facilities are available, confirmation of Epstein–Barr virus infection in CSF can accurately confirm the lymphoma (Little 2006).

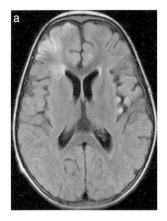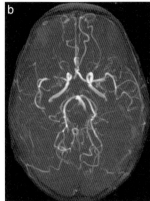

Fig. 11.4. (a) MRI (axial fluid attenuated inversion recovery) from a male child with HIV who presented with acute hemiplegia. Neuroimaging confirmed a subacute lesion in the right frontal region and evidence of an old infarct in the left parietal region. (b) Magnetic resonance angiography confirmed interruption of blood flow in the right middle cerebral artery.

Strokes, secondary to haemorrhage or ischaemia, are the most common cause of clinical focal neurological deficits in children with HIV-1 infection (Fig. 11.4) (Dickson et al. 1990, Park et al. 1990). Ischaemic strokes may be embolic, or secondary to infectious vasculitis (e.g. VZV). Acquired protein C and/or protein S deficiencies occur in patients with AIDS, leading to a hypercoagulable state (Mochan et al. 2005).

A characteristic vasculopathy also occurs in HIV-infected children, involving aneurysmal dilatation of vessels of the circle of Willis, with or without ischaemic infarction or haemorrhage. Some patients evolve a moyamoya-like syndrome. Whether the vasculopathy is caused by direct viral invasion, or by a secondary phenomenon, is not known (Connor 2007). Therapy and optimal intervention in these patients remains a challenge, and treatable causes must be excluded before HIV-1 alone is assumed to be the primary cause (Connor 2007).

Vacuolar myelopathy is relatively common in ART-naive adults, but rare in children (Wilmshurst et al. 2006). Myelopathies may be due to opportunistic infections (HSV, CMV, VZV) or tumours (Petito et al. 1985).

Peripheral neuropathies, once considered unusual complications in children infected with HIV-1, are probably underestimated (Floeter et al. 1997). Poor nutritional state and global wasting may dominate the clinical picture, masking focal wasting due to underlying peripheral neuropathy. Paraesthesiae and pain are the most common presenting complaints, followed by weakness and loss of motor milestones. The most recognized form is the distal sensory or axonal neuropathy, which is directly related to HIV-1 infection, and often compounded by ART, particularly the nucleoside reverse transcriptase inhibitors (NRTIs), didanosine and stavudine (d4T). This condition may be severe enough to warrant termination of the drug, but acetyl-L-carnitine or gabapentin may benefit some of these patients

(Phillips et al. 2010). Acute and subacute demyelinating neuropathy due to HIV-1 infection is relatively unusual in children with HIV, occurring either at the time of seroconversion, or as part of an immune reconstitution syndrome (Brannagan and Zhou 2003, Wilmshurst et al. 2006).

Myopathies may occur as part of an HIV myopathy, zidovudine- and stavudine-induced mitochondrial myopathy, or secondary myopathies (due to opportunistic infections or lymphoma). Muscle weakness usually dominates, but pain and raised creatine kinase enzyme levels can occur as well.

Mitochondrial toxicity is well described in children with HIV-1 infection and is related to NRTI exposure, especially didanosine and stavudine (Foster and Lyall 2008). Complications attributed to mitochondrial dysfunction include lactic acidosis, cardiomyopathy, neuropathy, myopathy, lipoatrophy, pancreatitis and bone marrow suppression. There remains debate as to whether direct involvement of HIV-1 might affect mitochondrial function (Foster and Lyall 2008). Data from HIV-negative infants, who were part of the mother-to-child transmission programmes, has reinforced concerns of drug-induced mitochondrial toxicity (Blanche et al. 1997).

Dyslipidaemia and lipodystrophy syndrome may occur as a side-effect of ART. Lipodystrophy is characterized by peripheral fat wasting, central fat accumulation, and metabolic disorders such as hypercholesterolaemia and insulin resistance (Resino et al. 2008). It is suggested that children with rapid immunological recovery experience higher rates of lipodystrophy (Resino et al. 2008). This association is difficult to explain, and the finding may be more closely related to the length of prior exposure than rapidity of recovery. Children with lipodystrophy are at increased risk of atherosclerosis and associated cardiovascular and cerebrovascular disease (Giuliano Ide et al. 2008).

Immune reconstitution inflammatory syndrome (IRIS) is a frequent complication in children and is seen most often within the first few weeks after initiating ART. A wide spectrum of microorganisms may precipitate IRIS, including mycobacteria, VZV, HSV and *Cryptococcus neoformans* (Puthanakit et al. 2006). Rarely, progressive multifocal leukoencephalopathy and non-infectious conditions, such as opisthotonus–myoclonus and acute inflammatory demyelinating polyradiculoneuropathy (AIDP), may manifest as IRIS events in children (Nuttall et al. 2004). Management is controversial and may include treatment of the specific reactivated opportunistic infection and the use of corticosteroids or both (Nuttall et al. 2004).

Epilepsy in children with HIV-1 infection may be related directly to viral damage, or may be secondary to acquired pathology. Aetiologies among adult patients with HIV-1 and seizures include incidental association, direct effects of HIV-1 disease, opportunistic infections, neoplasias, cerebrovascular disease, drug toxicity and metabolic derangements. The issue of therapy for seizures in HIV-1 infected children illustrates one of the major drug–drug and drug–disease interaction challenges. Phenytoin, phenobarbital and carbamazepine all increase metabolic activity of the cytochrome p450 complex, such that concurrent use with protease inhibitors may result in sub-therapeutic ART levels and treatment failure, as well as potential resistance to the protease inhibitor class of drugs (Birbeck et al. 2012).

TABLE 11.1
Drug–drug interactions[a]

Drug type	Protein binding %	Metabolism	Inhibits	Induces
Anticonvulsants				
Phenobarbital	45	Oxidative hydroxylation		CYP 3A4, 1A2, 2B6, 2C8, 2C9/19
Carbamazepine	45	CYP 3A4, 2C8		CYP 3A4
Phenytoin	90	CYP 2C9, CYP 2C19		CYP 3A4
Sodium valproate	90	50% glucuronidation 40% β-oxidation 10% CYP 2C9, 2C19, 2A6	CYP 2C9, 2C19, 3A4	
Lamotrigine	55–56	Glucuronidation CYP 450		
Topiramate	9–17	CYP 450		
Antiretrovirals				
NRTIs (e.g. zidovudine, stavudine, lamivudine, didanosine)	<38	Glucuronidation		
NNRTI – efavirenz	99	CYP 3A4, 2B6	CYP2C9, 2C19, 2B2	CYP 3A4
NNRTI – nevirapine	50–60	CYP 3A4	CYP3A4	
PI – ritonavir	>90	CYP 450	CYP 3A4, 2D6	CYP 3A4, 2C9, 2C19, 1A2
PI – lopinavir/ritonavir		CYP 450	CYP 3A4	CYP 2C19, 1A2, 2C9

[a]Adapted from Romanelli et al. (2000). CYP, cytochrome P; NRTI, nucleoside reverse transcriptase inhibitor; NNRTI, non-nucleoside reverse transcriptase inhibitor; PI, protease inhibitor.

Protease inhibitors may, in turn, cause toxic levels of anticonvulsants by inhibiting the cytochrome p450 system (Table 11.1).

Sodium valproate is the recommended first-line agent in South Africa for children with HIV-1, on ART, who have seizures requiring regular prophylaxis. However, it has potential interactions with ritonovir, lopinavir and efavirenz. Decreased valproate levels are described in combination therapy, with breakthrough seizures. We have seen this complication in several children, when converted from nevaripine to efavirenz, both non-nucleoside reverse transcriptase inhibitors (NNRTIs) but with different mechanisms of action (Table 11.1).

Other potential anticonvulsant agents include gabapentin, topiramate, tiagabine and pregabalin, which have limited protein binding and, theoretically, no effects on the cytochrome p450 system (Birbeck et al. 2012). Agents suggested in the USA include lamotrigine and levetiracetam. However, there are no large-scale studies that assess the efficacy of any of these anticonvulsants in combination with ART in children. The ketogenic diet, vigabatrin, carbamazepine, vagal nerve stimulation, phenobarbital and phenytoin are not considered to be viable alternatives.

Complexities of the disorder

The 'layering' effect of multiple comorbidities occurring in HIV-1 makes management particularly complex. HIV-associated infections (e.g. tuberculous or bacterial meningitis, CMV) are highly prevalent in resource-poor countries. Common conditions, such as epilepsy, may occur in isolation or be secondary to the sequelae of HIV-1 infection. There are significant drug–drug and drug–disease interactions that must be taken into account to avoid toxicity and treatment failure (Table 11.1). HIV-infected patients are prone to multiple pathophysiological alterations. Hypoalbuminaemia can occur due to drug–disease interactions; hypergammaglobulinaemia and gastrointestinal disorders with resultant impaired absorption also occur, as well as altered blood–brain barrier integrity and mitochondrial dysfunction.

Therapeutic and management issues

CNS penetration is a particular problem in the treatment of HIV-1. The NRTIs, zidovudine and abacavir have relatively good penetration (Brew et al. 2007). The NNRTI nevirapine has the best potential for treatment of CNS disease. However, with the exception of indinavir/ritonavir boosted and lopinavir, protease inhibitors generally have poor CNS penetration (Letendre et al. 2008, Letendre 2011).

The comprehensive management of children with HIV infection requires symptomatic treatment of pain, movement disorders, seizures, spasticity, ADHD and psychiatric/behavioural disorders. In most cases the same agents can be used in the HIV-infected child as in adults. However, numerous interactions can occur, so that caution is needed with respect to bone marrow suppression and liver and pancreatic toxicity. Patients with CNS involvement may be very sensitive to psychotropic medication (Civitello 2006).

Children with severe neurodevelopmental deficits may benefit from physical, occupational and speech therapy (Baillieu and Potterton 2008). Special support is needed for children with ADHD and learning difficulties. Nutrition must be optimized. Exclusion of other causes of neurodevelopmental disorders, e.g. endocrinological and metabolic disturbances (hypothyroidism, vitamin and cofactor deficiencies), is necessary.

Future directions and new interventions

Therapies targeting neuroprotection can be divided into those that are inhibitors of cell-signalling pathways, excitatory inhibitors, inhibitors of oxidative and nitrostative stress, neurotransmitter antagonists, biologics, vaccine strategies and erythropoietin (Rumbaugh et al. 2008, Webb et al. 2009). Some of these approaches are hypothetical, others are being tested in animal models, and only a few have reached the stage of human studies. Interventions specifically targeting attenuation of neuronal apoptosis, in the context of ART, include ABC transporter inhibitors and metallothionines. Agents that act independently of ART include promoters of GSK-3, minocycline, NMDAR (N-methyl D-aspartate receptor) antagonists, erythropoietin, specific chemokine antagonists and p38 MAPK (mitogen-activated protein kinase) inhibitors.

Conclusion

There is an urgent need for large-cohort studies to assess the prevalence of specific neurological complications of HIV-1, other than HIVE, in children. These studies would enhance our understanding of the impact of this disease and allow an evidence-based approach to management for disorders such as epilepsy. Childhood HIV-1 is becoming a rare condition in resource-rich countries, which demonstrates the success of health education and mother-to-child transmission programmes. It follows that studies of neurological complications of HIV-1 must be based in resource-poor, high HIV-1 prevalence regions, which bear the greatest disease burden. There is also a need for improved ARTs that target the neurological complications of the disease, since most current agents lack sufficient CNS penetration.

Specific genetic markers are being identified that begin to explain the heterogeneity in the disease patterns experienced by different patients with identical management. These genetic markers are being used to understand the pathophysiology of neurological complications of HIV-1 and to identify potential future drug targets in both adults and children. Much of our understanding of the mechanisms of neurological complications of HIV-1 is derived from studies in adults. While it is likely that many of these findings are directly relevant to the paediatric population, the HIV-1 infection of the maturing brain might result in hitherto unrecognized disease manifestations.

REFERENCES

Annunziato PW, Gershon AA (1998) Herpesvirus infections in children infected with HIV. In: Wilfert CM, Pizzo PA, eds. *Pediatric AIDS: the Challenge of HIV Infection in Infants, Children and Adolescents.* Baltimore: Williams & Wilkins, pp. 205–25.
Baillieu N, Potterton J (2008) The extent of delay of language, motor, and cognitive development in HIV-positive infants. *J Neurol Phys Ther* 32: 118–21.
Belman AL, Diamond G, Dickson D, et al. (1988) Pediatric acquired immunodeficiency syndrome. Neurologic syndromes. *Am J Dis Child* 142: 29–35.
Birbeck GL, French JA, Perucca E, et al. (2012) Antiepileptic drug selection for people with HIV/AIDS: evidence-based guidelines from the ILAE and AAN. *Epilepsia* 53: 207–14.
Blanche S, Newell ML, Mayaux MJ, et al. (1997) Morbidity and mortality in European children vertically infected by HIV-1. The French Pediatric HIV Infection Study Group and European Collaborative Study. *J Acquir Immune Defic Syndr Hum Retrovirol* 14: 442–50.
Brannagan TH, Zhou Y (2003) HIV-associated Guillain–Barré syndrome. *J Neurol Sci* 208: 39–42.
Brew BJ, Halman M, Catalan J, et al. (2007) Factors in AIDS dementia complex trial design: results and lessons from the abacavir trial. *PLoS Clin Trials* 2: e13.
Brouwers P, Belman AL, Epstein LG (1994) Central nervous system involvement: manifestations, evaluation, and pathogenesis. In: Pizzo PA, Wilfert CM, eds. *Pediatric AIDS: the Challenge of HIV Infection in Infants, Children and Adolescents, 2nd edn.* Baltimore: Williams & Wilkins, pp. 433–55.
CDC (1994) Revised classification system for human immunodeficiency virus infection in children less than 13 years of age. Official authorized addenda: Human immunodeficiency virus infection codes and official guidelines for coding and reporting ICD-9-CM (online: http://www.cdc.gov/mmwr/PDF/rr/rr4312.pdf).

CDC (2013) Managing drug interactions in the treatment of HIV-related tuberculosis (online: http://www.cdc.gov/tb/TB_HIV_Drugs/default.htm).

Chiriboga CA, Fleishman S, Champion S, et al. (2005) Incidence and prevalence of HIV encephalopathy in children with HIV infection receiving highly active anti-retroviral therapy (HAART). *J Pediatr* 146: 402–7.

Civitello L (2006) Neurologic problems. In: Zeichner SL, Read JS, eds. *Handbook of Pediatric HIV Care.* Cambridge: Cambridge University Press, pp. 503–18.

Connor M (2007) Stroke in patients with human immunodeficiency virus infection. *J Neurol Neurosurg Psychiatry* 78: 1291.

Cooper ER, Hanson C, Diaz C, et al. (1998) Encephalopathy and progression of human immunodeficiency virus disease in a cohort of children with perinatally acquired human immunodeficiency virus infection. *J Pediatr* 132: 808–12.

DeCarli C, Fugate L, Falloon J, et al. (1991) Brain growth and cognitive improvement in children with human immunodeficiency virus-induced encephalopathy after 6 months of continuous infusion zidovudine therapy. *J Acquir Immune Defic Syndr* 4: 585–92.

Dickson D, Llen AJF, Werdenheim KM, et.al (1990) CNS pathology in children with AIDS and focal neurologic signs: stroke and lymphoma. In: Kozlowski PB, Snider DA, Vietze PM, Wisniewski HM, eds. *Brain in Pediatric AIDS.* Basel: Karger, pp. 147–57.

Englund JA, Baker CJ, Raskino C, et al. (1996) Clinical and laboratory characteristics of a large cohort of symptomatic, human immunodeficiency virus-infected infants and children. AIDS Clinical Trials Group Protocol 152 Study Team. *Pediatr Infect Dis J* 15: 1025–36.

Floeter MK, Civitello LA, Everett CR, et al. (1997) Peripheral neuropathy in children with HIV infection. *Neurology* 49: 207–12.

Foster CJ, Biggs RL, Melvin D, et al. (2006) Neurodevelopmental outcomes in children with HIV infection under 3 years of age. *Dev Med Child Neurol* 48: 677–82.

Foster C, Lyall H (2008) HIV and mitochondrial toxicity in children. *J Antimicrob Chemother* 61: 8–12.

Giuliano Ide C, de Freitas SF, de Souza M, Caramelli B (2008) Subclinic atherosclerosis and cardiovascular risk factors in HIV-infected children: PERI study. *Coron Artery Dis* 19: 167–72.

Govender R, Eley B, Walker K, et al. (2011) Neurologic and neurobehavioral sequelae in children with human immunodeficiency virus (HIV-1) infection. *J Child Neurol* 26: 1355–64.

Kampmann B, Tena-Coki GN, Nicol MP, et al. (2006) Reconstitution of antimycobacterial immune responses in HIV-infected children receiving HAART. *AIDS* 20: 1011–8.

Koekkoek S, de Sonneville LM, Wolfs TF, et al. (2008) Neurocognitive function profile in HIV-infected school-age children. *Eur J Paediatr Neurol* 12: 290–7.

Kozlowski PB, Sher JH, Dickson D, et al. (1990) CNS infections in paediatric HIV infection: a multicentre study. In: Kozlowski PB, Snider DA, Vietze PM, Wisniewski HM, eds. *Brain in Pediatric AIDS.* Basel: Karger, pp. 132–46.

Letendre S, Marquie-Beck J, Capparelli E, et al. (2008) Validation of the CNS Penetration-Effectiveness rank for quantifying antiretroviral penetration into the central nervous system. *Arch Neurol* 65: 65–70.

Letendre S (2011) Central nervous system complications in HIV disease: HIV-associated neurocognitive disorder. *Top Antivir Med* 19: 137–42.

Little R (2006) Neoplastic disease in pediatric HIV infection. In: Zeichner SL, Read JS, eds. *Handbook of Pedaitric HIV Care.* Cambridge: Cambridge University Press, pp. 637–49.

Madhi SA, Madhi A, Petersen K, et al. (2001) Impact of human immunodeficiency virus type 1 infection on the epidemiology and outcome of bacterial meningitis in South African children. *Int J Infect Dis* 5: 119–25.

McKinney RE Jr, Johnson GM, Stanley K, et al. (1998) A randomized study of combined zidovudine–lamivudine versus didanosine monotherapy in children with symptomatic therapy-naive HIV-1 infection. The Pediatric AIDS Clinical Trials Group Protocol 300 Study Team. *J Pediatr* 133: 500–8.

Mellins CA, Smith R, O'Driscoll P, et al. (2003) High rates of behavioral problems in perinatally HIV-infected children are not linked to HIV disease. *Pediatrics* 111: 384–93.

Mellins CA, Brackis-Cott E, Dolezal C, Abrams EJ (2006) Psychiatric disorders in youth with perinatally acquired human immunodeficiency virus infection. *Pediatr Infect Dis J* 25: 432–7.

Melvin D, Krechevsky D, Divac A, et al. (2007) Parental reports of emotional and behavioural difficulties on the SDQ for school-age children with vertically acquired HIV infection living in London. *Psychol Health Med* 12: 40–7.

Mintz M (1994) Clinical comparison of adult and pediatric NeuroAIDS. *Adv Neuroimmunol* 4: 207–21.

Mitchell W (2001) Neurological and developmental effects of HIV and AIDS in children and adolescents. *Ment Retard Dev Disabil Res Rev* 7: 211–6.

Mochan A, Modi M, Modi G (2005) Protein S deficiency in HIV associated ischaemic stroke: an epiphenomenon of HIV infection. *J Neurol Neurosurg Psychiatry* 76: 1455–6.

Molyneux EM, Tembo M, Kayira K, et al. (2003) The effect of HIV infection on paediatric bacterial meningitis in Blantyre, Malawi. *Arch Dis Child* 88: 1112–8.

Nuttall JJ, Wilmshurst JM, Ndondo AP, et al. (2004) Progressive multifocal leukoencephalopathy after initiation of highly active antiretroviral therapy in a child with advanced human immunodeficiency virus infection: a case of immune reconstitution inflammatory syndrome. *Pediatr Infect Dis J* 23: 683–5.

Park YD, Belman AL, Kim TS, et al. (1990) Stroke in pediatric acquired immunodeficiency syndrome. *Ann Neurol* 28: 303–11.

Petito CK, Navia BA, Cho ES, et al. (1985) Vacuolar myelopathy pathologically resembling subacute combined degeneration in patients with the acquired immunodeficiency syndrome. *N Engl J Med* 312: 874–9.

Phillips TJ, Cherry CL, Cox S, et al. (2010) Pharmacological treatment of painful HIV-associated sensory neuropathy: a systematic review and meta-analysis of randomised controlled trials. *PLoS One* 5: e14433.

Puthanakit T, Oberdorfer P, Akarathum N, et al. (2006) Immune reconstitution syndrome after highly active antiretroviral therapy in human immunodeficiency virus-infected Thai children. *Pediatr Infect Dis J* 25: 53–8.

Ramey CT, Ramey SL (1998) Prevention of intellectual disabilities: early interventions to improve cognitive development. *Prev Med* 27: 224–32.

Ren Y, Nuttall JJ, Egbers C, et al. (2008) Effect of rifampicin on lopinavir pharmacokinetics in HIV-infected children with tuberculosis. *J Acquir Immune Defic Syndr* 47: 566–9.

Resino S, Micheloud D, Larru B, et al. (2008) Immunological recovery and metabolic disorders in severe immunodeficiency HIV type 1-infected children on highly active antiretroviral therapy. *AIDS Res Hum Retroviruses* 24: 1477–84.

Romanelli F, Jennings HR, Nath A, et al. (2000) Therapeutic dilemma: the use of anticonvulsants in HIV-positive individuals. *Neurology* 54: 1404–7.

Rumbaugh JA, Steiner J, Sacktor N, Nath A (2008) Developing neuroprotective strategies for treatment of HIV-associated neurocognitive dysfunction. *Futur HIV Ther* 2: 271–80.

Scharko AM (2006) DSM psychiatric disorders in the context of pediatric HIV/AIDS. AIDS Care 18: 441–5.

Schwartz L, Major EO (2006) Neural progenitors and HIV-1-associated central nervous system disease in adults and children. *Curr HIV Res* 4: 319–27.

Simmonds RJ, Gonzalo O (1998) Pneumocystis carinii pneumonia and toxoplasmosis. In: Wilfert CM, Pizzo PA, eds. *Pediatric AIDS: The Challenge of HIV Infection in Infants, Children and Adolescents.* Baltimore: Williams & Wilkins, pp. 251–65.

Sonza S, Crowe SM (2001) Reservoirs for HIV infection and their persistence in the face of undetectable viral load. *AIDS Patient Care STDS* 15: 511–8.

Tardieu M, Le Chenadec J, Persoz A, et al. (2000) HIV-1-related encephalopathy in infants compared with children and adults. French Pediatric HIV Infection Study and the SEROCO Group. *Neurology* 54: 1089–95.

Tardieu M, Boutet A (2002) HIV-1 and the central nervous system. *Curr Top Microbiol Immunol* 265: 183–95.

Van der Weert EM, Hartgers NM, Schaaf HS, et al. (2006) Comparison of diagnostic criteria of tuberculous meningitis in human immunodeficiency virus-infected and uninfected children. *Pediatr Infect Dis J* 25: 65–9.

Watkins JM, Cool VA, Usner D, et al. (2000) Attention in HIV-infected children: results from the Hemophilia Growth and Development Study. *J Int Neuropsychol Soc* 6: 443–54.

Weakly M, Vries A, Reichmuth KL, et al. (2009) HIV infection, tuberculosis and workload in a general paediatric ward. *SAJCH* 3: 55–9.

Webb KM, Mactutus CF, Booze RM (2009) The ART of HIV therapies: dopaminergic deficits and future treatments for HIV pediatric encephalopathy. *Expert Rev Anti Infect Ther* 7: 193–203.

WHO (2007) WHO case definitions of HIV for surveillance and revised clinical staging and immunological classification of HIV-related disease in adults and children (online: http://www.who.int/hiv/pub/guidelines/HIVstaging150307.pdf).

WHO (2011) Global HIV/AIDS response. Epidemic update and health sector progress towards universal access. Progress report 2011. Geneva: World Health Organization (online: http://whqlibdoc.who.int/publications/2011/9789241502986_eng.pdf).

Wilmshurst JM, Burgess J, Hartley P, Eley B (2006) Specific neurologic complications of human immunodeficiency virus type 1 (HIV-1) infection in children. *J Child Neurol* 21: 788–94.

Wolters P, Brouwers P (1998) Evaluation of neurodevelopmental deficits in children with HIV infection. In: Gendelman HE, Lipton SA, Epstein LG, Swindells S, eds. *The Neurology of AIDS*. New York: Chapman & Hall, pp. 425–42.

ACKNOWLEDGEMENTS

We wish to thank K Walker, K Donald, R Govender, R Petersen and R Nassen for providing clinical data, T Kilborn for neuroradiological images, and M Hatherill for proof-reading the manuscript.

12
ACUTE BACTERIAL MENINGITIS

Pratibha Singhi and Sunit Singhi

Bacterial meningitis is a devastating infection of the central nervous system (CNS) that has a high mortality and morbidity in spite of the availability of several new potent antimicrobials. CNS damage in meningitis is caused not only by the bacterial invasion, but also largely by the severe inflammatory response and its consequences. Early diagnosis, prompt antimicrobial therapy and supportive management are the keys to improving outcome.

Aetiology
Bacterial meningitis beyond the neonatal period is caused in more than 90% of cases by the three major meningeal pathogens, *Haemophilus influenzae*, *Neisseria meningitidis* and *Streptococcus pneumoniae*. The incidence of *H. influenzae* type b (Hib) and *S. pneumoniae* meningitis decreased after the introduction of vaccines, and *S. pneumoniae* predominates in many parts of the world. Neonatal meningitis is caused mainly by group B streptococci, gram-negative bacilli and *Listeria monocytogenes*, and occasionally by other organisms. Group B streptococci are the main causative organisms in resource-rich countries, gram-negative bacilli in resource-poor ones (Zaidi et al. 2009). *Listeria* is rarely reported from resource-poor countries (Furyk et al. 2011). The aetiological organisms vary mainly with the age, the nutritional and immune status of the child, and the coexistence of other clinical conditions. The common pathogens that cause meningitis in various age groups and with specific predisposing conditions are shown in Tables 12.1 and 12.2.

Epidemiology
Bacterial meningitis is essentially a disease of infants and children, although it can occur at any age. According to the World Health Organization (WHO), about 170 000 deaths per year are due to meningitis; the fatality rate is as high as 50% in untreated cases (WHO 2011). Widespread use of effective bacterial conjugate vaccines against Hib and pneumococci in resource-rich countries has resulted in a substantial reduction as well as a change in the epidemiology of bacterial meningitis in these countries. In the USA there has been a reduction in the incidence of meningitis from 2.00 cases per 100 000 population in 1998–9 to 1.38/100 000 in 2005–7; with a substantial decrease in both Hib and pneumococcal meningitis in young children, the burden of meningitis is now borne more by adults (Thigpen et al. 2011). A 7-year surveillance study of meningitis in France conducted after the introduction of immunization showed that about half (46%) of the cases were meningococcal, a third (28%) pneumococcal, and only 3% were due to *H. influenzae*. In infants under 1 year of

TABLE 12.1
Common causative organisms for bacterial meningitis in various age-groups

Age	Causative organisms	Antibiotics and doses (mg/kg)
<1mo	Group B streptococci, gram-negative bacilli (*E. coli, Pseudomonas*), *Listeria monocytogenes*	Ampicillin 50–100, every 6–8h, plus aminoglycoside (gentamycin/amikacin) 2–2.5, every 8h; *or* cefotaxime[a] 100, every 8h
1–3mo	Gram-negative bacilli, *Listeria monocytogenes, Streptococcus pneumoniae, Neissera meningitidis*	Ceftriaxone 100, every 24h, or 50, every 12h; *or* cefotaxime 100, every 8h, plus ampicillin 50–100, every 6–8h
>3mo	*Streptococcus pneumoniae, H. influenzae, Neissera meningitidis*	Ceftriaxone 100, every 24h, or 50, every 12h; *or* cefotaxime 75 every 6–8h plus vancomycin[b] 15, every 6h

[a]In places with aminoglycoside-resistant gram-negative organisms.
[b]In places with penicillin-resistant pneumococci.

TABLE 12.2
Causes of bacterial meningitis in special predisposing conditions

Underlying condition	Causative organisms
CSF shunt, neurosurgery	*Staphylococcus aureus, S. epidermidis, Pseudomonas* spp.
Neural-tube defects	*S. aureus, S. epidermidis, Pseudomonas* spp.
Head injury	
Basilar fractures	Pneumococcus, *Haemophilus influenzae, S. aureus*
Penetrating wounds	*S. aureus, S. epidermidis, Pseudomonas* spp.
Sickle-cell disease, asplenia	Pneumococcus, *H. influenzae, Salmonella* spp.
Immune suppression/malnutrition	Gram-negative organisms (*Escherichia coli, Klebsiella* spp., *Proteus* spp., *Pseudomonas* spp., *Citrobacter* spp.); other unusual organisms
Endocarditis	*Streptococcus viridans*
Pyoderma, cellulitis	*S. aureus*
Otitis media, sinusitis, pneumonia	Pneumococcus

age, the most common organism was pneumococcus, whereas in those over 1 year it was meningococcus (Levy et al. 2008).

The burden of bacterial meningitis including Hib and pneumococcal meningitis continues to be high in resource-poor countries because of lack of immunization, poor socio-economic conditions, overcrowding, high prevalence of malnutrition and human immuno-deficiency virus (HIV), and the occurrence of epidemics of meningococcal disease. Geographical variations in aetiology are possibly also related to differences in environment and populations – most cases of meningococcal meningitis in developed countries are caused by serogroups B and C, whereas serogroup A is responsible for large-scale epidemics in many resource-poor countries of Africa and Asia. Seasonal variations of meningitis are reported; pneumococcal meningitis is more common in winters, possibly because of the association of bacterial and viral respiratory cofactors. Most cases of meningitis are sporadic; however, secondary cases in vulnerable contacts occur particularly in crowded places such as day care centres, schools and camps because of the high transmission of organisms. Most cases of secondary meningitis are caused by *H. influenzae* and meningococci, rarely by pneumococci.

HAEMOPHILUS INFLUENZAE

Hib meningitis continues to account for a large proportion of cases of meningitis in many resource-poor countries, where Hib vaccination is not widely used. It is the most common cause of meningitis in non-immunized children between 3 months and 3 years of age. Hib meningitis is rarely seen in children over 5 years of age, except in high-risk children such as those with sickle-cell anaemia, splenectomy, cerebrospinal fluid (CSF) fistulas, and chronic pulmonary infections.

STREPTOCOCCUS PNEUMONIAE

Pneumococcal meningitis occurs throughout childhood. It is the most common meningitis in children under 2 years of age in countries where Hib immunization is routinely used. It is particularly seen in children with pneumonia, otitis media, sinusitis, CSF fistulas or leaks, head injury, sickle-cell disease and thalassaemia major. Pneumococcus is the most common cause of bacterial meningitis in HIV-infected patients (Scarborough and Thwaites 2008) and causes the most severe form of meningitis.

NEISSERIA MENINGITIDIS

Meningococcal meningitis is both an epidemic and an endemic disease, and it affects primarily school-age children and young adults. Recurrent or chronic meningococcal infections are occasionally seen in children with deficiencies of terminal complement components or properdin. Meningitis caused by Hib, pneumococcus and meningococcus is rare in the first 3 months of life, because of transplacental transfer of protective maternal antibodies.

GROUP B STREPTOCOCCAL MENINGITIS

This occurs mostly in neonates, rarely in older children. The organisms colonize the maternal genital tract and can infect the neonate during passage through the birth canal. Early-onset meningitis (within 7 days of birth) affects mostly term infants; preterm birth is a possible risk factor for late-onset meningitis (Georget-Bouquinet et al. 2008). Universal screening of pregnant women for rectovaginal group B streptococci and administration of intrapartum antibiotic prophylaxis to carriers has led to a decrease in early group B streptococcal meningitis (Daily et al. 2009).

Pathogenesis

Bacterial meningitis is an inflammation of the meninges secondary to bacterial invasion of the subarachnoid space that progresses through the following phases: (1) nasopharyngeal colonization and vascular invasion; (2) meningeal invasion and multiplication in the subarachnoid space; (3) induction and progression of inflammation in the subarachnoid space with associated pathophysiological alterations; and (4) damage to the CNS.

NASOPHARYNGEAL COLONIZATION AND VASCULAR INVASION

Inhaled bacteria adhere to the nasopharyngeal mucosa through adhesins on the fimbriae or on the bacterial cell wall. The organisms evade mucosal host defense mechanisms by secretion of IgA proteases that cleave the protective secretory IgA, allowing the organisms to colonize and penetrate the mucosal barrier and enter the blood stream. Within the blood stream, the pathogens evade the host defense mainly through their polysaccharide capsule, which protects them from complement-mediated bacterial killing and neutrophil phagocytosis. Activation of the alternative complement pathway is the main host defense against encapsulated bacteria, hence children with impaired alternative complement pathway (asplenia, sickle-cell disease) are at high risk for meningitis by these encapsulated bacteria. Neonates have non-specific low immunity, particularly against gram-negative organisms, and are thus more vulnerable to gram-negative meningitis.

MENINGEAL INVASION

Meningeal invasion occurs when the bacteria penetrate the blood–brain barrier. This is facilitated by various neurotropic and virulence factors and perhaps a critical magnitude of bacteraemia. The choroid plexus and cerebral capillaries are the preferential sites of invasion into the CSF. Non-haematogenous spread of bacteria into the CSF can also occur from contiguous sites of infections such as otitis media, sinusitis and mastoiditis, or through direct communication of the subarachnoid space with the skin or mucosa as in head trauma, dermal sinuses and infected CSF shunts.

Because of a lack of resident macrophages and deficient opsonization in the CSF, the bacteria multiply rapidly and spread over the entire surface of the brain and spinal cord, along penetrating vessels.

INFLAMMATION OF THE SUBARACHNOID SPACE

Bacterial multiplication and autolysis in the subarachnoid space leads to the release of bacterial components including fragments of cell wall and lipopolysaccharides. These trigger a strong inflammatory response by inducing the production and release of several inflammatory cytokines and chemokines including interleukin-1B, interleukin-6 and tumour necrosis factor. Cytokines further induce the release of other inflammatory mediators, including other interleukins, chemokines, platelet-activating factor, matrix metalloproteinases, nitric oxide and free oxygen radicals. Increase in cytokines disrupts the blood–brain barrier and recruits leukocytes from the blood into the CSF leading to CSF pleocytosis.

Leukocytes in the CSF release various toxic mediators that affect the cerebral blood flow and cerebral metabolism, and contribute to the development of cerebral oedema and neuronal damage.

Pathophysiology

CHANGES IN CEREBRAL BLOOD FLOW

In the early phase, the cerebral blood flow (CBF) increases due to the vasodilatory effect of nitric oxide, and later it decreases, probably due to vasospasm, causing a global cerebral hypoperfusion. Because of loss of autoregulation, cerebral perfusion becomes directly dependent on the systemic blood pressure. Vasculitis of large and small arteries traversing through the inflamed subarachnoid space can cause focal ischaemic damage including stroke, with permanent neurological sequelae.

CEREBRAL OEDEMA

Cerebral oedema is caused by several mechanisms. Vasogenic oedema occurs as a consequence of increased permeability of the blood–brain barrier. Cytotoxic oedema is caused by cell membrane injury and loss of cellular homeostasis with influx of potassium and calcium. Interstitial oedema occurs because of increased CSF production secondary to increased blood flow in the choroid plexus. Associated decreased re-absorption of the CSF secondary to increased outflow resistance across the arachnoid villi may cause hydrocephalus. Severe brain oedema may cause a marked increase in intracranial pressure (ICP), with resultant cerebral herniation and brainstem compression. Obstructive hydrocephalus, cerebritis, cerebral infarction, cerebral venous thrombosis and status epilepticus can aggravate the raised ICP.

Neuropathology

The brain and cerebral blood vessels are covered with inflammatory exudate; vasculitis and associated thrombosis may be seen. Parenchymal brain damage includes brain oedema that may be severe enough to cause cerebral herniation, and ischaemia that may lead to cerebral infarction. Loss of neurons, generally focal, occurs throughout the brain, particularly in the dentate gyrus of the hippocampus, and is commonly seen in cases with a late mortality (Hofer et al. 2011). On neuroimaging, grey-matter volume loss in the limbic system including the hippocampus, thalamus and cingulate gyri and in the temporal lobe has been demonstrated in patients after bacterial meningitis (Focke et al. 2013).

Clinical presentation

The clinical presentation of meningitis varies considerably with the age of the child. It is also determined by the infecting organism, immune status of the child, duration of illness at the time of presentation, and associated clinical conditions.

Neonates present with non-specific symptoms of sepsis with poor feeding, lethargy, fever, vomiting, irritability, high-pitched cry and at times seizures; low-birthweight infants may not have fever, and neck rigidity is rare. The anterior fontanelle may be level or full, and in some cases there may be enlargement of the head with separation of sutures.

In older children, meningitis usually presents as an acute illness in a previously healthy child, typically with fever, headache, vomiting, altered consciousness, stiff neck, and in some cases seizures and photophobia. *H. influenzae* and pneumococcal meningitis may start as non-specific sepsis, respiratory illness or pneumonia, and then progress to meningitis. A fulminant course with sepsis, shock, rapidly progressive cerebral oedema and raised ICP, evolving over a few hours, is often seen with meningococcal meningitis.

Fever is the single most common presenting feature and is a sensitive (83%) but not a specific (44.5%) indicator in children over the age of 1 year (Berkley et al. 2004, Best and Hughes 2008). It is less frequent in infants, and may be absent in very small infants, in severely malnourished or immunocompromised children, and in children on antibiotic therapy. Impairment of consciousness at presentation may be minimal, but worsens gradually with progression of the disease. Headache is a common non-specific feature in older children. Younger children may not be able to complain of headache but may be irritable. Seizures are the presenting feature in almost a third of children with meningitis and may recur. Seizure outside the age range for febrile convulsions, particularly if focal, is a reasonably specific (88.5%) but not a sensitive (55%) indicator (Best and Hughes 2008). Meningitis is a common cause of convulsive status epilepticus with fever, and the classic symptoms and signs of meningitis may be absent in such children (Chin et al. 2005).

The classic signs of meningitis are those that reflect meningeal irritation and include the following.

1 *Neck rigidity:* flexion of neck is either painful, or not possible because of neck stiffness. Neck stiffness is uncommon in infants but becomes a predominant feature as the child grows older.
2 *Kernig sign:* with thighs flexed on abdomen, passive extension of the knee produces pain in the back.
3 *Brudziński sign:* passive flexion of the neck produces flexion of both lower limbs.
4 *Tripod sign:* in the sitting position, the child supports him- or herself with both arms extended behind the back, which is kept straight.
5 *Knee-kiss sign:* the child cannot bend forward to kiss his or her knees.

Meningeal signs may be minimal or absent in neonates and young infants, and in malnourished and deeply comatose children. In infants, a bulging fontanelle is a reasonably specific sign of meningitis.

Symptoms and signs of raised ICP (headache, vomiting, hypertension, bradycardia, respiratory abnormalities) may be present at the time of admission/hospitalization in some patients or may appear in the ensuing 24–48 hours. Papilloedema at presentation is uncommon in the absence of complications, and if present, computerized tomography (CT) must be conducted to exclude a mass lesion or a complication. Focal signs are seen in about 14% of cases and may be due to subdural collection, cortical infarction or cerebritis.

Depending on the pathogen, there may be associated findings such as a maculopapular or petechial rash in meningococcal infections, otitis media or pneumonia in pneumococcal infections, and pustular skin lesions in staphylococcal infections. Rapid development of multiple haemorrhagic rashes and/or purpura with shock is almost pathognomonic of meningococcaemia (Waterhouse–Friderichsen syndrome). Rashes can occasionally be seen with *H. influenzae* or pneumococcal meningitis.

Diagnosis

A high index of suspicion is necessary for early diagnosis. No single clinical feature is robust enough to make a diagnosis of bacterial meningitis. However, fever, seizures, meningeal signs and altered consciousness are consistently associated with bacterial meningitis (Best and Hughes 2008). The absence of meningeal signs should not exclude the diagnosis of meningitis. The World Health Organization Integrated Management of Childhood Illness (IMCI) referral criteria for meningitis include lethargy, unconsciousness, inability to feed, stiff neck and seizures. These were found to have a sensitivity of 98% and a specificity of 72% to predict meningitis (Weber et al. 2002). However, they were not found to be very helpful in the first week of life (Mwaniki et al. 2011).

A good clinical history and detailed examination, particularly in the presence of predisposing factors, are essential for diagnosing bacterial meningitis.

Differential diagnosis

In neonates and very young infants meningitis can occur without any symptoms and signs of CNS involvement – they often present with non-specific sepsis; meningitis has therefore to be excluded by CSF examination. In older infants who present with fever and seizures, meningitis must be considered seriously, particularly if the child looks ill; in the absence of meningeal signs, meningitis may be missed. In older children with acute-onset fever and meningismus, the differential diagnoses include aseptic meningitis, pneumonia (especially with involvement of the right upper lobe), retropharyngeal abscess, cervical lymphadenitis, and rarely spinal epidural abscess. Clinical parameters such as a viral prodrome, with the child not looking very toxic, a rash, and lymph node or parotid enlargement may favour the diagnosis of viral meningitis. In children with rapidly progressive alteration of consciousness, viral encephalitis, cerebral malaria, Reye syndrome, metabolic problems, hepatic encephalopathy, intoxication and other causes of coma need to be considered. Cerebral malaria is an important differential diagnosis in endemic regions, particularly if there is associated splenomegaly and anaemia; however, malarial parasites can be seen in the blood film of children with meningitis, and their presence should not distract the clinician from the diagnosis of bacterial meningitis. In the presence of focal signs, especially with raised ICP, cerebral abscess, herpes encephalitis, intracranial haemorrhage and other space-occupying lesions need to be excluded with urgent neuroimaging. If the disease onset is subacute, a history of contact with an individual with tuberculosis and of prior administration of antibiotics is important, especially in resource-poor countries where chronic meningitis such as tuberculous meningitis is common. Tuberculous meningitis may occasionally have an acute presentation, but usually the symptoms are more prolonged; evidence of tuberculosis elsewhere in the body should be looked for. Other CSF tests for tuberculous meningitis may be helpful in doubtful cases.

Laboratory tests

CEREBROSPINAL FLUID

The diagnosis of meningitis is confirmed by analysis and culture of the CSF. Lumbar puncture should be done as early as possible in all cases of suspected meningitis, unless contraindicated. Delay in lumbar puncture often leads to delay in starting antibiotics, which is
associated with increased mortality and morbidity.

*Appropriate antibiotics should be administered early in all cases of suspected meningitis
even if the lumbar puncture is delayed.* Early antibiotic administration may decrease the yield
on culture and occasionally on Gram stain, but does not significantly alter the CSF cellular
response; some increase in CSF sugar and decrease in protein may occur (Nigrovic et al. 2009).

In bacterial meningitis the CSF is under pressure and characteristically shows polymorphonuclear leukocytosis, decreased glucose and increased protein concentration. The cell
count may vary from a few to over a thousand leukocytes. Almost 90% of patients have a
CSF cell count over 100/mm^3 and about 60% have counts greater than 1000/mm^3 (Tunkel
et al. 2004); however, this is not so in resource-poor countries where the reported CSF cell
counts are lower in most cases. A cloudy CSF under pressure is almost diagnostic of bacterial meningitis. In neonates, meningitis can be present even when the CSF shows a normal
cell count. The CSF glucose levels are less than 40mg/dL in more than half the cases; a CSF
to serum glucose ratio of 0.4 or less is 80% sensitive and 98% specific in children above 2
months of age. In neonates a CSF to serum glucose ratio of 0.6 or less is considered abnormal (Tunkel et al. 2004). The CSF can at times be completely normal in the early stages of
bacterial meningitis, more so in neonatal meningitis; a repeat lumbar puncture after a few
hours may show abnormalities; antibiotic therapy must therefore be started in all cases with
a strong suspicion of bacterial meningitis.

If the lumbar puncture is mildly traumatic, correction methods have been used for interpretation. A predicted CSF white blood cell (WBC) count is calculated using the formula
(where RBC = red blood cells): CSF WBC (predicted) = CSF RBC × (blood WBC/blood RBC).
The observed (O) WBC count divided by the predicted (P) count gives the O:P ratio. The
specificity and positive predictive value of an O:P ratio of 0.01 or less and a WBC:RBC
ratio of 0.01 or less were 100% in predicting the absence of disease in children over 1 month
of age (Mazor et al. 2003). However, none of the proposed correction methods is perfectly
accurate; this is particularly true for neonates where such correction does not help in the
diagnosis of bacterial meningitis (Greenberg et al. 2008). A grossly traumatic CSF can be
used for culture alone. In a child with a traumatic lumbar puncture, the clinician should
carefully consider the clinical condition and other laboratory parameters of the child for
deciding treatment.

Organism identification

Gram stain of the CSF is moderately sensitive (61%) and highly specific (99%) (Neuman
et al. 2008, Nigrovic et al. 2008), and is quick and inexpensive. The positivity of the Gram
stain depends on the number of organisms in the CSF. The lower limit for detection is about

10^5 colony-forming units per millilitre of CSF, which corresponds to a positive smear in 70%–80% cases of untreated bacterial meningitis. The Gram stain can be obtained directly from a cloudy CSF, but if the CSF is clear, the yield is markedly increased by examining fresh centrifuged sediment.

Acridine orange is a fluorochrome that stains the nucleic acid of some bacteria so that they appear bright red-orange when seen under a fluorescence microscope. It stains the intracellular bacteria better than the Gram stain and may be positive even when the Gram stain is negative.

A positive *CSF culture* is the criterion standard for organism identification. In untreated cases of bacterial meningitis the CSF culture is positive in 70%–80% of cases provided it is directly plated from a fresh specimen. Delayed plating, inadequate storage and transport of CSF, and pretreatment with antibiotics are the main causes of low culture positivity reported from resource-poor countries.

A *blood culture* should be obtained in all cases; high positivity (around 75%) reported from resource-rich countries is not seen in resource-poor countries because pre-hospital antibiotic therapy is common. A positive blood culture helps in organism identification, especially if the CSF culture is negative. In neonates, culture-positive meningitis frequently occurs in the absence of bacteraemia and in the presence of normal CSF parameters; no single CSF value can reliably exclude the presence of meningitis (Garges et al. 2006).

Organism identification should also be attempted by obtaining samples from other sites of infection such as pleural fluid, cellulitis, otitis, aspiration of petechiae in suspected meningococcaemia, and urine in young infants.

Pre-hospital use of antibiotics seriously interferes with detection of bacterial aetiology. Such partially treated cases, wherein the organism cannot be identified and the CSF picture is altered, may be difficult to differentiate from aseptic and tuberculous meningitis. This has been discussed in Chapter 3.

Although most children with viral meningitis show a lymphocytic response, an initial polymorphonuclear response persisting for over 24 hours has been reported in almost half the cases of aseptic meningitis seen in the enteroviral season. On the other hand, about 10% of children with bacterial meningitis can have an initial lymphocytic predominance. The presence and number of band cells in the CSF is not helpful in distinguishing bacterial from aseptic meningitis. The CSF sugar is normal in most cases of viral meningitis, but may be low in some cases; however, it is rarely below 20mg/dL. The presence of a neutrophilic response with hypoglycorrhachia in an acutely sick and toxic-looking child favours the diagnosis of bacterial meningitis.

Several clinical decision rules have been proposed to distinguish bacterial from aseptic meningitis in children with CSF pleocytosis but with no identified organism (Bonsu et al. 2008, Dubos et al. 2009, Nigrovic et al. 2009). However, they should be applied judiciously with a holistic view of the overall clinical condition of the child, and to populations in which they have been validated.

In cases where it is difficult to differentiate between viral and bacterial meningitis, *rapid diagnostic tests* that detect bacterial antigens by countercurrent immuno-electrophoresis

(CIEP), enzyme-linked immunosorbant assay (ELISA) and latex agglutination tests (LATs) are helpful in providing early diagnosis. LAT is more sensitive than CIEP. The LATs for *S. pneumoniae* and *N. meningitidis* have a specificity of 96% and 100% respectively, but a lower sensitivity varying from 69% to 100% for *S. pneumoniae* and from 37% to 70% for *N. meningitidis* (Roos 2000). A negative test does not exclude bacterial meningitis. Bacterial antigen tests are expensive and are not recommended for routine use.

Broad-range real-time bacterial DNA detection polymerase chain reaction (PCR) assays can rapidly detect a large number of viable and non-viable organisms with a sensitivity of 86%–100% and a specificity of 98% as compared to the criterion standard of bacterial culture (Deutch et al. 2006). They may also be helpful for determining the response to antibiotics (Chiba et al. 2009). False-positive tests may occur because of sample contamination, and false-negatives because of the presence of PCR inhibitors. The high cost and lack of availability of these tests limit their use in most resource-poor countries.

OTHER TESTS

• *C-reactive protein (CRP)*. Raised serum CRP above 50mg/dL is a non-specific indicator of bacterial infection. It falls to normal after 1–2 days of antibiotic therapy. Serum levels above 20mg/dL in children under 6 years of age and above 50mg/dL in older children in the presence of CSF pleocytosis indicate bacterial meningitis, but are not foolproof. CRP levels below 40mg/dL may be found in bacterial meningitis; however, where the serum CRP level is less than 10mg/dL, the diagnosis of acute bacterial meningitis is highly unlikely.

• *CSF cytokines*. Increased CSF levels of cytokines are highly sensitive and specific markers for bacterial infection, but have not been consistently proven to discriminate between bacterial and viral meningitis. They are not routinely used.

• *CSF lactate*. Elevated CSF lactate above 4.2mmol/L was reported to have a high sensitivity (96%) and positive predictive value (100%) for bacterial meningitis (Leib et al. 1999). However, it is not very specific and is not used routinely.

• *Procalcitonin (PCT)*. Elevated serum PCT (>5μg/L) has emerged as a sensitive and specific biological marker to differentiate bacterial from viral meningitis. PCT has a better sensitivity (99%), specificity (83%) and predictive value than CRP, leukocyte count, IL-6 and interferon-α (Dubos et al. 2008, Alkholi et al. 2011). However, this may not hold true in bacterial meningitis caused by unusual agents or of nosocomial origin. Elevated PCT level in CSF may be seen in patients with bacterial meningitis who do not have elevated serum PCT concentration. PCT estimation is still experimental and is not available in most resource-poor countries.

• *Other tests*. A CSF concentration of S100B above 3.1ng/mL has been reported to have 100% specificity for bacterial meningitis (Jung et al. 2011). Aquaporin-1 CSF concentrations

TABLE 12.3
Complications of bacterial meningitis

Early	*Long-term sequelae*
• Raised ICP	• Hydrocephalus
• Disseminated intravascular coagulation	• Cranial nerve palsies
• Seizures and status epilepticus	• Sensorineural deafness
• Subdural empyema	• Motor deficits
• Infarcts, cerebritis, brain abscess	
• Spread of infection to distant sites (pneumonia, pericarditis, arthritis, osteomyelitis)	
• Cranial nerve involvement	
• Diabetes insipidus	

have also been reported to be increased in bacterial meningitis (Blocher et al. 2011). However, these tests remain experimental.

Peripheral WBC count is elevated in most but not all cases of meningitis; it cannot be used as an indicator of meningitis.

Although useful, inflammatory markers (CRP, CSF lactate, PCT) by themselves cannot accurately discriminate bacterial from viral meningitis as they may not be elevated in the early stages of bacterial infection and may be elevated in some viral infections.

The *limulus amoebocyte lysate test* is a sensitive and specific test for detection of gram-negative endotoxin in CSF and can be used for diagnosis of gram-negative bacterial meningitis; however, it does not differentiate between specific gram-negative organisms, and can yield false negatives; it is not routinely used.

Course and complications

With appropriate antibiotic and supportive therapy, clinical improvement is generally seen within 48–72 hours, and the fever comes down within 4–5 days in uncomplicated cases. Fever may last for up to 10 days with *H. influenzae* meningitis. Persistent fever (lasting for over 10 days) in children with meningitis may be due to thrombophlebitis, subdural effusions, concomitant or distant spread of infection (such as pneumonia, arthritis or osteomyelitis), drug fever and, rarely, resistant organisms. Fever that recurs after 24 hours of an afebrile period may be caused by nosocomial infections or complications. Complications in meningitis may occur in the early phase when they are usually reversible, or as late events that usually cause permanent neurological damage. The common complications are listed in Table 12.3.

RAISED INTRACRANIAL PRESSURE
The majority of children requiring hospitalization for bacterial meningitis, particularly those with a Glasgow Coma Scale (GCS) score below 7, have raised ICP at the time of admission that needs aggressive management. In a study from India, almost half of the children with

meningitis who needed intensive care had signs of raised ICP either at or within 48 hours of admission (Singhi et al. 2004). The increase in ICP is associated with deepening coma and pupillary, respiratory and blood pressure changes. Cerebral herniation was seen on autopsy in 30% of children dying of meningitis. Early increase in ICP is primarily due to cytotoxic and vasogenic oedema; later in the disease, it may be because of obstructive or communicating hydrocephalus.

SEIZURES AND STATUS EPILEPTICUS

About one-third of affected children, particularly those with severe illness, have seizures. Early seizures (in the first 2–3 days) are due to cortical irritation secondary to the inflammatory process and fever, and at times because of electrolyte and other metabolic disturbances; they generally cease within 1–3 days and do not warrant prolonged anticonvulsant therapy, especially if the electroencephalogram recorded at the end of antibiotic therapy is normal. Late-onset seizures are associated with underlying structural damage such as infarct, and require anticonvulsant therapy for several months.

SUBDURAL EFFUSIONS

Benign subdural effusions are seen in almost 50% of affected children, especially infants, and in Hib meningitis; they resolve spontaneously and do not require any active intervention. Drainage is indicated in cases with persistent or recurrent fever, or raised ICP, focal signs or subdural empyema. Subdural effusion was found in 25% of children with meningitis; about a quarter of them required drainage (Singhi et al. 2004).

CEREBRITIS AND INFARCTION

These may occur secondary to vasculitis or direct spread of infection from the subarachnoid space to the brain. They present with new focal features and may progress to form a cerebral abscess.

VENTRICULITIS

Ventriculitis occurs particularly in neonates and infants; it presents with persistent fever and is diagnosed by ultrasound or CT and confirmed by a ventricular tap. Prolonged systemic antibiotics, and at times intraventricular antibiotics, are required. CSF drainage may be needed if there is associated hydrocephalus and raised ICP.

CRANIAL NERVE INVOLVEMENT

The cranial nerves may be involved directly in the inflammatory process or secondary to pressure and stretching because of the raised ICP; the VIIIth, VIth and IIIrd nerves are usually involved; palsies of the eye usually recover.

SENSORINEURAL DEAFNESS

Sensorineural deafness occurs in 5%–30% of affected children, especially those with pneumococcal meningitis. It is generally underestimated unless formal hearing evaluation is routinely done. It is often bilateral and occurs because of bacterial involvement of the cochlea through the internal auditory canal or via haematogenous spread. Low CSF glucose, use of ototoxic antibiotics and a low GCS score are reported high-risk factors. Abnormalities in the brainstem evoked responses (BSERs) occur within days and generally resolve at the end of the first 2 weeks but major deficits may persist. Formal hearing assessment by BSER or audiometry must be done at the time of discharge.

HYDROCEPHALUS

Ventriculomegaly with raised ICP can occasionally occur in the early phase of meningitis. It is caused by increased CSF production coupled with decreased CSF absorption by the arachnoid villi, and often decreases over a period of time. Persistent obstructive hydrocephalus requiring a shunt can occur in some children secondary to inflammatory obstruction of the CSF pathways.

DIABETES INSPIDUS

Dysfunction of the hypothalamic–pituitary axis secondary to ischaemia may complicate meningitis, and lead to diabetes insipidus. It generally occurs in severely ill children. The child may rapidly become hypovolaemic, with marked hypernatraemia and seizures.

DISSEMINATED INTRAVASCULAR COAGULATION

This may occur with fulminant meningococcal and gram-negative infections, and in neonates, and requires aggressive therapy.

OTHER COMPLICATIONS

Spread of infection leading to pneumonia, pericarditis, arthritis and osteomyelitis may rarely occur.

Neuroimaging in meningitis

Meningitis is diagnosed by CSF analysis in association with a suggestive clinical presentation. CT is not routinely required at presentation in a child with uncomplicated meningitis; it is primarily needed to exclude other pathologies in a child with focal neurological signs. In the early stage of meningitis, CT is often normal or may show cerebral oedema, meningeal enhancement and widening of basal cisterns. However, these findings do not affect therapeutic decisions. Later in the illness CT is conducted to look for complications in a child who does not show clinical improvement, has sudden unexplained deterioration, new onset seizures or focal neurological signs, signs of raised ICP, persistent fever or enlarging head. Common findings in such cases include subdural effusions, infarct, hydrocephalus, and at times cerebritis or cerebral abscess. MRI may be needed occasionally as it often detects parenchymal complications earlier than CT; if cerebral venous sinus thrombosis is suspected, magnetic resonance venography is required.

In neonates and in infants with open fontanelle, ultrasonography of the head plays an important role in initial evaluation and in early detection of complications; meningeal thickening, echogenic widening of sulci and hyperaemia suggest meningitis; extra-axial collections and hydrocephalus are easily detected. Intraventricular strands, loculations, debris and irregular echogenic ependyma suggest ventriculitis (Yikilmaz and Taylor 2008); further confirmation can be done by CT.

Treatment

Early institution of appropriate antimicrobial and supportive therapy is the cornerstone of management. In critically ill children, therapy needs to be started within minutes of hospitalization. Most deaths caused by bacterial meningitis occur during the first 48 hours of hospitalization. Coma, raised ICP, seizures and shock are significant predictors of death and morbidity. All children with meningitis must be observed and monitored so that acute life-threatening complications such as shock or raised ICP can be recognized and managed early. This is best done in a paediatric intensive care unit (PICU) until the child is haemodynamically and neurologically stable. In resource-poor situations with limited intensive-care facilities, prioritization of admission to the PICU can be done based on criteria that indicate a severe illness.

ANTIMICROBIAL THERAPY

Antibiotics are usually administered after obtaining CSF, blood, throat swab and other samples for bacterial culture. However, in critically ill children and in situations where there is a delay in obtaining samples, the initial dose(s) of antibiotics should be given and samples obtained later. Early antibiotic therapy prevents clinical deterioration and reduces mortality and morbidity. Antibiotics are given intravenously unless IV access is not possible, in which case they can be used intramuscularly until IV access is obtained. In a study on 723 African children with meningitis, continuous infusion of cefotaxime for the first 24 hours and paracetamol was reported to reduce mortality, particularly in pneumococcal meningitis (Pelkonen et al. 2011).

The initial empiric antibiotic therapy should be broad enough to cover all the likely pathogens according to the age of the child, any underlying predisposing conditions, and the prevalent epidemiology and resistance patterns of organisms. Bactericidal antibiotics that achieve high CSF concentration are preferred as they cause more effective sterilization of CSF and also improve survival in comparison to bacteriostatic drugs. The choice of antibiotics according to age is shown in Table 12.1. Other antibiotics may be added according to underlying risk factors (Table 12.2). Ceftriaxone has become affordable in most resource-poor countries and has been recommended by the WHO (1997) as first-line therapy for treatment of bacterial meningitis in Africa. A combination of ampicillin (300mg/kg/d, given 6 hourly) and chloramphenicol (100mg/kg/d given 6 hourly) may be used if financial constraints prevent the use of cephalosporins. An overview of Cochrane systematic reviews found no significant difference between cephalosporins and a combination of ampicillin and chloramphenicol in the combined end-points of death or deafness (Prasad et al. 2009). However, culture positivity of CSF at 10–48 hours was significantly higher in the conventional antibiotic group, and diarrhoea was significantly more common in the cephalosporin group. Also, most of the studies included were conducted in the 1980s when the incidence of penicillin and chloramphenicol resistance was low. *H. influenzae* resistant to ampicillin and chloramphenicol, and pneumococci resistant to penicillin and chloramphenicol and even to ceftriaxone, are being increasingly reported from Africa and Asia (Mwangi et al. 2002). Newer antibiotics such as meropenem and faropenem that have a good CSF penetration and are effective against gram-positive and gram-negative bacteria are being explored. Fluoroquinolones have been used in multi-drug-resistant meningitis but are best avoided in children because of their adverse effect on growing cartilage.

As soon as the organism is isolated on culture, and its susceptibility determined, antibiotic therapy is targeted accordingly (Table 12.4). If no organisms are isolated, the initial antibiotics should be continued for at least 7 days.

The duration of antibiotic therapy depends on the organism isolated. The standard recommendation is 10–14 days for *S. pneumoniae* and *H. influenzae*, 7 days for *N. meningitidis*, and a minimum of 3 weeks in gram-negative, group B streptococcus and *Listeria* meningitis. Shorter durations of antibiotic therapy have also been found effective. Ceftriaxone therapy was as effective when given for 7 days as for 10 days in children over 3 months of age with uncomplicated meningitis (Singhi et al. 2002). Ceftriaxone treatment given over 4 days was found to be as effective as 7 days' treatment in infants with signs of rapid recovery (Roine et al. 2000). A recent large randomized double-blind study of 5 versus 10 days of ceftriaxone treatment conducted in six resource-poor countries found no significant difference in outcome of children (beyond the neonatal period) with uncomplicated bacterial meningitis due to Hib, pneumococci or meningococci, who were stable on day 5 of treatment. According to this study ceftriaxone can be safely discontinued in such children after 5 days of treatment (Molyneux et al. 2011). However, the study did not assess organism-specific data, and about a third of the children in the study had no organisms grown. The results of the study cannot be generalized. Perhaps in resource-poor countries where the cost of therapy is an issue, there is a case for stopping ceftriaxone in a child who is 'clinically stable' on day 5 of therapy and has meningitis caused by Hib, pneumococci or meningococci; the same cannot be recommended universally.

With appropriate antibiotic therapy, the CSF culture and Gram stain become negative within 24–48 hours. The CSF glucose generally normalizes over 72 hours. The increase in cells and proteins may persist for several days. A repeat lumbar puncture either during treatment or at the end of therapy is not routinely needed if a child has improved and is afebrile. In cases of neonatal and gram-negative meningitis a repeat lumbar puncture may be required as a 'test of cure'.

Indications for repeat lumbar puncture on appropriate antibiotic therapy are as follows.

1 Lack of clinical improvement after 3–4 days.
2 Resistant/unusual organisms grown on initial CSF, and no clinical improvement within 24–48 hours of specific therapy.
3 Appearance of new symptoms or signs.
4 Unexplained persistent fever after several days.

TABLE 12.4
Targeted antibiotic therapy in bacterial meningitis

Organisms	Standard antibiotic	Other choices
Streptococcus pneumoniae		
Penicillin-sensitive	Penicillin (or ampicillin)	Ceftriaxone/cefotaxime
Penicillin-resistant		
Ceftriaxone/cefotaxime-sensitive	Ceftriaxone/cefotaxime	Cefipime, meropenem, fluoroquinolones, chloramphenicol
Partially sensitive to ceftriaxone	Vancomycin plus ceftriaxone/cefotaxime	Fluoroquinolones
Neissera meningitidis		
Penicillin-sensitive	Penicillin G (or ampicillin)	Ceftriaxone/cefotaxime
Penicillin-resistant	Ceftriaxone/cefotaxime fluoroquinolones, chloramphenicol	Meropenem
Haemophilus influenzae		
Ampicillin-sensitive	Ampicillin	Ceftriaxone/cefotaxime
Ampicillin-resistant		
Non-β-lactamase-producing	Ceftriaxone/cefotaxime	Cefipime, meropenem, fluoroquinolones, chloramphenicol
β-lactamase-producing	High-dose ceftriaxone with meropenem	Fluoroquinolones
Group B streptococcus (*Streptococcus agalactae*)	Penicillin G or ampicillin	Ceftriaxone/cefotaxime
Listeria monocytogenes	Ampicillin or penicillin G sulphamethoxazole, meropenem	Trimethoprim
Gram-negative bacilli		
E. coli, Klebsiella spp., others	Ceftriaxone/cefotaxime with aminoglycosides or meropenem	Ciprofloxacin, aztreonam, cefipime, meropenem, fluoroquinolones
Pseudomonas spp.	Cefipime, ceftazidime	Ciprofloxacin, aztreonam, meropenems
Staphylococcus aureus		
Methicillin-sensitive	Cloxacillin, oxacillin, flucloxacillin, nafcillin	Vancomycin, meropenem, linezolid, trimethoprim
Methicillin-resistant	Vancomycin, rifampin	Sulphamethoxazole
Staphylococcus epidermidis	Vancomycin	Linezolid

Note: In countries where facilities for measuring minimal inhibitory concentration are available, antibiotic therapy can be decided accordingly (Tunkel et al. 2004).

SUPPORTIVE MANAGEMENT

This is of vital importance and is described in detail in Chapter 3. To summarize, in all children with meningitis, urgent attention towards airway, breathing and circulation (ABCs) is needed to ensure haemodynamic stability. The level of supportive care depends upon the severity of illness. About a third of children need endotracheal intubation and supplemental oxygen (Singhi et al. 2004) for indications such as GCS score below 8, pharyngeal hypotonia, poor gag reflex and loss of swallowing reflex.

Immediate management of shock, raised ICP, seizures and status epilepticus is warranted whenever any of these occur. Refractory status epilepticus is common in severe meningitis and needs meticulous management.

FLUID AND ELECTROLYTE THERAPY

Enough fluids should be given to maintain normovolaemia and normal blood pressure and thereby adequate cerebral perfusion. Restriction of fluids should be done only if there is evidence of inappropriate secretion of antidiuretic hormone.

Hyponatraemia, if present, should be corrected slowly over 36–48 hours with normal saline; occasionally 3% saline may be needed. Hypokalaemia may occur secondary to gastrointestinal losses, haemodilution, osmotherapy, diuretic therapy and associated septicaemia. Early recognition and prompt treatment are essential.

CORTICOSTEROID THERAPY

The American Academy of Pediatrics Committee on Infectious Diseases (1990), the Canadian Pediatric Society (2008), the European Federation of Neurological Sciences (Chaudhuri et al. 2008) and the National Institute for Health and Clinical Excellence (NICE 2010) recommend the use of dexamethasone in *H. influenzae* and pneumococcal meningitis in children over 3 months of age (over 6 months of age in the USA). A dose of 0.4mg/kg given 12 hourly for 2 days has been found to be as effective as one of 0.15mg/kg given every 6 hours for 4 days (Odio et al. 1991). To be effective, steroids must be given before or with the first dose of antibiotics. However, the use of corticosteroids has been debated (see details in Chapter 3). Although corticosteroids have been found to reduce hearing loss and neurological sequelae, they do not reduce overall mortality. No beneficial effect of corticosteroid therapy has been found in resource-poor countries (Sankar et al. 2007, Brouwer et al. 2013). Also, when dexamethasone is used, clinicians must be vigilant because the presentation of underlying infections such as brain abscess, tuberculous meningitis or meningitis due to resistant bacteria may be masked by steroids. Hence steroids cannot be recommended for routine use in resource-poor countries (Singhi and Singhi 2008). With a dramatic decrease of Hib and pneumococcal meningitis in resource-rich countries following immunization, the routine use of corticosteroids in these countries also needs re-evaluation.

GLYCEROL

The use of oral glycerol for the first 48 hours (6g/kg/d given 6 hourly) has been found to reduce neurological sequelae in children with bacterial meningitis in a large, multicentre, randomized trial (Peltola et al. 2007, Peltola and Roine 2009). The effect was clearest in Hib meningitis. However, it did not prevent profound hearing loss. A Cochrane analysis of the use of osmotic agents in bacterial meningitis concluded that glycerol does not reduce mortality but may reduce hearing loss; however, glycerol is not routinely recommended (Wall et al. 2013).

OTHER THERAPIES FOR MODULATING INFLAMMATORY PATHWAYS

Various novel interventions – e.g. iNOS (inducible nitric oxide synthase) inhibition, endothelin agonists, antioxidants, neurotrophins, glutamate antagonists, tumour necrosis factor neutralization, matrix metalloproteinase inhibition and caspase inhibition – have been tried to improve the outcome of bacterial meningitis. However, all the agents used are still experimental (Woehrl et al. 2011).

The role of intravenous immunoglobulin is limited to children with immune-deficient states and in some cases of neonatal meningitis.

Prognosis

The mortality rates of meningitis continue to be high, at 15%–20%. Acute mortality from meningitis may occur because of critically raised ICP, extensive cerebral infarction, disseminated intravascular coagulation, and/or circulatory failure resulting from septic shock and refractory status epilepticus. Neurological sequelae are common and include hearing loss, hydrocephalus, spasticity, visual and cognitive deficits, and developmental delay. A GCS score below 7 and complicated meningitis with abnormal neuroimaging are associated with a higher risk of sequelae (Singhi et al. 2007). Hearing deficits and neurological sequelae correlated with high serum cortisol and high blood pressure (Singhi and Bansal 2006, Holub et al. 2007).

Coma, raised ICP, status epilepticus, shock and respiratory depression are important predictors of mortality and morbidity in children with acute bacterial meningitis (Singhi et al. 2004, Peltola and Roine 2009). Early diagnosis and urgent management can prevent and/or minimize the mortality and morbidity.

Prevention

INFECTION CONTROL

To prevent secondary meningitis, children with Hib or meningococcal meningitis should be isolated until they have received 24 hours of appropriate antibiotics.

CHEMOPROPHYLAXIS

For Hib meningitis, rifampicin prophylaxis (20mg/kg/d given once daily for 4 days) is recommended for all household contacts if there is at least one unvaccinated contact under 4 years old. Rifampicin prophylaxis before discharge is also needed for the index child if ampicillin and/or chloramphenicol were used, as they do not eradicate *H. influenzae*; it is not needed if ceftriaxone was used.

For meningococcal disease, rifampicin prophylaxis (10mg/kg every 12 hours for 2 days) is recommended for household and day-care contacts to prevent secondary cases and to reduce nasopharyngeal carriage. Ceftriaxone as a single intramuscular dose (125mg for children under 12 years and 250mg for older children and adults) has been found to be better than oral rifampicin for eliminating meningococcal group A nasopharyngeal carriage. Ciprofloxacin 500mg or azithromycin 500mg, in a single dose, may be used for adults. Chemoprophylaxis of pregnant women (found to be carriers of group B streptococci on screening) with amoxicillin is recommended to reduce the incidence of early-onset neonatal group B streptococcal disease (Daily et al. 2009).

VACCINATION

Universal immunization against *H. influenzae*, *Pneumococcus* and *Meningococcus* group C still needs to be implemented in many resource-poor countries. The Hib conjugate vaccines have a 70%–100% protective efficacy against meningitis and have virtually eradicated Hib meningitis in countries where Hib is a part of the routine immunization programme.

For meningococcus, several types of vaccines are available: polysaccharide vaccines – available in bivalent (groups A and C), trivalent (groups A, C and W135) and tetravalent (groups A, C, W135 and Y) forms; and conjugate vaccines against groups A and C (WHO 2011). The tetravalent vaccine is poorly immunogenic in children under 2 years of age. Since 2005 it has been used routinely in the USA and Canada for immunization of adolescents and persons at high risk of meningococcal meningitis. Conjugate serogroup C vaccine has been successfully used in several universal immunization programmes in resource-rich countries. It is strongly immunogenic and also confers herd immunity. It has significantly decreased the meningococcal C meningitis and nasopharyngeal carrier rates in areas where it has been used. A low-cost conjugate meningococcal serogroup A vaccine was introduced in December 2010 for use in Africa, and in 2011 the lowest number of confirmed meningitis cases ever were recorded during an epidemic season (WHO 2011). Serogroup B vaccine is poorly immunogenic. An outer membrane vesicle (OMV) vaccine against serogroup B has been found to be effective. The OMV vaccines are useful for epidemics as they can be specifically targeted against the predominant strain during an epidemic.

Two types of pneumococcal vaccines are currently available: (1) a 23-valent polysaccharide vaccine (PPV23); and (2) conjugate vaccines, which are either 10-valent (PPV10) or 13-valent (PPV13). The 7-valent vaccine is gradually being removed from the market (WHO 2012).

The 10-valent and 13-valent pneumococcal vaccines are equally effective for their respective serotypes and have been licensed for use in the USA and UK since 2010, and are included in their universal immunization programmes. The 23-valent polysaccharide pneumococcal vaccine is poorly immunogenic in children under 2 years of age; it is used in some resource-rich countries for immunocompromised patients at high risk of pneumococcal meningitis. Further development of vaccines that cover more serotypes is in the pipeline. In resource-poor countries, these vaccines could be used in special high-risk situations until such time as widespread immunization becomes feasible. Conjugate group B streptococcal vaccines are being tried in women of childbearing age to prevent neonatal infections.

Concerted global effort at implementing mass immunization programmes against the common pathogens causing meningitis is essential for prevention. The WHO has introduced a new vaccine policy to improve vaccine availability in resource-poor countries as a part of the United Nations Millennium Development Goal 4 and recommends the use of Hib and pneumococcal conjugate vaccine for all children in these countries (WHO 2008, 2012).

REFERENCES

Alkholi UM, Abd Al-Monem N, Abd El-Azim AA, Sultan MH (2011) Serum procalcitonin in viral and bacterial meningitis. *J Glob Infect Dis* 3: 14–18.

American Academy of Pediatrics Committee on Infectious Diseases (1990) Dexamethasone therapy for bacterial meningitis in infants and children. *Pediatrics* 86: 130–3.

Berkley JA, Versteeg AC, Mwangi I, et al. (2004) Indicators of acute bacterial meningitis in children at a rural Kenyan district hospital. *Pediatrics* 114: e713–9.

Best J, Hughes S (2008) Evidence behind the WHO Guidelines: hospital care for children—what are the useful clinical features of bacterial meningitis found in infants and children? *J Trop Pediatr* 54: 83–6.

Blocher J, Eckert I, Elster J, et al. (2011) Aquaporins AQP1 and AQP4 in the cerebrospinal fluid of bacterial meningitis patients. *Neurosci Lett* 10: 23–7.

Bonsu BK, Ortega HW, Marcon MJ, Harper MB (2008) A decision rule for predicting bacterial meningitis in children with cerebrospinal fluid pleocytosis when Gram stain is negative or unavailable. *Acad Emerg Med* 15: 437–44.

Brouwer MC, McIntyre P, Prasad K, van de Beek D (2013) Corticosteroids for acute bacterial meningitis. *Cochrane Database Syst Rev* 6: CD004405. doi: 0.1002/14651858.CD004405.pub4.

Canadian Pediatric Society (2008) Therapy of suspected bacterial meningitis in Canadian children six weeks of age and older – summary. *Pediatr Child Health* 13: 309.

Chaudhuri A, Martinez-Martin P, Kennedy PG, et al. (2008) EFNS guidelines on the management of community-acquired bacterial meningitis: report of an EFNS task force on acute bacterial meningitis in older children and adults. *Eur J Neurol* 15: 649–59.

Chiba N, Murayama SY, Morozumi M, et al. (2009) Rapid detection of eight causative pathogens for the diagnosis of bacterial meningitis by realtime PCR. *J Infect Chemother* 15: 92–8.

Chin RF, Neville BG, Scott RC (2005) Meningitis is a common cause of convulsive status epilepticus with fever. *Arch Dis Child* 90: 66–9.

Daily P, Aragon D, Burnite S, et al. (2009) Trends in perinatal group B streptococcal disease – United States, 2000–2006. *MMWR Morb Mortal Wkly Rep* 58: 109–12.

Deutch S, Pedersen LN, Pødenphant L, et al. (2006) Broad-range real time PCR and DNA sequencing for the diagnosis of bacterial meningitis. *Scand J Infect Dis* 38: 27–35.

Dubos F, Korczowski B, Aygun DA, et al. (2008) Serum procalcitonin level and other biological markers to distinguish between bacterial and aseptic meningitis in children: a European multicenter case cohort study. *Arch Pediatr Adolesc Med* 162: 1157–63.

Dubos F, Martinot A, Gendrel D, et al. (2009) Clinical decision rules for evaluating meningitis in children. *Curr Opin Neurol* 22: 288–93.

Focke NK, Kallenberg K, Mohr A, et al. (2013) Distributed, limbic gray matter atrophy in patients after bacterial meningitis. *AJNR Am J Neuroradiol* 34: 1164–7.

Furyk JS, Swann O, Molyneux E (2011) Systematic review: neonatal meningitis in the developing world. *Trop Med Int Health* 16: 672–9.

Garges HP, Moody MA, Cotten CM, et al. (2006) Neonatal meningitis: what is the correlation among cerebrospinal fluid cultures, blood cultures, and cerebrospinal fluid parameters? *Pediatrics* 117: 1094–100.

Georget-Bouquinet E, Bingen E, Aujard Y, et al. (2008) Group B streptococcal meningitis: clinical, biological and evolutive features in children. *Arch Pediatr* 15 Suppl 3: S126–32.

Greenberg RG, Smith PB, Cotten CM, et al. (2008) Traumatic lumbar punctures in neonates: test performance of the cerebrospinal fluid white blood cell count. *Pediatr Infect Dis J* 27: 1047–51.

Hofer S, Grandgirard D, Burri D, et al. (2011) Bacterial meningitis impairs hippocampal neurogenesis. *J Neuropathol Exp Neurol* 70: 890–9.

Holub M, Beran O, Dzupová O, et al. (2007) Cortisol levels in cerebrospinal fluid correlate with severity and bacterial origin of meningitis. *Crit Care* 11: R41.

Jung K, Goerdt C, Lange P, et al. (2011) The use of S100B and Tau protein concentrations in the cerebrospinal fluid for the differential diagnosis of bacterial meningitis: a retrospective analysis. *Eur Neurol* 66: 128–32.

Leib SL, Boscacci R, Gratzl O, Zimmerli W (1999) Predictive value of cerebrospinal fluid (CSF) lactate level versus CSF/blood glucose ratio for the diagnosis of bacterial meningitis following neurosurgery. *Clin Infect Dis* 29: 69–74.

Levy C, Bingen E, Aujard Y, et al. (2008) Surveillance network of bacterial meningitis in children, 7 years of survey in France. *Arch Pediatr* 15 Suppl 3: S99–S104.

Mazor SS, McNulty JE, Roosevelt GE (2003) Interpretation of traumatic lumbar punctures: who can go home? *Pediatrics* 111: 525–8.

Molyneux E, Nizami SQ, Saha S, et al. (2011) 5 versus 10 days of treatment with ceftriaxone for bacterial meningitis in children: a double-blind randomised equivalence study. *Lancet* 377: 1837–45.

Mwangi I, Berkerly J, Lowe B, et al. (2002) Acute bacterial meningitis in children admitted to a rural Kenyan hospital: increasing antibiotic resistance and outcome. *Ped Infec Dis J* 21: 1042–8.

Mwaniki MK, Talbert AW, Njuguna P, et al. (2011) Clinical indicators of bacterial meningitis among neonates and young infants in rural Kenya. *BMC Infect Dis* 11: 301.

Neuman MI, Tolford S, Harper MB (2008) Test characteristics and interpretation of cerebrospinal fluid Gram stain in children. *Pediatr Infect Dis J* 27: 309–13.

NICE (2010) Management of bacterial meningitis and meningococcal septicaemia in children and young people younger than 16 years in primary and secondary care. Clinical Guideline 102 (online: http://www.nice.org.uk/guidance/CG102).

Nigrovic LE, Malley R, Macias CG, et al. (2008) Effect of antibiotic pretreatment on cerebrospinal fluid profiles of children with bacterial meningitis. *Pediatrics* 122: 726–30.

Nigrovic LE, Malley R, Kuppermann N (2009) Cerebrospinal fluid pleocytosis in children in the era of bacterial conjugate vaccines: distinguishing the child with bacterial and aseptic meningitis. *Pediatr Emerg Care* 25: 112–7.

Odio CM, Faingezicht I, Paris M, et al. (1991) The beneficial effects of early dexamethasone administration in infants and children with bacterial meningitis. *N Engl J Med* 324: 1525–31.

Pelkonen T, Roine I, Cruzeiro ML, et al. (2011) Slow initial β-lactam infusion and oral paracetamol to treat childhood bacterial meningitis: a randomised, controlled trial. *Lancet Infect Dis* 11: 613–21.

Peltola H, Roine I (2009) Improving the outcomes in children with bacterial meningitis. *Curr Opin Infect Dis* 22: 250–5.

Peltola H, Roine I, Fernández J, et al. (2007) Adjuvant glycerol and/or dexamethasone to improve the outcomes of childhood bacterial meningitis. A prospective, randomized, double-blind, placebo-controlled trial. *Clin Infect Dis* 45: 1277–86.

Prasad K, Karlupia N, Kumar A (2009) Treatment of bacterial meningitis: an overview of Cochrane systematic reviews. *Respir Med* 103: 945–50.

Roine I, Ledermann W, Foncea LM, et al. (2000) Randomized trial of four vs. seven days of ceftriaxone treatment for bacterial meningitis in children with rapid initial recovery. *Ped Infect Dis J* 19: 219–22.

Roos KL (2000) Acute bacterial meningitis. *Semin Neurol* 20: 293–306.

Sankar J, Singhi P, Bansal A, et al. (2007) Role of dexamethasone and oral glycerol in reducing hearing and neurological sequelae in children with bacterial meningitis. *Indian Pediatr* 44: 649–56.

Scarborough M, Thwaites GE (2008) The diagnosis and management of acute bacterial meningitis in resource-poor settings. *Lancet Neurol* 7: 637–48.

Singhi P, Kaushal M, Singhi S, Ray M (2002) Seven days vs ten days therapy for bacterial meningitis in children. *J Trop Pediatr* 48: 273–9.

Singhi P, Bansal A, Geeta P, Singhi S (2007) Predictors of long term neurological outcome in bacterial meningitis. *Indian J Pediatr* 74: 369–74.

Singhi S, Singhi P (2008) Glycerol and dexamethasone in bacterial meningitis in low-income countries: response to the editorial commentary by Sáez-Llorens and McCracken Jr. *Clin Infect Dis* 47: 732–3; author reply 733–4. doi: 10.1086/590971.

Singhi S, Khetarpal R, Baranwal AK, Singhi PD (2004) Intensive care needs of children with acute bacterial meningitis: a developing country perspective. *Ann Trop Pediatr* 24: 133–40.

Singhi SC, Bansal A (2006) Serum cortisol levels in children with acute bacterial and aseptic meningitis. *Pediatr Crit Care Med* 7: 74–8.

Thigpen MC, Whitney CG, Messonnier NE, et al. (2011) Bacterial meningitis in the United States, 1998–2007. *N Engl J Med* 364: 2016–25.

Tunkel AR, Hartman BJ, Kaplan SL, et al. (2004) Practice guidelines for the management of bacterial meningitis. *Clin Infect Dis* 39: 1267–84.

Wall EC, Ajdukiewicz KM, Heyderman RS, Garner P (2013) Osmotic therapies added to antibiotics for acute bacterial meningitis. *Cochrane Database Syst Rev* 3: CD008806. doi: 10.1002/14651858.CD008806.pub2.

Weber MW, Herman J, Jaffar S, et al. (2002) Clinical predictors of bacterial meningitis in infants and young children in The Gambia. *Trop Med Int Health* 7: 722–31.

WHO (1997) Guidelines for research and management of non epidemic meningitis in children. Recommendations from a WHO meeting, Geneva, June 16–19. Geneva: World Health Organization.

WHO (2012) Pneumococcal vaccines: WHO position paper – 2012. Wkly Epidemiol Rec 87: 129–44 (online: http://www.who.int/wer/2012/wer8714.pdf).

WHO (2008) Progress introducing *Haemophilus influenza* type b vaccine in low-income countries, 2004–2008. *Wkly Epidemiol Rec* 83: 61–8.

WHO (2011) Meningococcal meningitis (online: http://www.who.int/immunization/topics/meningitis/en).

Woehrl B, Klein M, Grandgirard D, et al. (2011) Bacterial meningitis: current therapy and possible future treatment options. *Expert Rev Anti Infect Ther* 9: 1053–65.

Yikilmaz A, Taylor GA (2008) Sonographic findings in bacterial meningitis in neonates and young infants. *Pediatr Radiol* 38: 129–37.

Zaidi Ak, Thaver D, Ali SA, Khan TA (2009) Pathogens associated with sepsis in newborns and young infants in developing countries. *Pediatr Infect Dis J* 28 (1 Suppl): S10–8.

13
FOCAL INTRACRANIAL SUPPURATION

Pratibha Singhi

Collections of pus can occur in all compartments of the central nervous system (CNS). Focal intracranial suppuration in children is commonly seen in resource-poor countries. Although it is potentially lethal and has a high morbidity, particularly when the diagnosis is delayed, the increased availability of potent antibiotics and newer neuroimaging techniques has reduced the incidence, mortality and morbidity of intracranial suppuration especially in resource-rich countries. However, increasing survival of immune-compromised children vulnerable to such infections has to some extent nullified the decrease in incidence. In this chapter, the common bacterial suppurative lesions of the CNS are discussed.

Brain abscess
Brain abscesses are focal infections of the brain parenchyma that may be bacterial, tubercular, fungal or parasitic; only bacterial brain abscess will be discussed in this chapter. The mortality and morbidity of brain abscess continues to be high in spite of potent antibiotics, particularly in cases with delayed diagnosis.

Epidemiology
Bacterial brain abscesses have become rare in most developed countries (0.3–1.3 per 100 000 people per year), because of prompt treatment of orofacial, ear and sinus infections; however, they are not uncommon in resource-poor countries.

Aetiology
The common pathogens include streptococci, staphylococci, gram-negative organisms and anaerobic bacteria; several unusual aerobic and anaerobic organisms may also cause brain abscess. In neonates, gram-negative organisms, particularly *Citrobacter diversus* and *Proteus mirabilis*, are common pathogens. The causative organisms of the abscess are determined mainly by the underlying/predisposing condition, which is present in almost 80% of patients (Table 13.1). Polymicrobial sepsis is seen in about a third of patients.

Pathogenesis
Brain abscess usually develops in a compromised area of the brain. The organisms reach the brain parenchyma by haematogenous route, by contiguous spread from an adjacent infected focus, or by direct implantation secondary to trauma or a neurosurgical procedure. Haematogenous spread may occur in any child with bacteraemia; it is common in children with

TABLE 13.1
Likely pathogens and location of bacterial brain abscesses according to underlying condition or predisposing factor

Underlying condition/ predisposing factor	Number and location of abscess(es)	Likely pathogens
Neonate	Multiple, bilateral	Gram-negative organisms (*Escherichia coli, Citrobacter, Proteus, Klebsiella* spp.)
Cyanotic congenital heart disease	Multiple, region of middle cerebral artery	*Streptococcus viridans, Staphylococcus aureus*, microaerophillic streptococci, *Haemophilus* spp.
Endocarditis	Multiple, region of middle cerebral artery	*Streptococcus viridans, Staphylococcus aureus*, microaerophillic streptococci, *Haemophilus* spp.
Otitis media	Single, temporal (in older children), cerebellar (in younger children)	Streptococci (aerobic and anaerobic), *Bacteroides fragilis, Staphylococcus aureus, Haemophilus* spp., *Proteus* spp., anaerobic bacteria, *Pseudomonas* spp.
Sinusitis	Single, frontal	Streptococci (aerobic and anaerobic), *Bacteroides* spp., *Staphylococcus aureus, Haemophilis* spp., anaerobic bacteria, *Pseudomonas* spp.
Pulmonary infections	Multiple, any lobe	Streptococci, staphylococci, anaerobic bacteria
Facial and scalp infections	Single/multiple frontal	*Staphylococcus aureus*
Dental infections/ operations	Single/multiple frontal	Anaerobic bacteria, streptococci (aerobic and anaerobic), *Staphylococcus aureus*
Ventriculoperitoneal shunts	Near site of insertion	*Staphylococcus aureus, Staphylococcus epidermidis*
Penetrating skull injury	Near site of injury	*Staphylococcus aureus, Staphylococcus epidermidis*, streptococci, Enterobacteriaceae
Meningitis	Single or multiple, any location	Organisms causing the underlying meningitis
Malnutrition and immunosuppressed states	Multiple, scattered	*Staphylococcus aureus*, gram-negative organisms, anaerobic organisms, unusual organisms

cyanotic congenital heart disease, particularly tetralogy of Fallot. Microinfarcts secondary to polycythaemia with increased blood viscosity make the cerebral parenchyma vulnerable to bacterial seeding. Subacute bacterial endocarditis, chronic pulmonary infection, malnutrition and an immune-compromised state are other predisposing factors. Haematogenous spread may also occur via the draining veins; this occurs with orofacial infections and occasionally with sinus infections. Direct spread of infection may occur from chronic otitis, mastoiditis, sinusitis, and rarely from infected dermal sinuses, epidermoid cysts and encephaloceles. Although brain abscess secondary to meningitis is uncommon, it can be seen in children with gram-negative meningitis and in those with delayed treatment.

Following haematogenous infection, the pathogens localize in the poorly vascularized areas of the brain such as the grey–white junction and cause cerebritis. The inflammation and oedema progress through four stages (Britt et al. 1981): (1) 'early cerebritis' (1–3 days), which consists of leukocytic infiltration and focal brain oedema; (2) 'late cerebritis' (4–9 days), wherein there is central liquefaction necrosis surrounded by an area of neovascularization and fibroblastic infiltration; (3) early fibroblastic capsule formation (10–14 days); and (4) late capsule formation (>14 days) in which a dense fibrous capsule is surrounded by reactive astrocytes and glial cells, marked oedema and neovascularization. Progression from the onset of early focal cerebritis to late capsule formation may take 2–6 weeks. In some cases, however, the progression may be rapid and the abscess may rupture into the ventricular system. The capsule formation is more complete on the cortical than on the ventricular side of the abscess, possibly because of better vascularization of the grey matter. Encapsulation is more common in abscesses secondary to contiguous spread of infection than in those secondary to haematogenous spread.

Brain abscesses are most often seen in the cerebral hemispheres (Nathoo et al. 2011), with an almost equal distribution in the frontal, parietal and temporal lobes. However, they may also occur in the cerebellum and brainstem. The site of abscess is often determined by the underlying factors (Table 13.1). In children with a cardiac source, abscesses are generally seen in the distribution of the middle cerebral artery. With venous spread from the face and sinuses, the abscesses are commonly seen in the frontal lobe; otogenic abscesses are commonly seen in the temporal lobes.

Abscesses may be single or multiple. Multiple abscesses are common with haematogenous infections, particularly gram-negative and *Staphylococcus aureus* infections, and in neonates. The expanding abscess acts as a mass lesion and causes increase in intracranial pressure (ICP), focal deficits and, in some patients, obstructive hydrocephalus.

CLINICAL PRESENTATION

The clinical presentation varies with the age of the child and the origin and location of the abscess. Neonates and young infants present with non-specific features of irritability, lethargy, poor feeding, bulging fontanelle and, in some patients, enlargement of the head. Seizures may occur; fever and focal signs are uncommon. Older children generally have a subacute presentation with fever, headache, vomiting, altered consciousness, seizures, neck rigidity and focal neurodeficitis. The classic triad of fever, headache and vomiting seen in adults is encountered in less than half of childhood cases. Fever is not always present. Seizures may be focal or generalized and occur in almost half the patients. Papilloedema and VIth nerve palsy and occasionally cerebral herniation syndromes may occur secondary to raised ICP. Focal deficits, when present, are determined by the site of the abscess. Frontal lobe abscess may remain silent until it becomes quite large and then may present with frontal release signs, personality changes and hemiparesis. Occasionally the presentation may be acute or even sudden if the abscess ruptures in the ventricles or if there is haemorrhage in the abscess cavity. Symptoms and signs of the underlying source of infection are often present.

DIAGNOSIS
A high index of suspicion is essential, particularly in children with risk factors.

Neuroimaging
Prompt computed tomography (CT) or magnetic resonance imaging (MRI) should be done in suspected cases. A non-contrast CT shows a hypodense lesion, often with mass effect. Contrast-enhanced CT shows a characteristic ring-enhancing lesion with central hypodensity and surrounding oedema, usually with mass effect and midline shift. In early cerebritis, the ring enhancement may be incomplete, and double-contrast CT may be helpful in defining the capsule (Erdogan and Cansever 2008). MRI is more sensitive than CT for diagnosing cerebritis. MRI findings depend on the stage of the abscess. In the early phase, the lesion appears hypointense on T1- and hyperintense on T2-weighted images. In later stages these findings become prominent, and the cavity shows a rim that is hyperintense on T1- and hypointense on T2-weighted images. Contrast enhancement of the rim occurs with gadolinium. Abscesses tend to grow towards the poorly vascular white matter, with thinning of the medial wall (Karampekios and Hesselink 2005). Differential diagnosis of a ring-enhancing lesion includes tumour, toxoplasmosis, cerebral infarction and demyelination. It may be difficult to differentiate pyogenic abscesses from fungal and tubercular abscesses on MRI alone; a diffusion-weighted MRI and proton magnetic resonance spectroscopy (PMRS) may be helpful. Tubercular abscesses are generally seen at the base of the brain, especially in the cerebellum. Pyogenic and tubercular abscesses have smooth or lobulated walls, whereas fungal abscesses have irregular walls with intracavitary projections on MRI. On in-vivo PMRS, normal brain metabolites such as N-acetylaspartate, choline and creatine are not seen because the abscess is necrotic; the presence of amino acids is a sensitive marker of pyogenic abscess, but their absence does not rule out a pyogenic aetiology (Pal et al. 2010). The presence of acetate with or without succinate suggests anaerobic bacterial aetiology. Cytosolic amino acids, acetate and succinate are seen in pyogenic and tubercular abscesses, whereas lipids, lactate, amino acids and trephalose are seen in fungal abscesses. On diffusion-weighted MRI, the apparent diffusion coefficient (ADC) is low in the walls of all three types of abscesses, and in the cavity of pyogenic and tubercular abscesses; however, ADC is high in the cavity of fungal abscesses (Luthra et al. 2007).

Cerebrospinal fluid (CSF)
Lumbar puncture is contraindicated in a child with brain abscess because of the risk of cerebral herniation. If it is done inadvertently, the CSF is generally under pressure and shows a mild to moderate pleocytosis, elevation of protein and normal glucose. While there may be no cells in some cases, marked pleocytosis (in the thousands of cells per cubic millimeter) may be seen if the abscess has ruptured into the ventricles. Gram stain and culture are generally negative, unless the abscess has ruptured.

Organism identification
Confirmation of the aetiological organism is done by analysis and culture of the aspirated contents. Culture positivity is reduced in patients who have received pre-aspiration anti-biotics; 34% of aspirates from surgical patients were sterile in one series (Xiao et al. 2005). In endemic countries and in suspected cases, the aspirate should be sent for acid-fast bacilli and fungal cultures to exclude tubercular and fungal brain abscess. Other sources of organism identification such as blood culture and aspiration from mastoiditis should also be obtained. Blood cultures are useful in patients with haematogenous infections even though the positivity rates are low (10%–25%).

Electroencephalography
Electroencephalography usually shows focal slowing or occasionally spikes over the region of the abscess. Periodic lateralizing discharges or diffuse slowing may also be seen. The electroencephalogram may be normal in some cases.

DIFFERENTIAL DIAGNOSIS
In the presence of focal features, the differential diagnosis includes fungal and tubercular brain abscess, neoplasms, focal encephalitis such as herpes, subdural collections and other mass lesions.

MANAGEMENT
Prompt administration of antibiotics with surgical drainage or excision of the abscess and treatment of the underlying source of infection are required. Urgent decompression is required in cases with critically raised ICP. Delay in aspiration after antibiotic administration significantly reduces culture positivity; hence aspiration should be done as soon as possible (at the latest within 3 days) after starting antibiotic therapy (Arlotti et al. 2010, Gadgil et al. 2013). In children, aspiration under CT guidance is used more frequently because of the low mortality and morbidity associated with the procedure. Stereotactic burr-hole aspiration is safe and is particularly useful for deep-seated abscesses such as those in the thalamus, basal ganglia or brainstem and for abscesses located in eloquent areas (Arlotti et al. 2010). A single aspiration may suffice in some cases. Multiple aspirations may be needed when there is continued abscess growth in spite of appropriate antibiotic therapy. External drainage may be considered in select large abscesses.

Drainage by craniotomy (or craniectomy) is indicated in (1) patients who do not respond to multiple aspirations (wherein the abscess continues to enlarge after 2 weeks or does not shrink after 3–4 weeks of appropriate antibiotics); (2) multiloculated abscesses; (3) large superficial abscesses in non-eloquent areas (Mut et al. 2009); (4) cerebellar abscesses where recurrent pus collections can cause significant worsening (Moorthy and Rajshekhar 2008); and (5) periventricular abscesses to avoid risk of rupture into the ventricles. At the time of craniotomy, adequate evacuation and debridement should be done and the capsule should be microsurgically removed. If a foreign body such as a shunt is associated with the abscess, it should be removed. In case of multiple abscesses, all abscesses over 2.5cm in size or with mass effect should be aspirated (or excised). If the abscesses are all below 2.5cm, the largest one should be aspirated for diagnostic purpose. Excision is often used in posttraumatic, postoperative patients and in those with a poor response to repeated aspiration (Arlotti et al. 2010, Ratnaike et al. 2011). Complications of surgical intervention include haemorrhage, CSF leakage, seizures and stroke.

Antibiotics alone may be used in children with early cerebritis, very small abscesses (<2cm), or abscesses in deep-seated/critical areas of the brain provided the child has a good initial clinical condition (Glasgow Coma Scale [GCS] score >12) (Arlotti et al. 2010). Medical treatment alone is more successful if started in the early stages, with duration of symptoms over 2 weeks. If the child does not show clinical improvement within the first week, surgical intervention should be reconsidered. The decision to use antibiotics only, without surgical intervention, needs to be individualized, keeping in mind the condition of the child and the characteristics of the abscess as well as balancing the risks of a surgical approach and of not being able to get a specific microbiological diagnosis.

Empiric antibiotic therapy before organism identification typically consists of a broad-spectrum combination of agents to cover anaerobic, gram-negative, gram-positive and staphylococcal species. Ceftriaxone/cefotaxime or any other third- or fourth-generation cephalosporin, metronidazole and vancomycin are generally used. Penicillin and chloramphenicol can be used if cephalosporins are not affordable. Modifications may be made according to the underlying predisposing condition and the immune status of the child. In posttraumatic and postsurgical cases, a good antistaphylococcal antibiotic is recommended; linezolid or vancomycin in high doses may be used. Definitive antibiotic therapy is determined by the organism identified. Intravenous antibiotics in highest doses are required for at least 6 weeks in most cases and longer in immunocompromised patients. As anaerobic organisms are often difficult to isolate, anaerobic cover is continued in most cases. If no organisms are identified, empiric antibiotic therapy is continued for 6 weeks. Management of patients with intraventricular rupture of abscess remains controversial. A combination of intravenous and intrathecal antibiotics, urgent evacuation with debridement of abscess, and intraventricular antibiotics have been used.

Corticosteroids may be given intravenously at initial presentation for a short period to help reduce cerebral oedema and raised ICP in children with marked cerebral oedema. The fear that they may reduce penetration of antibiotics in the abscess cavity has not been substantiated. They may, however, decrease the contrast enhancement of the capsule, which may be mistaken for improvement. Follow-up scans are done periodically (weekly/biweekly) after surgical drainage/excision, to determine the response. Recurrence rates of 10%–50% are reported. Follow-up should ensure that the oedema has resolved and the rim has disappeared; this can take up to 6 months.

Principles of supportive management for raised ICP, seizures and general intensive care are the same as for any critically ill child and are discussed in Chapter 3. There is no scientific evidence to recommend the use of prophylactic anticonvulsants; this practice is influenced by individual preference. The source of the infection should be treated medically or surgically to prevent recurrences.

COMPLICATIONS

The most important complications of brain abscess are (1) seizures, (2) obstructive hydro-cephalus, and (3) intraventricular rupture.

PROGNOSIS

Increasing availability of imaging procedures has helped in early identification and better management of brain abscess, and has led to significant decreases in mortality and mor-bidity. Cure rates of about 90% are reported with early medical and surgical therapy (Bernardini 2004). Mortality continues to be high in newborn infants, in children with mul-tiple large abscesses, and in those with cyanotic heart disease. Rupture of abscess into the ventricular system can be life threatening unless managed immediately and aggressively. A low GCS score at presentation is associated with a poor outcome (Tseng and Tseng 2006). An imaging severity index based on the number, location and size of abscesses and the extent of perilesional oedema and mass effect was found to have a strong correlation with outcome (Demir et al. 2007). Significant neuromorbidity occurs in children with late detec-tion of abscess. The residual deficits depend on the site of the abscess and may include hemiparesis, cranial nerve palsies, cognitive deficits and epilepsy.

PREVENTION

Children with predisposing conditions such as otitis, sinusitis, meningitis or dental infections should be treated adequately to prevent complications including brain abscess. Children with cyanotic congenital heart disease should be given antibiotic prophylaxis for procedures associated with bacteraemia; early corrective surgery should be considered. Prophylactic antibiotics after penetrating skull injury and after craniotomy should be started as soon as possible and continued for at least 5 days to reduce the incidence of brain abscess.

Subdural empyema

A subdural empyema (SDE) is a suppurative collection in the subdural space of the brain or spinal canal. In young children, most SDEs occur as a complication of meningitis and are most frequently (>80%) seen in infants (Wu et al. 2008, Legrand et al. 2009, Gupta et al. 2011). SDEs secondary to sinusitis and otitis media are common in older children and adults.

AETIOLOGY

When SDE occurs as a complication of meningitis, the organisms are those that cause meningitis. SDE is common with pneumococcal and Hib meningitis, and may occasionally occur with salmonella and meningococcal infection; group B streptococci have been re-ported in infants aged under 4 months (Wu et al. 2008). In other SDEs the organisms are in general similar to those that cause brain abscess. Spinal SDEs are rarely seen in children; the causative organisms are mainly streptococci and staphylococci.

PATHOGENESIS

The subdural space is a potential space between the dura and the arachnoid that may get infected as a complication of meningitis, by haematogenous spread from a distant source of infection, or by direct spread from otitis media, infected sinuses, osteomyelitis of skull bones or head trauma. Spread from the sinuses is usually through the mucosal veins of the sinus to the emissary veins that link the facial and dural venous system. The emissary veins that traverse the subdural space get infected, and since the subdural space is not limited by an attachment, the pus collection can be large. Most SDEs are seen over the cerebral hemispheres, where the brain does not approximate the skull closely and the subdural space can be found easily by collections. Some may involve the parafalcine region. Infratentorial SDEs are rare (<10%), are usually secondary to untreated middle-ear infections, and are often associated with hydrocephalus (Madhugiri et al. 2011). The majority are unilateral; infants may have bilateral involvement. Large collections behave like space-occupying lesions and may cause dangerous elevations of ICP, as well as extensive involvement of brain parenchyma.

CLINICAL PRESENTATION

The onset is subacute with fever (>90%), seizures (about 70%) and focal neurological signs (about 60%). Infants present with poor feeding, irritability, fever, bulging fontanelle and an enlarging head. Older children often have fever, headache, vomiting and neck rigidity. Focal seizures and focal deficits are seen in about one-third to one-half of patients. Persistent or recurrent fever with focal seizures or other focal neurological signs in a child with bacterial meningitis suggests an SDE.

DIAGNOSIS

This is done by neuroimaging. In infants with an open fontanelle, ultrasound can detect the subdural collection in most (but not all) cases, and should be done within 1 week in all infants with meningitis. Non-contrast CT shows a crescentic hypodense collection over one or both cerebral hemispheres. Contrast-enhanced CT shows a crescent-shaped hypodense lesion, with peripheral enhancement, at times with loculations. The enhancement is generally linear, along the dura, with or without enhancement of underlying brain parenchyma. In cases of a parafalcine SDE, CT shows the collection as well as parenchymal changes such as thickening and hyperdensity of the white matter, indicating the presence of oedema and ischaemia. Further progression leads to infarcts, cerebritis and abscess. Venous sinus thrombosis is common in patients with SDE as the venous sinuses are the route of spread of infection. MRI is more sensitive than CT for detection of small collections, distinguishing extraaxial collections from associated intra-axial complications, and sterile effusions from purulent ones. On T1-weighted images, empyema is seen as a collection mildly hyperintense to CSF, whereas on T2-weighted images it is markedly hyperintense to the CSF. A hypodense medial rim representing the dura is seen with an epidural empyema but not with a subdural empyema. Use of contrast defines this as an enhancing rim. In difficult cases, diffusion-weighted imaging (DWI) is helpful in differentiating SDEs from reactive subdural effusions commonly seen in meningitis (Wong et al. 2004). SDEs show high signal intensity on DWI and low signal intensity on ADC maps. The ADC values are lower than those of normal cortical grey matter, and are much lower than those of reactive subdural effusions.

Most collections (>80%) are in the frontal region, the next most common site being the temporoparietal region; occipital SDEs are uncommon.

Analysis of the subdural fluid obtained by subdural tap or surgical drainage reveals a purulent fluid with marked leukocytosis. Organism identification can be done by Gram stain and culture.

A lumbar puncture is often contraindicated. If done, the CSF shows leukocytosis, with elevated protein and low sugar. Peripheral blood leukocytosis is not specific.

TREATMENT

Prompt removal of pus and appropriate antibiotic therapy intravenously in high doses for 3–6 weeks is warranted. Removal can be done by aspiration through burr holes or craniotomy. Burr-hole drainage is less invasive, and a good outcome equivalent to that of craniotomy is reported in infants with postmeningitic SDEs (Liu et al. 2010). However, a slightly better outcome with craniotomy was reported in another series (Banerjee et al. 2009). In infants with open fontanelle, a careful transcutaneous needle aspiration can be done. Antibiotics are chosen according to the suspected source of infection. Surgical removal of an adjacent source of infection such as chronic otitis media or osteomyelitis is required. Repeat scans are needed periodically to look for recollection and to monitor the course. Supportive therapy is provided on the same principles as for meningitis or brain abscess.

PROGNOSIS

The mortality and morbidity associated with SDEs have declined significantly with the use of early appropriate medical and surgical intervention. The GCS score at the time of presentation correlates well with the outcome (Mat Nayan et al. 2009). However, high mortality (11%–12%) and morbidity (12%–26%) have been reported from resource-poor countries (Banerjee et al. 2009, Nathoo et al. 2011). Common residual deficits after large SDEs include hemiparesis and focal seizures.

SPINAL SUBDURAL EMPYEMA

Spinal SDEs are extremely rare in children. They usually occur in children with spinal dysraphism (Sandler et al. 2013). The common causative agent is *S. aureus*. Presentation is with fever, back pain and signs of spinal cord involvement. In contrast to spinal epidural abscess, a spinal SDE is not associated with localized tenderness.

Epidural abscess

An epidural abscess is a collection of pus between the dura and the cranium, or the dura and the vertebral periosteum in the spinal canal.

INTRACRANIAL EPIDURAL ABSCESS

Aetiology

The common causative organisms include staphylococci, streptococci, gram-negative organisms and some anaerobic organisms such as *Bacteroides fragilis*.

Pathogenesis
The usual spread of infection is from a contiguous source such as sinusitis, otitis or mastoid-itis, or secondary to penetrating head injury, and in about 2% of patients as a complication of neurosurgical procedures. The infection progresses slowly and dissects the dura away from the skull, forming an abscess.

Clinical presentation
The presentation is subacute with fever, focal seizures and focal neurodeficits including hemiparesis. Headache, vomiting and neck rigidity are seen in older children. Papilloedema may occur with increasing ICP. Children with sinusitis and any neurological finding or sign of complicated sinusitis such as a Pott puffy tumour (frontal subgaleal abscess), orbital cellulitis, or persistent fever, headache or vomiting on appropriate antibiotics should be investigated for sinogenic intracranial empyemas (Adame et al. 2005).

Diagnosis
The diagnosis is by neuroimaging. MRI is more sensitive than CT and shows an enhancing lenticular collection between the dura and the cranium. On MRI the abscess is slightly hyperintense to CSF on T1-weighted images and markedly hyperintense to CSF on T2-weighted images. The enhancing rim is thick medially, representing the inflamed dura, and it is more irregular than that seen in SDE. A large epidural abscess can cause a mass effect. Epidural abscess and SDE often coexist.

Complications
Continuous progression of the epidural abscess may lead to associated SDE, brain abscess or meningitis.

Treatment
Treatment includes prompt surgical drainage through burr holes or craniotomy, appropriate intravenous antibiotics and supportive management.

Prognosis
Early appropriate management is associated with a good outcome. The presence of enceph-alopathy and significant neurodeficits at presentation is associated with a poor outcome.

SPINAL EPIDURAL ABSCESS
Although uncommon in children, a spinal epidural abscess represents a medical emergency that requires prompt intervention to prevent lifelong disability.

Aetiology
The most common causative organism is *S. aureus* (>60%) in both children and adults

(Chen et al. 2011); other uncommon organisms include pneumococci, streptococci, salmonellae and other gram-negative and anaerobic organisms.

Pathogenesis

Infection usually occurs by the haematogenous route from skin, orodental or pharyngeal infections, but may occasionally spread from an adjacent source of infection or be secondary to spinal trauma or a spinal procedure. Haematogenous spread from a distant source of infection is much more common in children than in adults. Most abscesses (>50%) are located in the lumbar, lumbosacral or thoracic regions, often on the posterior aspect of the cord (Chao and Nanda 2002). This is because of the anatomical configuration of the spinal cord wherein the epidural space is limited anteriorly because of the attachment to the vertebral canal, whereas posteriorly there is a large potential space; also the extensive venous plexuses in the dorsal space facilitate bacterial contamination (Pradilla et al. 2010). The epidural space is smaller in the cervical region than in the thoracolumbar region. Cervical epidural abscesses are therefore uncommon; they are generally seen in adolescent and adult drug abusers who take intravenous injections in the upper extremities. The extent of involvement may vary from a small segment to multiple segments, and even to the entire length of the cord. Progression of inflammation leads to vasculitis and venous thrombophlebitis, spinal-cord ischaemia, and even infarction; increase in size of the abscess causes spinal compression. All these factors cause the ensuing spinal cord dysfunction.

Clinical presentation

The initial presentation is non-specific with fever and back pain, so the diagnosis may be missed. Later there are symptoms and signs of spinal-cord compression, generally paraplegia. The child looks toxic and has localized pain and, at times, a tender swelling at the site of the abscess. Root pains and paraesthesiae occur in some children. However, all the symptoms and signs are not necessarily present, and absence of some of these may cause delay in diagnosis. A sensory level is seen in late cases. Progression may lead to bladder and bowel involvement. The rate of progression is variable; generally there is an interval of a few days from the onset of symptoms to complete paraplegia. However, in some cases the child may be paralysed within hours, resembling acute transverse myelitis. In general, haematogenous infections present acutely, whereas those due to a contiguous source present subacutely.

Although rare, epidural abscesses have been described in neonates and infants (Tang et al. 2001, Hazelton et al. 2012). They generally have a non-specific presentation that may cause delay in diagnosis.

Differential diagnosis

In the early stage when there are subtle signs and symptoms, an epidural abscess may be mistaken for meningitis, urinary tract infection, or some other cause of back pain.

Diagnosis

An urgent contrast MRI of the spine should be obtained in suspected cases; the whole spine should be scanned as there may be multiple abscesses. Abscesses appear isointense or hypotense on T1- and hyperintense on T2-weighted images. The MRI in the early stage shows a homogenous enhancement of the abnormal area; in the late stage it shows liquefaction with peripheral enhancement of the abscess. CT is not a good modality for diagnosis as it picks up only a third of cases. Plain radiographs of the spine and contrast myelography have no role in diagnosis. CT with myelography can be done if MRI is not available. A lumbar puncture is contraindicated as there is a risk of accidental spread of infection to the CSF, and spinal herniation in cases of complete spinal block. If done inadvertently, CSF shows predominantly polymorphonuclear leukocytosis, elevated protein and hypoglycorrhachia in most cases. Unless there is associated meningitis, the CSF Gram stain and culture show a low positivity (10%–15%).

Other markers of infection such as peripheral leukocytosis, raised erythrocyte sedimentation rate (ESR) and elevated serum C-reactive protein (CRP) are often present. Blood-culture positivity varies from 60% to 80%, and there is a high concordance between organisms grown on blood culture and aspirated pus culture.

Treatment

Urgent decompression (endoscopic assisted surgery, percutaneous drainage or laminectomy) should be done and appropriate intravenous antibiotic therapy started. As *S. aureus* is the most common pathogen, the initial antibiotic therapy should consist of a combination of antibiotics to cover staphylococci and gram-negative organisms (generally ceftriaxone or meropenem and cloxacillin or vancomycin). Once the abscess is drained and the organism identified, appropriate antibiotic therapy is administered intravenously for 4–6 weeks. Medical therapy alone may be used in the very early stages in patients with minimal or no neurodeficit. However, a close clinical laboratory analysis (ESR and CRP) and MRI monitoring should be done in such cases, as the rate of progression of neurological impairment is unpredictable (Chen et al. 2008). There is no scientific evidence to support the use of corticosteroids.

Surgery may not be feasible in extensive spinal involvement and may not be helpful in recovery of the neurodeficit if paralysis is present for more than 48 hours.

Prognosis

Early appropriate management has led to a significant decrease in mortality, as well as morbidity. Formulation of clinical decision guidelines with risk-factor assessment in the emergency department, along with determination of ESR and CRP, has helped in early diagnosis and thereby in improving outcome of spinal epidural abscesses (Davis et al. 2011). The outcome is determined by the extent of involvement, the severity of neurodeficits, especially paralysis present at the time of presentation, the urgency with which decompression is done, and many underlying risk factors such as diabetes mellitus or immunosuppression. Paralysis for over 36 hours before intervention is associated with a poor prognosis. Complete recovery may be expected in children who do not have paralysis at presentation.

TABLE 13.2
Source of infection and clinical presentation in suppurative intracranial phlebitis

Involved sinus	Source of infection	Clinical presentation
Cavernous sinus	Facial or dental infections, otitis media, sphenoid and ethmoid sinusitis	Acute onset of fever, headache, proptosis, chemosis, painful external ophthalmoplegia that starts in one eye and usually progresses within 24–48 hours to involve the other eye; periorbital swelling, violaceous discoloration of the eye, pupillary abnormalities (dilation in parasympathetic paralysis, constriction with sympathetic paralysis), papilloedema, decreased visual activity, at times decreased corneal reflex, internal ophthalmoplegia, decreased sensation in trigeminal area, occasionally seizures, hemiparesis
Superior sagittal sinus	Bacterial meningitis, subdural or epidural empyema, frontal and maxillary sinusitis	Fever, seizures, hemiparesis; occasionally raised ICP, encephalopathy
Lateral sinus	Otitis media, mastoiditis, pharyngitis	Subacute onset of fever, unilateral headache, diplopia, vertigo, involvement of Vth and VIth cranial nerves

Suppurative intracranial phlebitis

Inflammation of the intracranial veins can occur as a primary process or secondary to other intracranial suppuration such as brain abscess and subdural and epidural empyemas. The condition has become rare in resource-rich countries but is not uncommon in resource-poor ones.

AETIOLOGY

The most common responsible pathogen is *S. aureus* (>70%). Other organisms such as streptococci, pneumococci, gram-negative and anerobic organisms may occasionally be involved.

PATHOGENESIS

Infection may spread from skin infections of the face, ear or scalp, or from the sinuses, or occasionally from dental infections (Lazow et al. 2011) (Table 13.2). The venous drainage of the face and skull goes through emissary veins into the dural sinuses, which empty into the internal jugular veins. There are no valves in the venous system of the head and brain, thus there is easy retrograde spread of thrombophlebitis from the infected venous sinuses into the dural and cortical venous channels. The extensive vascular connections of the cavernous sinuses make them vulnerable to septic thrombosis from infective sources at multiple sites.

CLINICAL PRESENTATION

The child usually presents with fever and headache, and may look toxic. Other symptoms and signs vary according to the sinus(es) involved (Table 13.2). Symptoms and signs of raised ICP are present in most cases of cavernous and lateral sinus thrombosis whereas they are uncommon with sagittal sinus thrombosis; seizures are common with saggital sinus thrombosis.

DIAGNOSIS

Thin-cut contrast MRI of the suspected sinus is often diagnostic (Jonas Kimchi et al. 2007, Agostoni et al. 2009). Magnetic resonance venography may be required in some cases. High-resolution contrast-enhanced CT shows irregular filling defects; in sagittal sinus thrombosis it shows the 'empty delta sign' in many cases. Lumbar puncture is contraindicated in the presence of raised ICP. If done, CSF shows neutrophilic leukocytosis but culture is positive in less than 20% of cases. Blood culture is positive in most (>70%), especially in fulminant cases.

DIFFERENTIAL DIAGNOSIS

Cavernous sinus thrombosis needs to be differentiated mainly from orbital cellulitis, which also causes fever, proptosis, chemosis (conjunctival oedema), painful opthalmoplegia and decreased vision. Bilateral involvement, papilloedema, pupillary dilation and trigeminal sensory loss favour the diagnosis of cavernous sinus thrombosis.

TREATMENT

High-dose intravenous antibiotics primarily to cover staphylococcus are given; initial therapy includes gram-negative and anaerobic cover until culture results are available. Antibiotics are given for at least 3–4 weeks.

The use of anticoagulants is controversial because of the risk of bleeding. Anticoagulants have become part of standard therapy in sinus venous thrombosis of non-infective origin (Lebas et al. 2012, Weimar 2014). Their safety and efficacy in septic venous thrombosis is gaining acceptance (Bhatia and Jones 2002) but is not yet well established (Kojan and Al-Jumah 2006). If used (after excluding significant haemorrhage), low molecular weight heparin followed by warfarin are used. There are no definite guidelines regarding duration of anticoagulant therapy in children, particularly in those with septic phlebitis. In general, anticoagulants are given for 3–6 months or until the thrombus resolution is confirmed by neuroimaging.

The role of corticosteroids is not established. Appropriate management of the primary source of infection is important.

PROGNOSIS

Although the mortality and morbidity are considerably reduced because of the use of potent antibiotics, they are still quite high for sagittal sinus and cavernous sinus thrombosis (20%–30%), and are determined by the severity of the involvement at presentation (Ebright et al. 2001). Permanent neurological sequelae are seen in number of cases. However, in a small case series, neither death nor severe permanent deficits were found in the majority of patients (Visudtibhan et al. 2001). Early recognition and appropriate antibiotic therapy can prevent mortality and morbidity to a large extent.

Ventriculoperitoneal shunt infection

Shunt infection is a common complication of shunt surgery, more so in resource-poor countries. A diagnosis of shunt infection requires the following conditions: (1) no meningitis or ventriculitis, and a sterile CSF culture at the time of shunt placement; (2) the shunt should have been in place for at least 24 hours; and (3) a positive CSF culture obtained from the shunt/lumbar puncture.

EPIDEMIOLOGY

Over the last two decades the operative incidence of shunt infection has ranged from 2.8% to 14%. A drop in infection rates to 4.2% (NNIS 2002) was attributed to changes in the type of shunt materials, reduction in pre-shunt invasive studies such as pneumoencephalography, and better operative facilities. Almost 70%–85% of shunt infections occur within 6 months, usually within one month of surgery.

AETIOLOGY

Most shunt infections (>80%) are caused by staphylcococcal species. The relative frequency of *S. epidermidis* and *S. aureus* varies in different studies; in a study from Korea, the most common causative microorganisms were coagulase-negative staphylococci (45.7%) followed by *S. aureus* (22.9%) (Lee et al. 2012). Other organisms include gram-negative bacteria such as *Escherichia coli* and *Klebsiella*, *Proteus*, *Pseudomonas* and streptococcal species; multiple organisms account for 10%–15% of infections. The common meningitis pathogens (*Haemophilus influenzae*, *Streptococcus pneumoniae*, *Neisseria meningitidis*) have been found in 5% of shunt infections. Rarely, fungi, diphtheroids and other commensal microbes may cause shunt infections. Infection usually occurs within 2 months of insertion (Lee et al. 2012).

PATHOGENESIS

The most common mechanism of shunt infections is introduction of infection at the time of surgery. Occasionally, direct spread from breakdown of the surgical wound or of the skin overlying the shunt assembly may be responsible. Retrograde infection from the distal end because of transluminal passage of bacteria, or secondary to delayed perforation of the bowel, may account for some cases. Haematogenous seeding from a distant source of infection is rare.

A shunt acts as a foreign body and interferes with the host defense mechanisms, particularly chemotaxis and phagocytosis. In addition, staphylococci form an extracellular biofilm termed 'slime' that increases adherence to shunt and decreases the effect of antibiotic therapy. Higher rates of infection in young infants have been attributed to a higher skin bacterial density and a relatively poor immune status.

CLINICAL PRESENTATION

Fever, headache, vomiting and drowsiness are the usual presenting features, though not all of them necessarily co-occur in a given child. The symptoms are those of shunt malfunction; fever is often the clue to infection but may be absent in about a third of cases. Drowsiness has been found to be the best clinical predictor of ventriculoperitoneal shunt block; headache and vomiting are less predictive (Barnes et al. 2002). Atypical presentations with seizures, cranial nerve palsies and neck rigidity may occur. Occasionally, inflammation along the shunt tube may produce pain and erythema.

Shunt infection leads to ventriculitis in about a third of cases, and to meningitis in some cases; intracranial empyemas may occur occasionally. Infection of the distal end of the shunt can cause peritonitis.

DIAGNOSIS

A high index of suspicion is essential for early diagnosis. Any child with a shunt in place and who has fever, change in level of consciousness, or vomiting and headache must be considered to have shunt infection unless proven otherwise.

A diagnostic shunt tap should be done and CSF obtained for analysis and culture. The CSF shows a high white blood cell count in most cases; however, sometimes counts may be normal even in the presence of infection. On the other hand an elevated CSF white cell count after shunt placement may occur owing to a hypersensitivity reaction to the presence of shunt tubing (chemical meningitis), and may remain elevated for a prolonged period. Eosinophilia defined as 5% or above reportedly has a 96% positive predictive value for shunt pathology (McClinton et al. 2001). However, the aetiology of eosinophilia in the CSF can be multifactorial; latex allergy, delayed hypersensitivity to the shunt materials, and IV gentamicin which is often used to sterilize shunt material, have all been implicated as causes of increased CSF eosinophils. Although ventricular fluid eosinophilia is an excellent positive predictor of ventriculoperitoneal shunt pathology, its absence is not helpful. The combination of fever history and ventricular fluid neutrophils in excess of 10% had a 99% specificity, and a 93% and 95% positive and negative predictive value, for shunt infection (McClinton et al. 2001).

Laboratory studies are helpful when positive, but may be negative in the face of shunt pathology. Typical findings of infection such as the number of white blood cells and presence of neutrophils in the ventricular fluid show a degree of overlap between the infection and malfunction groups. CSF glucose may be low and protein levels increased but they are often within normal range in spite of obvious infection. Organism identification may be done by Gram stain but the criterion standard for diagnosis of shunt infection is the isolation of organisms on culture of the shunt or of any fluid in contact with it. Culture of the CSF obtained from the shunt is more often positive than that obtained from a lumbar puncture. The peripheral WBC count is usually high but has a poor correlation with shunt infection. In a group of high-risk patients, a correlation with raised CRP above 10mg/dL was reported in a recent study (Lolak and Bunyaratavej 2013). Blood culture is seldom positive. CSF cyst detected on ultrasonography strongly suggests infection. In neonates, ventriculitis associated with shunt infection can be diagnosed by ultrasound, which shows increased echogenicity of ventricular fluid with strands. CT or MRI often shows an increase in ventricular size because of shunt blockage. Wherever possible, CT findings should be interpreted in the context of previous imaging; it must be remembered that not all cases of proven shunt blockage present with an increase in ventricle size (Barnes et al. 2002).

DIFFERENTIAL DIAGNOSIS

Differentiation of ventriculoperitoneal shunt infection from malfunction without infection may be difficult in children who present with constitutional signs and symptoms of illness, with equivocal signs and symptoms of shunt infection and/or malfunction. Younger age (especially preterm birth), postoperative CSF leak, presence of fever, frequent shunt manipulation, and shorter time interval from prior manipulation to current presentation have been linked to ventriculoperitoneal shunt infection, whereas a history of vomiting has been associated with shunt malfunction. However, in some studies no statistically significant relationship was found between age, interval between prior and current manipulations or number of shunt revisions, and shunt infection; presence of fluid accumulation along the shunt tract was associated with a significant increase in incidence of shunt infection (Davis et al. 1999, McClinton et al. 2001). Also, no difference in infection rate has been found between shunts with or without a valve.

MANAGEMENT

The infected shunt should be removed, appropriate antibiotics started and an external drainage device (EVD) inserted. Ventriculitis related to shunt infection responds well to antibiotics and external drainage. The EVD is useful also for daily CSF examination, which helps in monitoring infection and in administration of intraventricular antibiotics. Initial antibiotics are started to cover staphylococcus and gram-negative organisms. Once organisms are grown on CSF culture, definitive antibiotics are accordingly decided. The antibiotics usually used for staphylococcal coverage include cloxacillin (or vancomycin in areas with high prevalence of methicillin-resistant staphylococci), often in conjunction with an aminoglycoside. Rifampicin can be added to augment the therapy. In cases with resistant organisms, linezolid could be used. Third-generation cephalosporins and aminoglycosides are used for gram-negative bacteria. Intraventricular therapy with vancomycin and aminoglycosides (gentamicin and amikacin) has also been used. The duration of therapy is determined by the organisms isolated and the persistence of infection as determined by CSF analysis and cultures obtained after externalization. Generally 2–3 weeks of therapy is required; once the CSF has been sterile for several consecutive days, a new shunt assembly is inserted. Shunt infection following treatment and replacement of an infected shunt occurs in some cases.

PREVENTION

Prophylactic antibiotic administration before and after shunt surgery reduces the rate of shunt infection regardless of the patient's age and the type of shunt used (Ratilal et al. 2008).

In a randomized trial, ceftriaxone and trimethoprim sulfamethoxazole were equally effective in preventing shunt infection (Nejat et al. 2008). Use of antibiotic-impregnated shunts also reduces the incidence of shunt infections (Kandasamy et al. 2011). However, concern has been raised about infection with antibiotic-resistant strains in cases with antibiotic-impregnated shunts (Demetriades and Bassi 2011). Simple techniques such as changing gloves before insertion of shunt (Rehman et al. 2010) and the use of standardized protocols for shunt surgery incorporating proper sterile techniques, use of antimicrobial sutures and antibiotic-impregnated shunt material have been shown to reduce the infection rate significantly (Kestle et al. 2011).

REFERENCES

Adame N, Hedlund G, Byington CL (2005) Sinogenic intracranial empyema in children. *Pediatrics* 116: e461–7.

Arlotti M, Grossi P, Pea F, et al. (2010) Consensus document on controversial issues for the treatment of infections of the central nervous system: bacterial brain abscesses. *Int J Infect Dis Suppl* 4: S79–92.

Banerjee AD, Pandey P, Devi BI, et al. (2009) Pediatric supratentorial subdural empyemas: a retrospective analysis of 65 cases. *Pediatr Neurosurg* 45: 11–8.

Barnes NP, Jones SJ, Hayward RD, et al. (2002) Ventriculoperitoneal shunt block: what are the best predictive clinical indicators? *Arch Dis Child* 87: 198–201.

Bernardini Gl (2004) Diagnosis and management of brain abscess and subdural empyema. *Curr Neurol Neurosci Rep* 4: 448–56.

Bhatia K, Jones NS (2002) Septic cavernous sinus thrombosis secondary to sinusitis: are anticoagulants indicated? A review of the literature. *J Laryngol Otol* 116: 667–76.

Britt RH, Enzmann DR, Yeager AS (1981) Neuropathological and computerized tomographic findings in experimental brain abscess. *J Neurosurg* 55: 590–603.

Chao D, Nanda A (2002) Spinal epidural abscess: a diagnostic challenge. *Am Fam Physician* 65: 1341–6.

Chen SH, Chang WN, Lu CH, et al. (2011) The clinical characteristics, therapeutic outcome, and prognostic factors of non-tuberculous bacterial spinal epidural abscess in adults: a hospital-based study. *Acta Neurol Taiwan* 20: 107–13.

Chen WC, Wang JL, Wang JT, et al. (2008) Spinal epidural abscess due to Staphylococcus aureus: clinical manifestations and outcomes. *J Microbiol Immunol Infect* 41: 215–21.

Davis DP, Salazar A, Chan TC, Vilke GM (2011) Prospective evaluation of a clinical decision guideline to diagnose spinal epidural abscess in patients who present to the emergency department with spine pain. *J Neurosurg Spine* 14: 765–70.

Davis SE, Levy ML, McComb JG, Masri-Lavine L (1999) Does age or other factors influence the incidence of ventriculoperitoneal shunt infections? *Pediatr Neurosurg* 30: 253–7.

Demetriades AK, Bassi S (2011) Antibiotic resistant infections with antibiotic-impregnated Bactiseal catheters for ventriculoperitoneal shunts. *Br J Neurosurg* 25: 671–3.

Demir MK, Hakan T, Kilicoglu G, et al. (2007) Bacterial brain abscesses: prognostic value of an imaging severity index. *Clin Radiol* 62: 564–72.

Ebright JR, Pace MT, Niazi AF (2001) Septic thrombosis of the cavernous sinuses. *Arch Intern Med* 161: 2671–6.

Erdogen E, Cansever T (2008) Pyogenic brain abscess. *Neurosurg Focus* 24: E2.

Gadgil N, Patel AJ, Gopinath SP (2013) Open craniotomy for brain abscess: a forgotten experience? *Surg Neurol Int* 4: 34. doi: 10.4103/2152-7806.109522.

Gupta S, Vachhrajani S, Kulkarni AV, et al. (2011) Neurosurgical management of extraaxial central nervous system infections in children. *J Neurosurg Pediatr* 7: 441–51.

Hazelton B, Kesson A, Prelog K, et al. (2012) Epidural abscess in a neonate. *J Paediatr Child Health* 48: E132–5. doi: 10.1111/j.1440–1754.2011.02078.x.

Jonas Kimchi T, Lee SK, Agid R, et al. (2007) Cerebral sinovenous thrombosis in children. *Neuroimaging Clin N Am* 17: 239–44.

199

Kandasamy J, Dwan K, Hartley JC, et al. (2011) Antibiotic-impregnated ventriculoperitoneal shunts—a multi-centre British paediatric neurosurgery group (BPNG) study using historical controls. *Childs Nerv Syst* 27: 575–81.

Karampekios S, Hesselink J (2005) Cerebral infections. *Eur Radiol* 15: 485–93.

Kestle JR, Riva-Cambrin J, Wellons JC 3rd, et al. (2011) A standardized protocol to reduce cerebrospinal fluid shunt infection: the Hydrocephalus Clinical Research Network Quality Improvement Initiative. *J Neurosurg Pediatr* 8: 22–9.

Kojan S, Al-Jumah M (2006) Infection related cerebral venous thrombosis. *J Pak Med Assoc* 56: 494–7.

Lazow SK, Izzo SR, Vazquez D (2011) Do dental infections really cause central nervous system infections? *Oral Maxillofac Surg Clin North Am* 23: 569–78.

Lebas A, Chabrier S, Fluss J, et al. (2012) EPNS/SFNP guideline on the anticoagulant treatment of cerebral sinovenous thrombosis in children and neonates. *Eur J Paediatr Neurol* 16: 219–28. doi: 10.1016/j.ejpn.2012.02.005.

Lee JK, Seok JY, Lee JH, et al. (2012) Incidence and risk factors of ventriculoperitoneal shunt infections in children: a study of 333 consecutive shunts in 6 years. *J Korean Med Sci* 27: 1563–8.

Legrand M, Roujeau T, Meyer P, et al. (2009) Paediatric intracranial empyema: differences according to age. *Eur J Pediatr* 168: 1235–41.

Liu ZH, Chen NY, Tu PH, et al. (2010) The treatment and outcome of postmeningitic subdural empyema in infants. *J Neurosurg Pediatr* 6: 38–42.

Lolak S, Bunyaratavej K (2013) C-reactive protein in prediction of ventriculoperitoneal shunt-related infection in high-risk patients. *Surg Infect* 14: 192–5.

Luthra G, Parihar A, Nath K, et al. (2007) Comparative evaluation of fungal, tubercular, and pyogenic brain abscesses with conventional and diffusion MR imaging and proton MR spectroscopy. *AJNR Am J Neuroradiol* 28: 1332–8.

Madhugiri VS, Sastri BV, Bhagavatula ID, et al. (2011) Posterior fossa subdural empyema in children—management and outcome. *Childs Nerv Syst* 27: 137–44.

Mat Nayan SA, Mohd Haspani MS, Abd Latiff AZ, et al. (2009) Two surgical methods used in 90 patients with intracranial subdural empyema. *J Clin Neurosci* 16: 1567–71.

McClinton D, Carraccio C, Englander R (2001) Predictors of ventriculoperitoneal shunt pathology. *Pediatr Infect Dis J* 20: 593–7.

Moorthy RK, Rajshekhar V (2008) Management of brain abscess: an overview. *Neurosurg Focus* 24: E3.

Mut M, Hazer B, Narin F, et al. (2009) Aspiration or capsule excision? Analysis of treatment results for brain abscesses at single institute. *Turk Neurosurg* 19: 36–41.

Nathoo N, Nadvi SS, Narotam PK, van Dellen JR (2011) Brain abscess: management and outcome analysis of a computed tomography era experience with 973 patients. *World Neurosurg* 75: 716–26; discussion 612–7.

Nejat F, Tajik P, El Khashab M, et al. (2008) A randomized trial of ceftriaxone versus trimethoprim-sulfamethoxazole to prevent ventriculoperitoneal shunt infection. *J Microbiol Immunol Infect* 41: 112–7.

NNIS (2002) National Nosocomial Infections Surveillance (NNIS) System Report, data summary from January 1992 to June 2002, issued August 2002. *Am J Infect Control* 30: 458–75.

Pal D, Bhattacharyya A, Husain M, et al. (2010) In vivo proton MR spectroscopy evaluation of pyogenic brain abscesses: a report of 194 cases. *AJNR Am J Neuroradiol* 31: 360–6.

Pradilla G, Nagahama Y, Spivak AM, et al. (2010) Spinal epidural abscess: current diagnosis and management. *Curr Infect Dis Rep* 12: 484–91.

Ratilal B, Costa J, Sampaio C (2008) Antibiotic prophylaxis for surgical introduction of intracranial ventricular shunts: a systematic review. *J Neurosurg Pediatr* 1: 48–56.

Ratnaike TE, Das S, Gregson BA, Mendelow AD (2011) A review of brain abscess surgical treatment—78 years: aspiration versus excision. *World Neurosurg* 76: 431–6.

Rehman AU, Rehman TU, Bashir HH, Gupta V (2010) A simple method to reduce infection of ventriculoperitoneal shunts. *J Neurosurg Pediatr* 5: 569–72.

Sandler AL, Thompson D, Goodrich JT, et al. (2013) Infections of the spinal subdural space in children: a series of 11 contemporary cases and review of all published reports. A multinational collaborative effort. *Childs Nerv Syst* 29: 105–17.

Tang K, Xenos C, Sgouros S (2001) Spontaneous spinal epidural abscess in a neonate. With a review of the literature. *Childs Nerv Syst* 17: 629–31.

Tseng JH, Tseng MY (2006) Brain abscess in 142 patients: factors influencing outcome and mortality. *Surg Neurol* 65: 557–62.

Visudtibhan A, Visudhiphan P, Chiemchanya S (2001) Cavernous sinus thrombophlebitis in children. *Pediatr Neurol* 24: 123–7.

Weimar C (2014) Diagnosis and treatment of cerebral venous and sinus thrombosis. *Curr Neurol Neurosci Rep* 14: 417. doi: 10.1007/s11910-013-0417-5.

Wong AM, Zimmerman RA, Simon EM, et al. (2004) Diffusion-weighted MR imaging of subdural empyemas in children. *AJNR Am J Neuroradiol* 25: 1016–21.

Wu TJ, Chiu NC, Huang FY (2008) Subdural empyema in children – 20 year experience in a medical center. *J Microbiol Immunol Infect* 41: 62–7.

Xiao F, Tseng MY, Teng LJ, et al. (2005) Brain abscess: clinical experience and analysis of prognostic factors. *Surg Neurol* 63: 442–9.

14
TUBERCULOSIS

Johan F Schoeman and Ronald van Toorn

Tuberculous meningitis

Central nervous system (CNS) tuberculosis accounts for only approximately 1% of all disease caused by *Mycobacterium tuberculosis* but it kills or disables more people than any other form of tuberculosis. Tuberculous meningitis (TBM) is the most common and most devastating form of CNS tuberculosis and has become the most common form of chronic meningitis in poor communities affected by the human immunodeficiency virus/autoimmune deficiency syndrome (HIV/AIDS) epidemic. If diagnosed and treated early, most patients recover completely, but if the disease progresses untreated, death and disability are very common despite microbiological cure. TBM occurs most frequently in resource-poor countries, where the diagnosis and therefore antituberculosis treatment is often delayed because of the non-specific nature of the presenting symptoms. In resource-rich countries TBM occurs particularly in the elderly and in immune-compromised people, and the diagnosis is frequently missed because of unfamiliarity with the disease.

PATHOGENESIS

Understanding of the pathogenesis of CNS tuberculosis is still based on the investigations of Rich and McCordock, published more than 80 years ago (Rich and McCordock 1933). They showed that intravenous injection of virulent *M. tuberculosis* into experimental animals did not immediately lead to meningitis in any of the animals. At autopsy they demonstrated small granulomas in communication with the subarachnoid space in 77 of 82 people with fatal TBM. These granulomas were found predominantly within the brain parenchyma, rather than the meninges, and were believed to develop during a preceding bacteraemia. Rich and McCordock then postulated that meningitis occurred once bacteria contained within these granulomas (now called Rich foci) were released into the subarachnoid space, months or years after the initial bacteraemia. This model of CNS tuberculosis pathogenesis has remained largely unchallenged ever since. Direct spread from a tuberculous focus adjacent to the subarachnoid space such as otitis media or tuberculous spondylitis is a rare cause of TBM.

The role of bacterial and host genotype in the pathogenesis and outcome of TBM is currently being investigated. The first possible interaction between host and organism has recently been demonstrated when individuals with the C allele of TLR-2 T597C allele were found to be more likely to develop tuberculosis caused by the east-Asian/Beijing genotype (Caws et al. 2008). Another study showed that mycobacterial lineage may influence the intracerebral inflammatory response because adults with TBM infected with the Beijing strain had more rapid disease progression with fewer cerebrospinal fluid (CSF) leukocytes (Thwaites et al. 2008). In addition, a strong association between the Beijing genotype and drug resistance has been reported for HIV-infected Vietnamese adults with TBM (Caws et al. 2006). However, no definite relationship between mycobacterial genotype and clinical outcome has yet been demonstrated in either adults or children (Maree et al. 2007, Thwaites et al. 2008).

TBM is associated with defective immunity, including malnutrition and HIV (Sterling et al. 2007). In the acute phase the CSF pleocytosis and markedly raised CSF cytokine levels reflect the inflammatory response in the subarachnoid space. Concentrations of cytokines such as tumour necrosis factor (TNF), interferon gamma (INF-γ), and interleukins IL-8 and IL-10 are elevated and often remain persistently high during the first weeks of therapy (Donald et al. 1995). Elevated CSF inflammatory cytokines at baseline are not associated with death or disability in HIV-negative adults with TBM. The same study reported that low CSF IFN-γ concentrations were associated with death in HIV-positive adults with TBM, implying that this cytokine contributes to immunity.

PATHOLOGY

Central to the macropathology of TBM is the florid, basal meningeal exudate that obliterates the basal cisterns and encases the brainstem, cerebral arteries, cranial nerves and spinal roots (Dastur et al. 1995). Hydrocephalus results whenever the basal exudate blocks CSF flow. In about 70% of cases CSF can exit the fourth ventricle but is prevented from moving past the tentorium by the exudate blocking the basal cisterns (communicating hydrocephalus) (Van Well et al. 2009). In the remainder, obstruction of the outlet foramina of the fourth ventricle results in non-communicating hydrocephalus. Occasionally hydrocephalus results from obstruction of a foramen of Munro or the aqueduct of Sylvius.

Apart from obstructive hydrocephalus, brain damage in TBM is mainly the result of basal structures such as the arteries, cranial nerves and brainstem being encased by the exudate. These structures are affected from the outside inwards (e.g. peri-arteritis/perineuritis) and are damaged by inflammatory, ischaemic and/or compressive mechanisms. The anterior branches of the middle cerebral artery are most commonly involved, resulting in endarteritis and infarction of the caudate nucleus and internal capsule (Springer et al. 2009). Other common sites of infarction are the thalami and brainstem, the latter best demonstrated by magnetic resonance imaging (MRI) (Pienaar et al. 2009). Occlusion of the main branch of the middle cerebral arteries is much less common, and involvement of the other cerebral arteries is rare. Children with TBM have hypercoagulability (prothrombotic and antifibrinolytic), which may further increase the risk for thrombosis and infarction (Schoeman et al. 2007).

Border-zone encephalopathy is the term for the inflammatory changes that occur in brain tissue immediately adjacent to tuberculous exudate. This may present as blindness (optochiasmatic arachnoiditis), cranial nerve paresis (especially IIIrd and VIth cranial nerve palsy) and signs of brainstem dysfunction. An acute tuberculous encephalopathy was described in young children and infants with pulmonary tuberculosis (Udani and Dastur 1970). A recent review highlighted that this rare condition is most likely to be pathologically heterogeneous and not only the result of immune demyelination as originally suggested (Lammie et al. 2007). Intracranial tuberculomas are space-occupying masses of granulomatous tissue.

CLINICAL ASPECTS OF TUBERCULOUS MENINGITIS

Staging

Outcome in TBM relates closely to the stage of disease at the time treatment is begun. Apart from having prognostic value in the individual patient, staging is also important when treatment modalities in different studies are compared. Shortly after the introduction of streptomycin, the first antituberculosis drug, the British Medical Research Council introduced a three-stage classification system (Medical Research Council 1948). During the 1970s this staging was 'modified' to include the Glasgow Coma Scale (GCS) and more recently 'refined' to improve prognostic accuracy (van Toorn et al. 2012b). The refined MRC scale is as follows.

Stage 1: GCS score of 15/15 with no focal neurological signs.
Stage 2a: GCS score of 15 with neurological deficit or a GCS score of 13–14 with or without neurological deficit.
Stage 2b: GCS score of 10–12 with or without neurological deficit.
Stage 3: GCS score <10.

Clinical features

Tandon (1978) called TBM the "Great Imposter" of neurological illness because it may mimic any neurological disease. He emphasized that TBM may be "acute, subacute or chronic in nature, febrile or afebrile at onset, with or without evidence of raised intracranial pressure and associated with sudden or progressive neurological deficit". Tuberculosis of the CNS can present with almost every symptom and sign ever described in neurology.

TBM is a disease of young children with 40% of patients being under 2 years of age and about 70% under 5 years at the time of presentation (Van Well et al. 2009). The onset is mostly insidious (days to weeks), and the early symptoms are non-specific, such as cough, low-grade fever, vomiting, irritability and general listlessness. Over days to weeks the full-blown clinical picture of meningitis develops, and loss of consciousness, signs of raised intracranial pressure (ICP) and motor and cranial nerve palsies become apparent. The neurological picture is mostly the result of the combined effects of ICP and infarction. Occasionally, either hydrocephalus or infarction is demonstrated by neuroimaging as the only cause of the clinical features. The following are common neurological manifestations of childhood TBM.

(1) *Meningeal irritation* (neck stiffness) is the first manifestation of possible meningitis in

the majority of cases. Occasionally a seizure or acute paralysis (hemiparesis or cranial nerve palsy) is the first neurological manifestation of TBM. Most children are too young to complain of headache and will instead show their discomfort by excessive crying or irritability.

(2) *Coma* occurs when the midbrain and/or the cerebral hemispheres are dysfunctional. Possible pathological correlates of coma in TBM include stroke (hemispheres and/or brainstem), border-zone encephalopathy (brainstem), raised ICP (cerebral hemispheres and brainstem when herniation occurs) and strategically situated tuberculomas (brainstem). Onset of coma is usually gradual. Rapid progressive loss of consciousness is highly suggestive of impending herniation due to non-communicating hydrocephalus.

(3) *Raised ICP* manifestations in childhood TBM are determined by the patient's age and type of onset (acute or chronic). Tuberculous hydrocephalus is by far the most common and presents with a bulging fontanelle in the young infant. Sudden-onset strabismus (due to nervus abducens paresis) is common in all age groups. Chronically raised ICP presents with excessive head growth and widened skull sutures in young infants and papilloedema in older children (Udani et al. 1971).

(4) *Motor paralysis* is common and almost always the result of arterial stroke of the basal ganglia and internal capsule due to panarteritis of the perforating branches of the middle cerebral arteries (Udani et al. 1971). Other non-ischaemic causes of motor paralysis include a Todd's paresis following a focal seizure or a strategically situated tuberculoma or tuberculoma en plaque involving the motor cortex. The latter is a thick tuberculous exudate covering the sensorimotor cortex and is a form of border-zone encephalopathy (Bharucha et al. 1969). Udani et al. (1971) found hemiparesis in 98 (20%) and bilateral hemiplegia (quadriplegia) in 96 (19%) of 500 Indian children with TBM. A recent study found that 37% and 25% of 554 South African children with TBM respectively had hemiparesis and quadriparesis on admission (Van Well et al. 2009). Hemiparesis may develop early during the course of treatment, presumably as a result of the progressive inflammation, but rarely later or after completion of antituberculosis therapy. Possible causes for late-onset paralysis include new or enlarging tuberculomas, dilatation of one lateral ventricle due to obstruction of the foramen of Munro, and vascular constriction and infarction due to organization of the basal exudate (Udani et al. 1971). Mycobacterial drug resistance or bacteriological relapse should always be excluded in these late-onset cases.

(5) *Extrapyramidal movement disorders* such as tremor, chorea and dystonia commonly occur because of ischaemia of the basal ganglia. Hemiballismus, usually on the opposite side to the hemiplegia, results when the subthalamic nuclei are involved.

(6) *Brainstem dysfunction other than coma* can occur in stage 3 TBM and usually carries a poor prognosis. The signs include decerebrate posturing, absence of the oculocephalic reflex and neurogenic hyperventilation (Schoeman et al. 1985).

(7) *Cranial nerves*, especially the IIIrd and VIth, are commonly affected during the later stages of the disease due to inflammation (perineuritis) or compression as a result of raised ICP. Anisocoria is the result of selective involvement of the external (oculomotor) fibres of the IIIrd cranial nerve. Facial weakness is usually of an upper motor neuron type and part of a hemiplegia. Lower motor paralysis of the facial nerve is rare in TBM, and tuberculous infection of the middle ear should always be excluded as a possible cause.

DIAGNOSIS

TBM is a medical emergency and treatment should be initiated as soon as the condition is suspected because delay is associated with death and neurological disability. All currently available rapid diagnostic tests are of low sensitivity. Emperic antituberculosis treatment is therefore advocated as soon as TBM is suspected clinically. This is based on a number of clinical features and special investigations. A uniform definition for classifying children with TBM for clinical research has been proposed (Marais et al. 2010).

Clinical diagnosis

The early onset of TBM is characterized by *persistence of non-specific symptoms and signs*. A South African study describing the initial presentation in 554 children with TBM found the most common presenting complaints were fever (67%), vomiting (53%), poor feeding (46%) and cough (32%) (Van Well et al. 2009). A mean period of 12 days elapsed between the time of first complaint and correct diagnosis. One hundred and thirty-six children (66%) were seen once or more during this period and were mostly diagnosed as having gastro-enteritis or an upper respiratory tract infection. As a rule, TBM was diagnosed only after repeated visits to health workers. Incorrect diagnoses included viral meningitis, other forms of bacterial meningitis, encephalitis, tetanus and brain abscess.

A large retrospective study recently reported weight faltering, documented as *crossing of weight centiles*, in 90% of cases at the time of first presentation. Even though this is a non-specific finding, it has definite diagnostic value when acted on in the context of a chronically ill child with non-specific symptoms (Van Well et al. 2009). The same study showed that once a diagnosis of TBM is considered, the following features support a diagnosis of tuberculosis: tuberculosis contact (53%), positive Mantoux skin test (60%), chest radiograph suggestive of primary tuberculosis (60%), and positive culture from gastric aspirate (18.6%). Once the disease has evolved into the second and third stages, neck stiffness and the other neurological signs described above will almost invariably lead to a clinical diagnosis of meningitis and the request for lumbar puncture.

Lumbar puncture

The CSF in TBM is typically macroscopically clear because of the relatively low cell count. In cases with very high protein content (e.g. spinal block) the appearance may be xantho-chromic. CSF analysis characteristically shows a predominance of lymphocytes, decreased CSF glucose (CSF:plasma ratio <0.5) and increased CSF protein. Atypical results may be encountered, ranging from a lymphocytic response with normal CSF glucose and protein

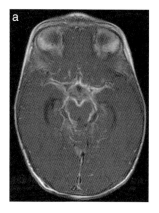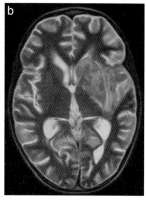

Fig. 14.1. (a) MRI: basal enhancement. Axial T1-weighted image with gadolinium in a 3-year-old male demonstrates marked basal enhancement typically seen in tuberculous meningitis, as evident by the linear, irregular and double-line enhancement as well as interpeduncular enhancement. (b) MRI: cerebral infarction. Axial T2-weighted image in a 6-year-old female demonstrates heterogeneous T2 hyperintense signal change in the left middle cerebral artery distribution involving almost the entire basal ganglia, in keeping with ischaemia.

values, to very high cell counts and a predominance of polymorphonuclear leukocytes. Failure to identify another causative organism when presented with one of these unusual CSF pictures must lead to consideration of TBM.

Neuroimaging

Cranial computerized tomography (CT) and more recently MRI are extremely helpful in diagnosing and managing TBM and its complications (Fig. 14.1) (Springer et al. 2009). The classic CT triad of TBM consists of basal meningovascular enhancement, obstructive hydrocephalus, and cerebral infarction, most commonly of the basal ganglia. One study found that the combination of hydrocephalus, basal enhancement and infarction is 100% specific and 41% sensitive for the diagnosis of childhood TBM (Andronikou et al. 2004). It should be noted that cryptococcal meningitis, toxoplasmosis, sarcoidosis, meningeal metastases and lymphoma can all produce similar radiological findings. Asymptomatic tuberculomas are often demonstrated in TBM. They may paradoxically enlarge or even develop on antituberculosis treatment and then become symptomatic. Follow-up CT often shows an increase in the degree of basal enhancement in spite of good clinical response to antituberculosis treatment. One study showed that MRI was superior to CT in demonstrating basal enhancement, infarction, morphology of tuberculomas and pathology of the posterior fossa structures, especially the brainstem (Pienaar et al. 2009).

Bacteriological diagnosis

Every effort should be made to confirm the diagnosis of TBM; this is particularly important in an era when drug-resistant tuberculosis is increasing. Demonstration of acid-fast bacilli is still the best rapid diagnostic test for CNS tuberculosis. Collecting adequate CSF volumes for culture and microscopy has been shown to improve diagnostic yield, and the recommendation for adults is that at least 6mL of CSF should be examined for at least 30 minutes (Thwaites et al. 2004). Collecting similar volumes of CSF in children with communicating hydrocephalus poses no danger to the patient. However, care should been taken in non-communicating hydrocephalus because of the possible danger of cerebral herniation. All other possible sources should also be sampled, and a positive gastric aspirate culture may be obtained even in the presence of a normal chest radiograph.

Molecular and immunodiagnosis

A systematic review and meta-analysis concluded that commercial nucleic acid amplification (NAA) assays can confirm TBM (98% specificity) but cannot rule it out (56% sensitivity) (Pai et al. 2003). One study showed that NAA was not diagnostically superior to microscopy and culture when large volumes of CSF were submitted for analysis (Thwaites et al. 2004). The greatest value of NAA may be in patients already commenced on treatment, a smaller proportion of whom may have a positive culture for *M. tuberculosis*. NAA assays that can detect rifampicin-resistant genotypes are valuable in the context of possible multidrug-resistant tuberculosis. There is some evidence that quantitative real-time polymerase chain reaction (PCR) may enhance bacterial detection in the CSF (Takahashi et al. 2008). Pre-treatment peripheral blood INF-γ enzyme-linked immunospot (ELISPOT) response has not shown any advantage over conventional bacteriological diagnosis in adults but has not been evaluated in children. The small CSF volumes obtained in children limit the use of INF-γ release assays, where much larger CSF volumes are required in order to obtain sufficient cells (Thwaites 2013). Adenosine deaminase activity is raised in the CSF of patients with TBM, but also in a number of other CNS infections including pyogenic and cryptococcal meningitis, malaria and brucellosis, and thus is not recommended as a routine diagnostic test for TBM. Recently, CSF protein electrophoresis has been suggested to differentiate TBM and pyogenic meningitis (Shekhar et al. 2013). Xpert MTB/RIF assay (Xpert; Cepheid, Sunnyvale, CA, USA) has been used for rapid diagnosis of TBM; sensitivities of 67%–85% and specificities of 94%–98% were obtained (Tortoli et al. 2012, Patel et al. 2013).

TREATMENT OF TUBERCULOUS MENINGITIS AND ITS COMPLICATIONS

Chemotherapy regimens for TBM are based on expert opinion rather than controlled randomized trials. Studies evaluating length of antituberculosis therapy for childhood TBM report similar relapse rates comparing 6-months treatment with 12-months treatment (Woodfield et al. 2008). Current WHO guidelines state that TBM should be treated with four antituberculosis drug therapy (RHZE, comprising rifampicin [R], isoniazid [H], pyrazinamide [Z] and ethambutol [E]) for 2 months followed by two-drug therapy (HR) for 10 months (WHO 2010). As the WHO has to consider the circumstances under which tuberculosis will be treated worldwide, this long duration of treatment was a compromise between the importance of preventing relapse, the unavailability of certain drugs (e.g. ethionamide)

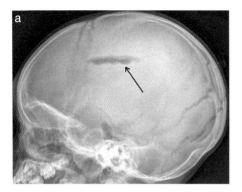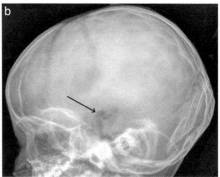

Fig. 14.2. (a) Lateral skull radiograph in a 4-year-old male showing air in the basal cistern and lateral ventricles. This indicates communicating hydrocephalus (arrow) due to basal cistern obstruction to the flow of cerebrospinal fluid. (b) Lateral skull radiograph in a 3-year-old male showing only air at the level of the basal cistern (arrow). This indicates non-communicating hydrocephalus due to obstruction of the fourth ventricle outlet foramen.

and an unwillingness to give pyrazinamide for more than 2 months in many settings (Donald 2010). Recently, short-course intensified treatment (6 months RHZE for HIV-uninfected and 9 months RHZE for HIV-infected patients) was found to be safe and effective in children with drug-susceptible TBM (van Toorn et al. 2013). The following single daily doses are suggested for the 6-month intensive treatment course: isoniazid 10–15mg/kg (maximum 300mg), rifampicin 10–20mg/kg (max. 600mg), pyrazinamide 30–40mg/kg and ethambutol (15–25mg/kg). Liver function should be monitored upon initiation of therapy and when clinically indicated thereafter. Adjunctive corticosteroids reduce death and disability from TBM by about 30% (Prasad and Singh 2008). Recently it was discovered that the beneficial effect of corticosteroids on survival might be augmented by aspirin and be predicted by screening for a polymorphism in LTA4H, which encodes an enzyme involved in eicosanoid synthesis (Thwaites 2013). Large doses of rifampicin and fluoroquinolones might improve outcome (Ruslami et al. 2013).

In practice, empirical treatment for TBM is usually completed unless a positive alternative diagnosis (e.g. bacterial meningitis) is made. A repeat lumbar puncture may be valuable in differentiating bacterial meningitis from TBM retrospectively. In TBM, CSF chemistry takes weeks or months to normalize and may even become more abnormal during the early weeks of antituberculosis treatment (Schoeman et al. 2001). However, the value of serial lumbar puncture results in stopping empirical treatment for TBM has not been tested in clinical practice.

Hydrocephalus
Treatment of tuberculous hydrocephalus is determined by the level of CSF obstruction. Air-encephalograpy (Fig. 14.2) is the most reliable way of determining the level of CSF

obstruction (Bruwer et al. 2004). The majority (80%) of children with communicating hydrocephalus will respond to medical therapy consisting of acetozolamide 50mg/kg/d and furosemide 1mg/kg/d (Lamprecht et al. 2001). Patients with non-communicating hydrocephalus are preferably treated surgically because of the risk of sudden death due to cerebral herniation. Endoscopic third ventriculoscopy is another surgical option offering the benefits of CSF diversion without the risk of shunt complications. This operation is not without risk as the anatomy of the floor of the third ventricle is often clouded by thick basal exudate (Jha et al. 2007). The high rate of survivors who have impairments despite active treatment of hydrocephalus underlines the important role of other mechanisms of brain damage, especially vasculitis, in TBM (Sil and Chatterjee 2008).

Stroke

Ischaemic brain damage is the most important reason for permanent neurological sequelae in TBM and also explains the poor response to treatment of hydrocephalus in some patients. About a third of all patients with advanced TBM will develop stroke (Van Well et al. 2009). Recent MRI studies show that the older CT-based literature vastly underestimated the extent of infarction and the incidence of brainstem infarcts in TBM (Pienaar et al. 2009). Infarcts are more common in younger children and those with advanced disease (Springer et al. 2009). Two randomized studies showed that adjunctive corticosteroids possibly reduce the risk of infarction in children and adults with TBM (Thwaites et al. 2007). The value of aspirin's antithrombotic, anti-ischaemic and anti-inflammatory properties in TBM was explored in two studies. An adult TBM study reported a significant reduction in mortality at 3 months (Misra et al. 2010). In contrast, a randomized controlled trial in children reported no significant benefit in morbidty or mortality at 6 months (Schoeman et al. 2011).

Hyponatraemia

Hyponatraemia is common in TBM and has been related to stage of disease, cerebral perfusion pressure and clinical outcome. Hyponatraemia may result from the syndromes of inappropriate antidiuretic hormone secretion (SIADH) or cerebral salt wasting (CSWS) (see Chapter 4). Patients with SIADH are euvolaemic or hypervolaemic and need fluid restriction, while CSWS is associated with hypovolaemia and requires fluid replacement. Evidence for CSWS in TBM is scanty and largely depends on case reports with poor documentation of hypovolaemia (Rivkees 2008).

A positive fluid balance in TBM is important because of the risk for stroke and also because of the associated hypercoagulability (Schoeman et al. 2007). Fluid intake should probably not be restricted because its dangers may outweigh the complications of hyponatraemia. In addition, diuretic treatment for tuberculous hydrocephalus should be initiated only once the patient's hydration status has normalized.

Multidrug-resistant tuberculous meningitis

Multidrug-resistant TBM in children has a poor clinical outcome and is associated with death (Seddon et al. 2012). Diagnosis of drug resistance depends on the recognition of risk factors (e.g. multidrug-resistant contact) and the results of susceptibility testing (molecular or conventional methods). Drug resistance should also be considered in cases of disease progression or relapse despite compliance on adequate drug dosages. Treatment regimes are determined by susceptibility results and include the use of pyrazinamide, a fluoroquinolone, ethionamide and an injectable agent such as amikacin.

HIV co-infection
The clinical, laboratory and radiological features of patients with TBM who are infected or uninfected with HIV are similar (Van der Weert et al. 2006). Diagnostic work-up for TBM should therefore always include an HIV test. The diagnostic sensitivity of cranial CT may be reduced in patients co-infected with HIV because of less prominent basal enhancement, presumably the result of a decreased inflammatory response (Katrak et al. 2000, Van der Weert et al. 2006).

The optimal time to initiate antiretroviral therapy (ART) in children with HIV-associated TBM is unknown. A randomized, double-blind, placebo-controlled trial of immediate versus deferred ART in adult patients found that HIV-associated TBM had such a poor prognosis that the timing of ART made no appreciable difference regarding survival probability. However, there were significantly more grade 4 adverse events in the immediate ART arm, providing some support for delaying the initiation of ART in HIV-associated TBM, especially in those patients with CD4 counts greater than 100 cells/mL (Torok et al. 2011). Drug interactions, toxicity and immune reconstitution disease are possible complications of treatment in these patients.

Tuberculous meningitis-associated immune reconstitution inflammatory syndrome (IRIS)
Clinical and neuroradiological deterioration may occur in TBM despite adequate treatment and drug-sensitive organisms. This phenomenon, the result of IRIS, is often more severe in the setting of HIV co-infection and may be life threatening. Paradoxical TBM-IRIS should be considered when new neurological signs develop shortly after initiation of ART in children. Neurological signs and symptoms include headache, seizures, meningeal irritation, decreased level of consciousness, ataxia and focal motor deficit (van Toorn et al. 2012a). Corticosteroids are the mainstay of treatment for TBM-IRIS with interruption of ART reserved for life-threatening complications. Other immune-modulatory agents that have been used to treat IRIS in a limited number of children include thalidomide, chloroquine, mycophenolatemofetil and cyclosporine (van Toorn et al. 2012a). Two case series of consecutive patients, one with large tuberculomas and the other with tuberculous abscesses and blindness due to optic arachnoiditis, showed dramatic clinical and neuroradiological improvement after low-dose thalidomide was added to the treatment regimen (Schoeman et al. 2010). Caution should be exercised, however, as thalidomide has serious side-effects.

PROGNOSIS
The combination of modern antituberculosis treatment regimens with adjunctive corticosteroids and active treatment of hydrocephalus has reduced mortality in TBM to below 15%

(Mahadevan et al. 2002, Van Well et al. 2009). The most important determinants of outcome are age and stage of disease at presentation (Van Well et al. 2009). In contrast to the improvement in mortality, neurological disability is still unacceptably high, with a recent study reporting mild neurological sequelae in 52% and severe sequelae in 18% of 412 South African children (mean age 28 months) with stage 2 and 3 TBM (Van Well et al. 2009). The main long-term sequelae of TBM relate to cognitive (80%) and behavioural (40%) impairments. Delayed diagnosis, drug resistance and HIV co-infection affect outcome adversely.

Tuberculoma
Intracranial tuberculomas are space-occupying masses of granulomatous tissue that result from haematogenous spread from a distant focus of tuberculous infection, usually the lung. Histologically, tuberculomas consist of a necrotic caseous centre surrounded by a capsule that contains fibroblasts, epithelioid cells, Langhans giant cells and lymphocytes. Liquefaction of the caseous centre may result in a tuberculous abscess.

CLINICAL PRESENTATION
Intracranial tuberculomas are often clinically silent and may occur in patients with or without other manifestations of tuberculosis. Asymptomatic tuberculomas are often an incidental finding on CT in children with TBM. The most common clinical presentation of a tuberculoma is that of a seizure in a child who is otherwise clinically well. Large tuberculomas can mimic a brain tumour with signs of chronically raised ICP and focal neurological deficit. The neurological presentation in these cases depends on the location of the lesion (Udani et al. 1971). Exceptionally, tuberculomas can present with hypopituitarism, extrapyramidal symptoms and brainstem syndromes.

DIAGNOSIS
Intracranial tuberculomas are usually not suspected before they present with neurological symptoms and signs. Constitutional symptoms vary, clinical findings suggestive of extraneural tuberculosis are frequently absent, and only a minority of patients have a history of a tuberculosis contact. Once a tuberculoma becomes symptomatic, neuroimaging confirms a mass lesion and tuberculoma is considered in the differential diagnosis. The CT and (T1-weighted) MRI appearance of a solid caseous tuberculoma is that of an isodense or mildly hyperdense brain lesion with marked surrounding low density that demonstrates vasogenic oedema (Fig. 14.3). Marked rim enhancement is always present after contrast administration. A hypodense centre indicates liquefaction and abscess formation. Unfortunely these radiological features are not specific for tuberculoma. The differential diagnosis of solid tuberculomas includes toxoplasmosis and cerebral tumours, while cystic tuberculomas cannot be differentiated from pyogenic brain abscess and neurocysticercosis on usual imaging alone. Other clinical or radiological evidence of tuberculosis (e.g. pulmonary tuberculosis or TBM) is helpful when present. The characteristic T2-hypointense appearance ('T2 black') of solid, caseous tuberculomas may help to differentiate them from other solid ring-enhancing lesions such as brain tumours (Fig. 14.4).

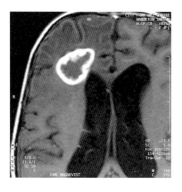

Fig. 14.3. MRI: tuberculoma. Axial T1-weighted image with gadolinium in an 8-year-old male demonstrates well-circum-scribed, irregular ring-enhancing lesion in the right frontal lobe with surrounding vasogenic oedema and minimal mass effect on the right frontal horn.

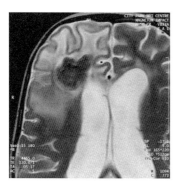

Fig. 14.4. MRI: tuberculoma. Axial T2-weighted image of the same patient as in Figure 14.3 demonstrates the characteristic hypointense T2 signal seen centrally in a solid caseous tuber-culoma, confirming the diagnosis.

Childhood tuberculomas may be located in the brain (parenchymal) or have their origin from the meninges or even ependyma (meningeal). Tuberculomas associated with TBM are often adjacent to the dense basal meningovascular enhancement. Intracranial tuberculomas may develop or increase in size on antituberculosis therapy (for either pulmonary tuberculosis or TBM). A small, single granuloma is a common CT finding in children who present with a first seizure, and may be caused by tuberculosis or neurocysticercosis. In the absence of other clinical or laboratory evidence, it is often impossible to discern between these two aetiologies without histology. One study on histologically proven single granulomas found that, on CT, tuberculomas tend to be larger (>20mm) and have a more irregular outline than cysticercus granulomas (Rajshekhar et al. 1993). In a small series the high lipid and choline content of tuberculomas differentiated them from cysticerci on magnetic resonance spectroscopy (Pretell et al. 2005). In contrast to the situation in adults, intracranial mass lesions other than tuberculomas are uncommon in HIV-infected children.

TREATMENT AND PROGNOSIS
The treatment of intracranial tuberculomas is similar to that of TBM and includes antituberculosis therapy and corticosteroids. Corticosteroids are generally believed to be beneficial

but the evidence for this is mainly anecdotal. Most tuberculomas will become smaller or even resolve within 3 months of medical treatment, although large tuberculomas may take years to heal. Secondary obstructive hydrocephalus should be treated surgically (usually by ventriculoperitoneal shunting or endoscopic third ventriculostomy), and debulking of huge tuberculomas may be clinically indicated. Tuberculous abscesses are notoriously resistant to medical treatment and should preferably be excised and not just drained. It has been shown that adjunctive thalidomide may enhance the resolution of tuberculous abscesses that are surgically inaccessible (Schoeman et al. 2006).

Spinal tuberculosis

Spinal tuberculosis is an ancient disease that has been demonstrated in a skeleton dating from around 5000 BC. The English surgeon Percival Pott (1714–1788) is credited as having recognized the tuberculous nature of this condition, and spinal tuberculosis is often referred to as Pott disease. It is the most common cause of tuberculous myelopathy, usually affecting the lower thoracic and upper lumbar vertebrae. It is predominantly a disease of children in resource-poor countries where tuberculosis is prevalent. Less common causes of tuberculosis-related spinal involvement include spinal tuberculomas (intra- or extradural) and tuberculous arachnoiditis (myeloradiculopathy).

Pathogenesis and Pathology

Spinal tuberculosis occurs secondary to lympho-haematogenous spread. The central type of vertebral tuberculosis spreads along the Batson plexus of veins, while paradiscal infection spreads through the arteries. The tubercle bacillus destroys cancellous bone and spreads to adjacent vertebrae via the disc space. Eventually vertebral collapse ensues, resulting in kyphosis and gibbus formation. Bony displacement, abscess or granulation tissue formation may all lead to spinal cord compression.

Tuberculomas compromise spinal cord function through mass effect and inflammation. Injury to the cord occurs mainly through oedema and ischaemia rather than frank infarction because the larger arteries are rarely involved (Dastur and Wadia 1969).

Tuberculous myeloradiculopathy arises primarily in the meninges. Occasionally it may be secondary to downward extension of tuberculous basal meningitis and rarely secondary to osteitis. The underlying pathological process responsible for cord and nerve-root damage is arachnoid adhesions that cause CSF flow obstruction, arteritis and border-zone encephalopathy.

Clinical Features

The onset is usually insidious because disease progression is slow. Pain overlying the vertebrae and non-specific constitutional symptoms (fever, malaise, weight loss) are most commonly encountered. Manifestations of extra-skeletal tuberculosis may also be present. Neurological complications occur in 10%–30% of children. Since tuberculosis can affect any part of the spinal cord, including the nerve roots, the clinical presentation may be that of upper or lower motor neuron involvement, or both. Children often present with either

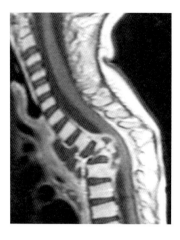

Fig. 14.5. Spinal MRI: tuberculous spondylitis. Sagittal T1-weighted image with gadolinium enhancement in a 5-year-old boy demonstrates thoracic gibbus formation secondary to destruction of T3 and T4 vertebral bodies with an associated extradural, ring-enhancing fluid collection (tuberculous abscess) causing compression of the spinal cord. The anterior subligamentous spread of the disease is typical for tuberculous spondylodiscitis.

flaccid or spastic paraparesis, often with associated sensory involvement. Cervical involvement (uncommon) should be considered in children presenting with hoarseness, dysphagia, respiratory stridor or torticollis. Examination of the spine may reveal localized tenderness and paravertebral muscle spasm. A kyphotic (gibbus) deformity due to prominence of spinous processes may be evident owing to collapse and anterior wedging of vertebral bodies.

DIAGNOSIS

Diagnostic imaging should begin with plain radiology (anteroposterior and lateral). Early changes include anterior vertebral body scalloping, loss of vertebral height or endplate changes in multiple vertebral bodies. Relative disc-space sparing distinguishes spinal tuberculosis from pyogenic osteomyelitis. Advanced disease changes include further vertebral collapse and the development of a kyphotic or gibbus deformity.

CT allows for earlier detection and is useful for demonstrating calcification within paraspinal abscesses and visualizing of small bone fragments in areas of destroyed bone. The best diagnostic modality for spinal tuberculosis is MRI with gadolinium administration (Fig. 14.5). It provides superior visualization of paraspinal and subligamentous disease and is best at detecting intramedullary tuberculomas, cord oedema and cavitation. The radiological signs of radiculomyelitis include enhancement, thickening and clumping of the nerve roots. The presence of cord atrophy or cavitation (syrinx) is associated with poor outcome (Wasay et al. 2003).

CSF analysis, blood investigations (erythrocyte sedimentation rate), chest radiography, tuberculin skin testing and gastric washings may also aid in the diagnosis. As skeletal tuberculosis is paucibacillary, cultures are usually negative.

TREATMENT

There is no consensus on the most appropriate management of spinal tuberculosis and little evidence on which to base guidelines. Antituberculosis medication of 12 months duration has been found to be effective in more than 90% of cases (Eisen 2012). Corticosteroids appear to have a beneficial effect but have not been subjected to randomized clinical trials.

Surgery is indicated when neurological complications develop and to prevent progressive scoliosis. Patients with relatively preserved cord size on MRI respond well to non-operative treatment in the presence of predominantly fluid compression. Early surgical decompression is indicated where MRI demonstrates extradural compression by granulation tissue with little fluid component compressing or constricting the spinal cord circumferentially.

REFERENCES

Andronikou S, Smith B, Hatherhill M, et al. (2004) Definitive neuroradiological diagnostic features of tuberculous meningitis in children. *Pediatr Radiol* 34: 876–85.

Bharucha PE, Iyer CG, Bharucha EP, et al. (1969) Tuberculous meningitis in children: a clinico-pathological evaluation of 24 cases. *Indian Pediatr* 6: 282–90.

Bruwer GE, van der Westhuizen S, Lombard CJ, et al. (2004) Can CT predict the level of CSF block in tuberculous hydrocephalus? *Childs Nerv Syst* 20: 183–7.

Caws M, Thwaites G, Stepniewska K, et al. (2006) Beijing genotype of *Mycobacterium tuberculosis* is significantly associated with human immunodeficiency virus infection and multidrug resistance in cases of tuberculous meningitis. *J Clin Microbiol* 44: 3934–9.

Caws M, Thwaites G, Dunstan S, et al. (2008) The influence of host and bacterial genotype on the development of disseminated disease with *Mycobacterium tuberculosis*. *PLoS Pathog* 4: e1000034.

Dastur DK, Wadia NH (1969) Spinal meningitides with radiculomyelopathy. Part II: Pathology and pathogenesis. *J Neurol Sci* 8: 261–97.

Donald P, Schoeman JF, Beyers N, et al. (1995) Concentrations of interferon gamma, tumour necrosis factor alpha, and interleukin-1 in the cerebrospinal fluid of children treated for tuberculous meningitis. *Clin Infect Dis* 21: 924–9.

Donald PR (2010) The chemotherapy of tuberculous meningitis in children and adults. *Tuberculosis* 90: 375–92.

Eisen S, Honywood L, Shingadia D, et al. (2012) Spinal tuberculosis in children. *Arch Dis Child* 7: 724–9.

Jha DK, Mishra V, Choudhary A, et al. (2007) Factors affecting the outcome of neuroendoscopy in patients with tuberculous meningitis hydrocephalus: a preliminary study. *Surg Neurol* 68: 35–41.

Katrak SM, Shembalker PK, Bijwe SR, et al. (2000) The clinical, radiological and pathological profile of tuberculous meningitis in patients with and without human immunodeficiency virus infection. *J Neurol Sci* 181: 118–26.

Lammie GA, Hewlett RH, Schoeman JF, et al. (2007) Tuberculous encephalopathy: a re-appraisal. *Acta Neuropathol* 113: 227–34.

Lamprecht D, Schoeman J, Donald P, et al. (2001) Ventriculoperitoneal shunting in childhood tuberculous hydrocephalus. *Br J Neurosurg* 15: 119–25.

Mahadevan B, Mahadevan S, Serane VT, et al. (2002) Prognostic factors in childhood tuberculous meningitis. *J Trop Pediatr* 48: 362–5.

Marais S, Thwaites G, Schoeman JF, et al. (2010) Tuberculous meningitis: a uniform case definition for use in clinical research. *Lancet Infect Dis* 10: 803–12.

Maree F, Hesseling AC, Schaaf HS, et al. (2007) Absence of an association between *Mycobacterium tuberculosis* genotype and clinical features in children with tuberculous meningitis. *Pediatr Infect Dis J* 26: 13–8.

Medical Research Council (1948) Streptomycin treatment of tuberculous meningitis. Streptomycin in Tuberculosis Trials Committee. *Lancet* 1: 582–96.

Misra UK, Kalita J, Nair PP (2010) Role of aspirin in tuberculous meningitis: randomized open label placebo controlled trial. *J Neurol Sci* 293: 12–7.

Pai M, Flores LL, Pai N, et al. (2003) Diagnostic accuracy of nucleic acid amplification tests for tuberculous meningitis: a systemic review and meta-analysis. *Lancet Infect Dis* 3: 633–43.

Patel VB, Theron G, Lenders L, et al. (2013) Diagnostic accuracy of quantitative PCR (Xpert MTB/RIF) for tuberculous meningitis in a high burden setting: a prospective study. *PLoS Med* 10: e1001536.

Pienaar M, Andronikou S, van Toorn R (2009) MRI to demonstrate diagnostic features and complications of TBM not seen with CT. *Childs Nerv Syst* 25: 941–7.

Prasad K, Singh MB (2008) Corticosteroids for managing tuberculous meningitis. *Cochrane Database Syst Rev* 1: CD 002244. doi: 10.1002/14651858.CD002244.pub3.

Pretell EJ, Martinot C Jr, Garcia HH, et al. (2005) Differential diagnosis between cerebral tuberculosis and neurocysticercosis by magnetic resonance spectroscopy. *J Comput Assist Tomogr* 29: 112–4.

Rajshekhar V, Haran RP, Prakash GS, et al. (1993) Differentiating solitary small cysticercus granulomas and tuberculomas in patients with epilepsy. Clinical and computerized tomographic criteria. *J Neurosurg* 78: 402–7.

Rich AR, McCordock HA (1933) The pathogenesis of tuberculous meningitis. *Bull Johns Hopkins Hosp* 52: 5–38.

Rivkees SA (2008) Differentiating appropriate antidiuretic hormone secretion, inappropriate antidiuretic hormone secretion and cerebral salt wasting: the common, uncommon, and misnamed. *Curr Opin Pediatr* 20: 448–52.

Ruslami R, Ganiem AR, Dian S, et al. (2013) Intensified regimen containing rifampicin and moxifloxacin for tuberculous meningitis: an open-label, randomised controlled phase 2 trial. *Lancet Infect Dis* 13: 27–35.

Schoeman JF, Le Roux D, Bezuidenhout PB, et al. (1985) Intracranial pressure monitoring in tuberculous meningitis: clinical and computerized tomographic correlation. *Dev Med Child Neurol* 27: 644–54.

Schoeman JF, Elshof JW, Laubsher JA, et al. (2001) The effect of adjuvant steroid treatment on cerebrospinal fluid changes in tuberculous meningitis. *Ann Trop Paediatr* 21: 299–305.

Schoeman JF, Fieggen G, Seller N, et al. (2006) Intractable intracranial tuberculous infection responsive to thalidomide: report of four cases. *J Child Neurol* 21: 301–8.

Schoeman JF, Andronikou S, Stefan DC, et al. (2010) Tuberculous meningitis-related optic neuritis: recovery of vision with thalidomide in 4 consecutive cases. *J Child Neurol* 25: 822–8.

Schoeman JF, Janse van Rensburg A, Laubsher JA, et al. (2011) The role of aspirin in childhood tuberculous meningitis. *J Child Neurol* 26: 956–62.

Seddon JA, Visser DH, Bartens M, et al. (2012) Impact of drug resistance on clinical outcome in children with tuberculous meningitis. *Pediatr Infect Dis* 7: 711–6.

Shekhar R, Rao JR, Devi KA, Rao RB (2013) CSF proteins as discriminatory markers of tubercular and pyogenic meningitis. *J Clin Diagn Res* 7: 1586–8. doi: 10.7860/JCDR/2013/6361.3226.

Sil K, Chatterjee S (2008) Shunting in tuberculous meningitis: a neurosurgeon's nightmare. *Childs Nerv Syst* 9: 1029–32.

Springer P, Swanevelder S, van Toorn R, et al. (2009) Cerebral infarction and neurodevelopmental outcome in childhood tuberculous meningitis. *Eur J Paediatr Neurol* 13: 343–9.

Sterling TR, Martire T, de Almeida AS, et al. (2007) Immune function in young children with previous pulmonary or miliary/meningeal tuberculosis and impact of BCG vaccination. *Pediatrics* 120: e912–21.

Takahashi T, Tamura M, Asami Y, et al. (2008) Novel wide-range quantitative nested real-time PCR assay for *Mycobacterium tuberculosis* DNA: development and methodology. *J Clin Microbiol* 46: 1708–15.

Tandon PN (1978) Tuberculous meningitis (cranial and spinal). In: Vinken PJ, Bruyn GW, eds. *Handbook of Clinical Neurology*. Amsterdam: Elsevier/North Holland Biomedical Press, pp. 195–262.

Thwaites GE (2013) Advances in the diagnosis and treatment of tuberculous meningitis. *Curr Opin Neurol* 26: 295–300.

Thwaites GE, Chau TT, Farrar JJ (2004) Improving the bacteriological diagnosis of tuberculous meningitis. *J Clin Microbiol* 42: 378–9.

Thwaites GE, Macmullen-Price J, Tran TH, et al. (2007) Serial MRI to determine the effect of dexamethasone on the cerebral pathology of tuberculous meningitis: an observational study. *Lancet Neurol* 6: 230–6.

Thwaites GE, Caws M, Chau TTH, et al. (2008) Relationship between *Mycobacterium tuberculosis* genotype and the clinical phenotype of pulmonary and meningeal tuberculosis. *J Clin Microbiol* 46: 1363–8.

Torok ME, Yen NT, Chau TT, et al. (2011) Timing of initiation of antiretroviral therapy in human immunodeficiency virus (HIV)-associated tuberculous meningitis. *Clin Infect Dis* 52: 1374–83.

Tortoli E, Russo C, Piersimoni C, et al. (2012) Clinical validation of Xpert MTB/RIF for the diagnosis of extrapulmonary tuberculosis. *Eur Respir J* 40: 442–7.

Udani PM, Dastur DK (1970) Tuberculous encephalopathy with and without meningitis. Clinical features and pathological correlations. *J Neurol Sci* 10: 541–61.

Udani PM, Parekh UC, Dastur DK (1971) Neurological and related syndromes in CNS tuberculosis. Clinical features and pathogenesis. *J Neurol Sci* 14: 341–57.

Van der Weert EM, Hartgers M, Eley B, et al. (2006) Comparison of diagnostic criteria of TBM in HIV-infected and -uninfected children. *Ped Infect Dis J* 25: 65–9.

van Toorn R, Rabie H, Dramowski A, et al. (2012a) Neurological manifestations of TB-immune reconstitution inflammatory syndrome. *Eur J Paediatr Neurol* 16: 676–82.

van Toorn R, Springer P, Laubsher JA, Schoeman JF (2012b) Value of different staging systems for predicting neurological outcome in childhood tuberculous meningitis. *Int J Tuberc Lung Dis* 16: 628–32.

van Toorn R, Schaaf HS, Laubscher JA, et al. (2013) Short intensified treatment in children with drug-susceptible tuberculous meningitis. *Pediatr Infect Dis J* Oct 28. [Epub ahead of print.]

Van Well GTJ, Paes BF, Terwee CB, et al. (2009) Twenty years of pediatric tuberculous meningitis: a retrospective cohort study in the Western Cape of South Africa. *Pediatrics* 123: e1–8.

Wasay M, Kheleani BA, Moolani MK, et al. (2003) Brain CT and MRI findings in 100 consecutive patients with intracranial tuberculoma. *Neuroimaging* 13: 240–7.

WHO (2010) *Rapid Advice. Treatment of Tuberculosis in Children.* Geneva: World Health Organization (online: http://whqlibdoc.who.int/publications/2010/9789241500449_eng.pdf).

15
FUNGAL INFECTIONS

Sunit Singhi

A large number of fungi can infect the CNS. The majority cause disease in immunocompromised hosts (e.g. *Candida* spp., *Aspergillus* spp., *Zygomycetes* spp. and *Trichosporon* spp.), others cause disease in a healthy host (*Cryptococcus* spp., *Histoplasma* spp., *Blastomyces dermatidis*, *Coccidioides immitis*, *Sporothrix* spp., etc.), while some (*Cryptococcus* and *Candida* spp.) cause disease in both healthy and immunocompromised hosts.

In recent years fungal infections of the CNS appear to be on the increase particularly in immunocompromised hosts. The predisposing conditions include neutropenia, leukaemia, lymphoreticular malignancy, lymphoma, malnutrition, use of immunosuppressive drugs, corticosteroid therapy, widespread use of potent broad-spectrum antibiotic therapy, or acquired immunodeficiency syndrome (AIDS) caused by human immunodeficiency virus (HIV). Diabetes mellitus, renal failure and solid organ transplantation are other predisposing conditions.

Epidemiology

The incidence of fungal CNS infections is unknown. Of the several thousand fungal species that exist, about a dozen yeasts and thirty moulds are common causes of human fungal infections. CNS infection can be caused by yeasts (*Candida*, *Cryptococcus*), moulds (*Aspergillus* spp., *Fusarium* spp.) zygomycetes (*Mucor* spp., *Rhizopus* spp.) and dematiaceous fungi (*Pseudallescheria* [*Scedosporium*] spp.) (Redmond et al. 2007). *Candida* and *Aspergillus* spp. are ubiquitous and disseminate from endogenous sources. Most cases of invasive aspergillosis are caused by *A. fumigatus*, others by *A. flavus*, *A. niger* and *A. terreus* (Perfect et al. 2001). *Cryptococcus neoformans*, an encapsulated yeast, is an environmental fungus that is found in soil and bird droppings and causes primary infection usually through inhalation. The incidence of cryptococcal meningitis has increased with the spread of HIV infection. Although the use of antiretroviral therapy has led to a decrease in the incidence of cryptococcosis in resource-rich countries, the condition still affects about 1 million patients globally every year and has an estimated mortality of 625 000 persons (Park et al. 2009). The majority of these deaths occur in HIV-positive patients in sub-Saharan Africa. *C. neoformans* and *C. gattii* are the main pathogens in humans. Recently two varieties of *C. neoformans* – *C. neoformans* var. *grubii* (formerly group A) and *C. neoformans* var. *neoformans* (formerly group D) – as well as *C. gattii* (formerly groups B and C) have been recognized as distinct species (Franzot et al. 1999). Varieties *grubii* (serotype A) and *neoformans* (serotype D) are found worldwide, whereas variety *gattii* (serotypes B and C) is found in tropical and subtropical regions (Australia, southeast Asia, central Africa and California), particularly on flowering eucalyptus trees. *Zygomycetes* and *Trichosporon* are ubiquitous in distribution. *Coccidioides*, *Histoplasma* and *Blastomycoses* have been reported only from different parts of the USA and rarely cause disease in children.

Pathogenesis

The primary site of fungal infection is usually in the lungs and rarely the skin, from where haematogenous spread occurs to the central nervous system (CNS). Pulmonary infection occurs mainly from inhalation of fungal particles (yeast, *Aspergillus*, basidiospores of *Cryptococci*, arthroconidia of *Coccidioides*, and spores of *Histoplasma* and *Blastomycoses*). *Scedosporium apiospermum* and its teleomorph, which are ubiquitous saprophytic fungi, may get into lungs during a near-drowning episode (Katragkou et al. 2007). The pulmonary infection often remains subclinical or asymptomatic, although in immunocompromised patients it may cause pneumonia of varying severity including diffuse interstitial pneumonia. *Candida* and *Aspergillus* spp. spread to the CNS primarily through the haematogenous route. Dissemination from lung may rarely occur with *Coccidioides*, *Histoplasma* and *Scedosporium*, causing CNS disease. *Blastomycoses* causes a granulomatous lung lesion, which may disseminate to the CNS in about a third of cases.

Zygomyces (*Mucor*) has a contiguous spread to the CNS from paranasal sinuses, ear or orbit through tissue planes and blood vessels. *Aspergillus* may also spread through this route causing invasive intracranial disease, which may sometimes remain confined to extradural space (Mohindra et al. 2008). *Candida* usually colonizes in the skin and gastrointestinal mucosa; haematogenous spread to the CNS can occur in immunocompromised patients. Direct inoculation of *Candida* may occur during head injury or neurosurgical procedures such as ventriculostomy and ventricular peritoneal shunt placement. Contiguous spread from osteomyelitis of skull or vertebrae can rarely occur.

Yeast forms (*Cryptococcus* and *Candida*) are prime pathogens in immunodeficient and HIV/AIDS patients. Hyphal forms (*Aspergillus* and *Zygomycetes*) are the most common organisms in non-HIV patients. In haematological malignancy, renal failure, prolonged steroid therapy and solid organ transplant, candidiasis and aspergillosis are common.

Spinal-cord involvement can occur in the form of epidural abscess, focal spinal meningitis (arachnoiditis) and frank fungal myelitis.

Pathology

CNS pathology is determined largely by the size of the fungus. Yeast forms, being small in size enter the microcirculation and tend to cause more diffuse disease. Hyphal forms or moulds generally cause focal disease with vascular invasion causing haemorrhagic necrosis. The pathological findings in children with fungal CNS infections can thus range from meningitis and meningoencephalitis to focal lesions, infarction and abscesses. Meningitis is the most frequent; *C. gattii* is the aetiological agent in healthy individuals, whereas *C. neoformans* mainly affects immunocompromised subjects. Occurrrence of chronic suppurative and granulomatous inflammation leads to thickening of meninges, hydrocephalus, arteritis, cranial nerve palsies and infarction. *Coccidioides immitis* causes widespread basal meningitis. *Candida* commonly causes meningitis in low-birthweight infants and immuno-deficient children.

C. neoformans and *Candida* spp. may also cause meningoencephalitis. In cryptococcosis, clusters of fungi spread through the brain, with little or no surrounding inflammatory response, forming partially cystic and partially solid lesions. These lesions predominantly involve the basal ganglia and cortical grey matter, and rarely the brainstem (Hong et al. 2008). The typical cystic lesions contain gelatinous polyscaccharide, which is detected in cerebrospinal fluid (CSF).

Disseminated candidiasis, especially *C. albicans* and *C. tropicalis*, may cause focal necrosis producing microabcesses mainly in the middle cerebral artery territory.

Aspergillus, zygomycetes (*Mucorales*), *Blastomyces*, and *Scedosporium* spp. more commonly cause focal lesions and brain abscess. *Aspergillus* (all species *A. fumigatus*, *A. flavus*, *A. terreus*) is the most common cause of focal CNS infections in organ transplant patients. Extensive angio-invasion occurs with *Aspergillus* spp. and mucormycoses. The resultant arteritis/vasculitis predisposes to thrombosis, infarction and haemorrhage. Zygomycosis causes invasive fungal infection of the base of the skull by contiguous spread from paranasal sinuses; involvement of adjoining parts of carotid arteries and their branches can present as complicated stroke with signs of meningitis.

Clinical features
There are no specific clinical features. The underlying clinical context of a predisposed host may give aetiological clues (Table 15.1). Clinical syndromes that are seen with various fungal infections (Murthy 2007) are shown in Table 15.2.

SEIZURES
New-onset seizures and altered consciousness in a child with an underlying predisposing condition should alert the clinician to the presence of CNS fungal infection including encephalitis and meningitis (Teive et al. 2008).

MENINGITIS
Fungal meningitis is commonly caused by *Cryptococcus* spp. and *Candida* spp., sometimes by *Histoplasma* spp., *Blastomyces* spp. and *Coccidioides* spp. Clinical manifestations of fungal meningitis are less stereotypical than the manifestations of bacterial meningitis (Fernandez et al. 2000, Chen et al. 2004). Cryptococcal meningitis is often acute or sub-acute in children infected with HIV (Gumbo et al. 2002) and in those with T-cell suppression (Shih et al. 2000). A combination of fever, headache, lethargy, nausea, vomiting, neck rigidity, impaired consciousness, convulsions and focal neurological deficits is often present (Shih et al. 2000, Gumbo et al. 2002). Raised intracranial pressure (due to encephalitis or hydrocephalus) may develop acutely or during progression of the disease. Children on high-dose corticosteroid therapy or those with underlying HIV infection may have severe symptoms and signs.

TABLE 15.1
Common fungal infections and their likely association with predisposing factors

Predisposing factor	Likely fungi
Preterm birth, low birthweight	*Candida albicans, Aspergillus*
Immune deficiency states (e.g. chronic granulomatous disease, severe combined immunodeficiency)	*Candida, Cryptococcus, Aspergillus*
HIV/AIDS	*Cryptococcus, Histoplasma, Candida coccidioides*
Corticosteroid therapy	*Cryptococcus, Candida*
Haematological malignancy	*Candida, Cryptococcus, Coccidioides*
Organ transplantation	*Candida, Cryptococcus*
Cytotoxic agents	*Aspergillus, Candida*
Ketoacidosis, renal acidosis	*Zygomycetes* (*Mucor*)
Iron chelator therapy	*Zygomycetes*
Intravenous drug abuse	*Candida, Zygomycetes*
Trauma, foreign body	*Candida*
Near-drowning	*Scedosporium*

HIV, human immunodeficiency virus; AIDS, autoimmune deficiency syndrome.

Fungal meningitis should always be considered in the differential diagnosis of a patient with a subacute or chronic meningitis syndrome.

RHINO-CEREBRAL SYNDROME

Rhino-cerebral syndrome consisting of orbital pain, serosanguinous or blackish nasal discharge and facial oedema (Fig. 15.1) is a major presentation of zygomycosis (*Rhizopus* and *Mucor*), especially in patients with poorly controlled diabetes (Sundaram et al. 2005), renal failure or neutropenia, and in infants who were born preterm (Zauotis et al. 2007). Affected children may have proptosis and visual loss; trigeminal nerve involvement often occurs as the disease progresses. This is classically seen in mucormycosis where blackish necrotic areas are seen in the palate and nasal turbinates.

Involvement of carotid arteries may cause extensive infarction and hemiparesis. Aspergillosis or mucormycosis may present with sudden onset of stroke, focal neurodeficit and seizures caused by vasculitis (arteritis or phlebitis), and rarely with cerebral or subarachnoid haemorrhage caused by rupture of mycotic aneurysms.

BRAIN ABSCESS

CNS aspergillosis occurs in 10%–15% of patients with invasive aspergillosis and most commonly presents as single or multiple brain abscesses with focal neurodeficits (Dotis et al. 2007) (Fig. 15.2). In the series reported by Dotis et al. (2007), leukaemia, most commonly acute lymphoblastic type, was the most frequent underlying disease. *Aspergillus fumigatus* was isolated from 76% of the patients.

TABLE 15.2
Fungal infection of the central nervous system – clinical syndromes

Fungal infection	Relative incidence	Meningitis	Intracranial mass lesions	Skull–base syndrome	Rhinocerebral form	Stroke syndrome	Spinal syndrome
Aspergillosis	Common	+	++	+++	+	+	+
Cryptoccocis	Common	+++	+	–	–	+	+
Candidiasis	Occasional	+	–	–	–	+	–
Zygomycosis	Occasional	+	++	–	+++	+	–
Scedosporiosis	Rare	+	++	–	–	+	–
Histoplasmosis	Occasional	+	++	–	–	–	–
Blastomycosis	Occasional	+	+++	–	–	–	–

223

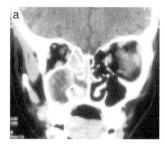
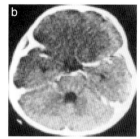

Fig. 15.1. (a) MRI in a 5-year-old child with rhino-orbito-cerebral mucormycosis and underlying diabetic ketoacidosis showing complete opacification of right maxillary sinus. Biopsy confirmed mucormycosis. (b) Extensive infarct caused by mucormycosis in the same patient. (Reproduced by permission from Singhi et al. 2011.)

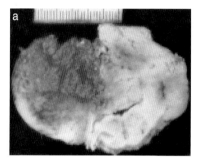
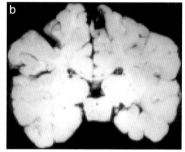

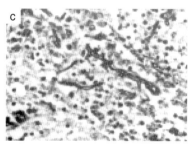

Fig. 15.2. (a,b) Cut sections of the brain showing necrotic lesions and abscesses caused by *Aspergillus* in a child with disseminated aspergillosis. (c) Photomicrograph showing acute-angle dichotomous branching fungal hyphae of *Aspergillus* in brain, as seen with periodic acid Schiff stain.

Fungal brain abscess can occasionally be caused by yeast (*Candida, Cryptococcus* spp.) and dimorphic fungi (*Histoplasma, Coccidiodes, Blastomycosis* spp.) in immunocompromised patients. Patients present with focal neurological signs, raised intracranial pressure or seizures, often accompanied by headache (Bariola et al. 2010).

Scedosporiosis of the CNS, seen in near-drowning cases, presents mainly as multiple brain abscesses. These patients also have clinical and radiographic evidence of a pulmonary focus (Katragkou et al. 2007).

SPINAL CORD SYNDROME

Fungal infections of the spinal cord are rare. They may present as myelopathy, myeloradiculopathy, intramedullary granuloma or epidural abscess, and frank myelitis. *Aspergillus* spp. may rarely cause aspergilloma, epidural abscess and spinal arachnoiditis. Arachnoiditis can also occur with cryptococcal infection.

Diagnosis

Fungal infections of the CNS should be suspected in children with underlying predisposing condition who present with fever and headache with or without CNS signs, or with orbital pain and serosanguinous nasal discharge. Computerized tomography (CT) or magnetic resonance imaging (MRI) should be conducted to exclude a mass lesion, and a lumbar puncture done for CSF analysis and culture.

CEREBROSPINAL FLUID EXAMINATION

CSF sampling must be coordinated with the laboratory personnel to ensure proper and prompt processing. The CSF usually reveals high proteins, low glucose and mononuclear (lymphocytic or monocytic) leukocytosis in the range of 20–500 cells/mm^3. Polymorphonuclear leukocytosis is more likely in infections with *Aspergillus*, *Zygomycetes* or *Blastomyces* spp. The presence of eosinophils should raise suspicion of *Coccidioides immitis*. Cell count may be normal or below 20 cells/mm^3 in patients with HIV/AIDS and in those on high-dose corticosteroid therapy. Protein levels in excess of 1g/dL tend to occur in HIV/AIDS-associated *C. neoformans* meningitis and are suggestive of a subarachnoid block.

Direct microscopic examination of an India ink preparation of the CSF is helpful in identification of encapsulated *Cryptococci* in more than 50% of cases; in patients with HIV/AIDS the yield may be 80%.

CSF cultures are frequently negative. Cisternal CSF may yield organism when lumbar CSF is negative. *C. neoformans* has the best yield on culture; it is positive in up to 90% of patients, especially among those with HIV/AIDS. *Blastomyces* and *H. capsulatum* rarely yield positive culture. In coccidioidal meningitis culture may be positive in about 50% of patients. Even when culture is positive for fungi it takes a long time to grow: *Candida* spp. take a few days, *Cryptococci* spp. 3–10 days; *Histoplasma* and *Coccidioides* spp. may take up to 6 weeks.

METHANAMINE SILVER STAIN

Methanamine silver stain of a direct aspirate or biopsy is very helpful in identification of *Aspergillus* and *Zygomycetes*, which cause tissue invasion and infarction.

IMMUNOLOGICAL TESTS

Detection of intrathecally produced antibodies has been the mainstay of diagnosis.

Latex agglutination test using CSF is positive (titre 1:8 or more) in up to 90% of cases of cryptococcal meningitis (Likasitwattanakul et al. 2004). The test is highly specific and may be positive early in the infection even when culture is negative. False-negative results are uncommon and repeated negative tests over 1 month rule out the diagnosis (Perfect 2004). Although antigen detection tests for cryptococcus are highly sensitive and specific, they are expensive and need technical expertise. A lateral-flow immunoassay for the detection of cryptococcal antigen (LFA CrAg) has been developed recently that gives results within 15 minutes and is both reliable and affordable (Lindsley et al. 2011) and is therefore very useful in resource-limited countries.

Complement fixating antibody (CFA) titre of 1:32 or more is found in the CSF of 90% of patients with coccidiodomycosis meningitis; in the absence of meningitis the test is negative in CSF (even if the serum CFA titres are high).

Serum or CSF galactomannan assay helps in the diagnosis of aspergillosis. Galactomannan is a polysaccharide marker on *Aspergillus* cell wall. Galactomannan index value greater than 0.5 in serum has a sensitivity and specificity exceeding 80% (Wheat 2003).

Immunological tests to detect specific antibodies in CSF are also available for *Histoplasma*, *Zygomycetes* and *Sporothrix*, but these are not very specific.

Serological tests that are available for diagnosis of *Candida* and *Aspergillus* have not been evaluated in CSF for the diagnosis of CNS infections. 1,3-beta-D-glucan assay may be helpful in the diagnosis of meningitis. Fungal polymerase chain reaction (PCR) tests for the diagnosis of fungal meningitis are still being evaluated.

Tissue biopsy for histopathology and culture is required for infections such as mucormycosis wherein immunological tests are generally negative and no standardized PCR is available (Skiada et al. 2013).

IMAGING

CT and MRI may show basal involvement, discrete mass lesions with or without contrast enhancement, associated abscess and areas of infarction. The findings are generally non-specific and are frequently mistaken for tuberculous meningitis, pyogenic brain abscess or brain tumour. Cryptococcomas may be seen as small enhancing lesions in intraventricular or intraparenchymal locations. Pseudocysts are seen as well-circumscribed, round to oval, low-density lesions on CT, and show CSF attenuation on both T1- and T2-weighted images. Clusters of these cysts in basal ganglia and thalami strongly suggest cryptococcal infection.

In rhino-cerebral mucormycosis, CT and MRI show opacification of paranasal sinuses with variable mucosal thickening, usually absence of fluid levels and bony erosion (Fig. 15.1a). Intracranial findings may include vascular thrombosis and infarct involving internal carotoid territory (Fig. 15.1b) mycotic emboli, frontal lobe abscess and involvement of cavernous sinus (Jain et al. 2007). In *Candida* CNS infections, CT usually underestimates the extent of the disease. Micro-abcesses appear isodense or hypodense on non-enhanced CT, and show multiple punctate enhancing nodules on contrast study. On MRI, granuloma and micro-abscesses may be hypointense on T2-weighted images and show ring enhancement on contrast administration. MRI shows features of meningitis, vasculitis and infarction (Jain et al. 2007).

Fungal brain abscesses are hypointense on T1- and hyperintense on T2-weighted images with well-defined enhancement on contrast administration in immunocompetent patients

(Saini et al. 2010). In immunocompromised patients abscesses appear patchy or as punctate hyperintense lesions on T2-weighted images without contrast enhancement, have irregular walls (lobulated or crenated) and high apparent diffusion coefficient (ADC) in contrast to low ADC seen in pyogenic and tuberculous abscesses. Proton magnetic resonance spectroscopy shows lipid, lactate, amino acids and trehalose (Luthra et al. 2007). Details of neuroimaging are discussed in Chapter 3.

Treatment

Optimal management of fungal CNS infections includes specific antifungal therapy (Table 15.3), measures to control raised intracranial pressure, supportive treatment, surgical intervention and management of risk factors for fungal disease, i.e. hyperglycaemia, acidosis, and elimination/minimization of immunosuppression.

Most antifungal agents are targeted towards specific fungal cell wall components, except flucytosine that has metabolic effects. Antifungal therapy is rather expensive and is often associated with significant toxicity. Commonly recommended regimens consist of an induction phase lasting for 2–6 weeks followed by a suppressive phase lasting from 3 months to life long (Blyth et al. 2010, Katragkou and Roilides 2011).

Amphotericin B given intravenously remains the most used and successful drug for most fungal infections of the CNS. It is a polyene antibiotic that binds to ergosterols in the cell wall of fungi and thereby disrupts the cell-wall integrity leading to cell death. It is highly protein-bound and has a poor penetration of the blood–brain barrier and thereby low CSF concentration. However, brain tissue concentration appears to be adequate and is related to the non-protein-bound (i.e. free) amphotericin levels. The main toxicity of amphotericin is renal impairment secondary to reduction in blood flow to the renal tubules and glomeruli. This toxicity is infusion-rate related and can be largely prevented by using continuous infusion through a dedicated peripheral line and by giving a saline infusion prior to the amphotericin infusion. Using this technique, the toxicity is reduced to the levels associated with the use of lipid-based amphotericin that is meant to be less toxic but is much more expensive than non-lipid-based amphotericin. Some clinicians use intrathecal amphotericin (0.25–0.5mg/kg daily to weekly), along with systemic amphotericin B through a reservoir or direct injection, in patients who do not respond to systemic amphotericin B or have a relapse. Hydrocortisone (1mg/kg) is added to the intrathecal dose to prevent side-effects of intrathecal use, which include vasculitis, arachnoiditis, paraplegia, paraesthesiae, headache and backache.

Flucytosine enters fungal cells via cytosine permease and inhibits DNA and mRNA synthesis. It penetrates well into the CSF, and achieves concentrations approaching 75% of simultaneous serum concentrations. However, if given alone for treatment of CNS fungal infections there is a high risk of treatment failure owing to development of in-vitro and in-vivo resistance. It is therefore used in combination with amphotericin B or fluconazole. Dose adjustment is required in the presence of renal insufficiency, to allow peak serum levels of 70–80µg/mL.

Fluconazole is effective against *Cryptococcus* and *Candida* but not against filamentous fungi. It is available in intravenous and oral preparations. The bioavailability of the oral

TABLE 15.3
Treatment recommendations for common fungal infections of the central nervous system in children

Indication	First-line treatment	Second-line treatment
CNS candidiasis[a]	Liposomal amphotericin B (3–5mg/kg/d) *with or without* Flucytosine (100mg/kg/d in four divided doses) PO Fluconazole (6–12mg/kg/d in two divided doses) PO as step-down therapy	Fluconazole (6–12mg/kg/d) *or* Voriconazole (6mg/kg/d in two divided doses followed by 3mg/kg/d) IV for patients unable to tolerate amphotericin B
Cryptococcus[b] Non-neutropenic (recommended therapy based on extrapolation of findings from adult studies)	1 Induction Amphotericin B (1mg/kg/d) IV plus flucytosine (100mg/kg/d PO in four divided doses) 2 Consolidation therapy Fluconazole (10–12mg/kg/d in two divided doses) PO 3 Maintenance therapy Fluconazole (6mg/kg/d) PO	Liposomal amphotericin B (5mg/kg/d) *or* Lipid complex (5mg/kg/d) plus flucytosine (100mg/kg/d PO in four divided doses)
Neutropenic (based on HIV-infected or organ transplant adult recipients)	1 Induction – 2 weeks Amphotericin B (1mg/kg/d) IV or liposomal amphotericin B (3–5mg/kg/d) IV or lipid complex (5mg/kg/d) IV plus flucytosine (100mg/kg/d PO in four divided doses) 2 Consolidation therapy, minimum 8 weeks Fluconazole (6–12 mg/kg/day in two divided doses) PO 3 Maintenance therapy Fluconazole (6 mg/kg/day) PO	Alternative regimens for induction and consolidation in case of amphotericin intolerance: fluconazole (12mg/kg/d in two divided doses) PO plus flucytosine (100mg/kg/d in four divided doses) PO
Aspergillosis[c]	Voriconazole (5–7mg/kg IV every 12 hours)	Lipid formulations of amphotericin B (3–5mg/kg/day) IV *or* Caspofungin (50mg/m^2/d)
Mucormycosis[d]	Amphotericin B 1.5mg/kg/d IV by continuous infusion *or* Lipid formulations of amphotericin B (3–5mg/kg/d) IV	Posaconazole (200mg PO four times a day or 400mg PO twice a day) (data for paediatric dosing not available)

[a]Pappas et al. (2009), [b]Perfect et al. (2010), [c]Walsh et al. (2008), [d]Spellberg et al. (2009).
PO, per os (oral); IV, intravenous; HIV, human immunodeficiency virus.
Data from paediatric dosing not available for children aged under 13 years.

preparation is high. It passes easily across the blood–CSF barrier and has a long half-life in the CNS. However, CSF sterilization is slower as compared to an amphotericin-B-containing regimen. As the clearance of fluconazole is rapid in children, a higher dosage is employed in children than in adults.

Itraconazole has potent antifungal activity against a broad spectrum of fungi including *Aspergillus* but has a limited oral bio-availability. It is highly protein-bound and has very limited penetration into CSF yet it has been successful in the treatment of cryptococcal meningitis in patients with HIV/AIDS, and in *Aspergillus* CNS infections.

Voriconazole has remarkable activity against yeast and filamentous moulds *Aspergillus*, *Fusarium* and *Scedosporium*, and dematiaceous fungi, but does not work against *Zygomycetes*. Oral bio-availability is almost 90%. It has good penetration into the CSF (CSF to plasma ratio is 0.5) with high CSF levels achieved rapidly. It also penetrates brain tissue, and brain tissue levels are higher than plasma levels. These pharmacokinetic properties and favourable clinical experience make voriconazole the preferred drug in CNS aspergillosis and scedosporiosis, and a reasonable alternative for other CNS fungal infections when amphotericin cannot be tolerated (Walsh et al. 2010, Schwartz et al. 2011). Higher doses are required in children than in adults to achieve similar levels (Table 15.3). Voriconazole is susceptible to numerous drug interactions; particularly important are interactions with rifampicin, phenytoin and carbamazepine.

Posaconazole has an extended spectrum with in-vitro activity against *Candida*, *Aspergillus*, *Zygomycetes* and *Fusarium* species. It is available as an oral suspension. It may be considered as an option in mucormycosis and amphotericin B refractory infections, particularly cryptococcal meningitis when other therapies have failed.

Echinocandins are not orally bio-available.

Caspofungin is fungicidal against *Candida* spp. and active against *Aspergillus*, but activity against *Fusarium*, *Rhizopus* and *Trichosporon* spp. is limited. It is effective alone or in combination with amphotericin in refractory invasive *Candida* infection and in combination with voriconazole in refractory aspergillosis of CNS. However, caspofungin has poor CNS penetration and is therefore not recommended as a single agent in CNS fungal infections. *Micafungin* is approved for use in children, including infants born before the 29th week of gestation. Transaminase monitoring is recommended during treatment. In neonates, higher doses (10–15mg/kg/d) of micafungin should be used when CNS involvement is suspected (Caudle et al. 2012).

ANTIFUNGAL THERAPY IN SOME IMPORTANT CENTRAL NERVOUS SYSTEM INFECTIONS

Cryptococcal meningitis
Amphotericin B combined with flucytosine is used as induction therapy (Table 15.3). This combination usually sterilizes CSF within 2 weeks. It is followed by oral fluconazole for 8–10 weeks. In patients with HIV a repeat lumbar puncture should be performed 2 weeks after starting amphotericin to ensure that CSF pressure is normal and CSF is sterile before switching to maintenance fluconazole. In patients without neutropenia or HIV infection,

fluconazole is given for 6–12 months, whereas in patients with HIV it is continued indefinitely as suppressive therapy to prevent relapses. Intraventricular amphotericin B has been used successfully in cases with a poor prognosis. In many resource-limited settings, amphotericin and flucytosine are not available. High-dose oral fluconazole (12mg/kg/d) has been tried in such situations. Adjunctive use of interferon along with amphotericin and flucytosine has better outcome in some studies but is too expensive to be used in resource-limited countries. In patients with HIV who have cryptococcal meningitis, antiretroviral therapy is usually initiated after a clinical response to antifungal therapy is obtained.

Cryptococcoma
Antifungal chemotherapy alone is generally successful in small lesions. Large cryptococcomas (>3cm) located in accessible areas should be removed surgically. For multiple cryptococcomas, antifungal therapy may be needed for an extended period up to 2 years.

In patients with CNS cryptococcal infections, corticosteroid administration should be discontinued; if it is not possible to do so, the dose should be minimized as much as possible. Relapse rate is above 50% in patients with underlying HIV/AIDS, and about 15%–25% in non-HIV-infected patients. Most relapses occur in the first 3–6 months after cessation of therapy, hence there is a need for prolonged suppressive therapy in patients with HIV/AIDS. Data in adults suggest that patients with control of their HIV infection (CD4 count >100 cells/µL on highly active antiretroviral therapy regimen) and who have been asymptomatic after 2 years of treatment may be considered for cessation of antifungals (Mussini et al. 2004). In some patients with HIV/AIDS and cryptococcal meningitis, sudden deterioration with dramatic increase in intracranial pressure (Graybil et al. 2000), loss of vision and even death have been reported during the first 1–2 weeks of treatment. The pathogenesis of such an event is not fully understood and prompt management of raised intracranial pressure is warranted.

Coccidioidal meningitis
Isolated coccidioidal meningitis is treated with oral fluconazole. If a patient does not respond to fluconazole within a few weeks, itraconazole can be tried. In disseminated disease, both amphotericin B and fluconazole are used (Bariola et al. 2010). Intrathecal amphotericin B injection followed by a lumbar, cisternal or ventricular reservoir is used as an alternative regimen, beginning with 0.01mg/d and increasing as tolerated up to 0.5mg/d. The need for continuing therapy may be guided by monitoring CSF cells and glucose; 10 cells/mm^3 or less with normal CSF glucose concentrations for at least 1 year is the target. A lowering of the CSF antibody titre is considered a good prognostic sign. The infection is rarely cured and thus therapy may be needed for life.

Candida meningitis
In *Candida* meningitis (except *C. lusitanal* and *C. krusei*) amphotericin B is the primary therapeutic agent and is preferably used in combination with flucytosine as the two have synergistic activity against *Candida*. However, clinical superiority of the combination

remains to be confirmed. It is followed by fluconazole. Voriconazole may also be effective. Treatment is continued until all symptoms and signs, CSF abnormalities and radiological abnormalities have resolved. In neonates if flucytosine is used, its serum levels need to be monitored as very high levels may accumulate because of renal immaturity.

If *Candida* or cryptococcal meningitis develops in a patient with a shunt in place, eradication of infection is best achieved by removing the shunt, placing an external drain, and treating with antifungal agents for at least 4–6 weeks.

Aspergillus infection

Aspergillus infections of the CNS warrant early aggressive therapy. Until recently, the usual treatment was high-dose amphotericin B even though it has rarely been successful in arresting the infection. Voriconazole in children aged 2–11 years is now considered the first-choice treatment for CNS aspergillosis, as it has a better outcome as compared to amphotericin B (Traunmüller et al. 2011). Itraconazole or posaconazole are used in patients who are intolerant to voriconazole. Caspofungin (for children >3 months) or micafungin (Amador et al. 2011) are recommended as alternatives. Combination therapy with voriconazole and caspofungin has also been used (Marr et al. 2004). In desperate cases addition of amphotericin has been proposed by the Infectious Diseases Society of America guidelines (Walsh et al. 2008). Simultaneous management of contiguous infections of the paranasal sinuses or vertebral bodies is essential. Any underlying immune deficits should be corrected. Corticosteroids are not recommended and may in fact be deleterious. Intrathecal use of amphotericin may induce severe arachnoiditis, headache and seizures and is therefore not recommended (Walsh et al. 2008).

Zygomycetes infection

In patients with *Zygomycetes* (*Rhizopus*, *Mucor*), liposomal amphotericin or lipid preparations of amphotericin are considered first-line therapy. Voriconazole or posaconazole and combination therapy of liposomal amphotericin B with caspofungin may be used as second-line therapy (Skiada et al. 2013). Prompt surgical debridement in rhino-orbito-cerebral mucormycosis is essential. Metabolic factors (ketoacidosis, iron overload) should be corrected (Hamilton et al. 2003, Sunderam et al. 2005).

The management of fungal brain abscesses is not fully standardized. In scedosporiosis, voriconazole along with neurosurgical intervention is an effective option. *Aspergillus*, *Blastomyces* and *Histoplasma* abscesses have been successfully drained or removed surgically, with concomitant amphotericin B treatment. Surgical debridement was independently associated with survival in *Aspergillus* brain abscesses (Dotis et al. 2007). Brain abscesses caused by dematiaceous fungi are surgically removed and antifungal agents are simultaneously administered.

Clinical guidelines for treatment of fungal infections of the CNS by the Infectious Diseases Society of America are freely available on the internet. However, local susceptibility testing should guide the choice of appropriate therapy.

Prognosis

The outcome of fungal CNS infections depends upon several factors, most importantly the causative fungus and the patient's underlying condition, particularly their immune status. The outcome of cryptococcal CNS infection is usually better than that of other forms of fungal meningitis. In cryptococcal meningitis, convulsions and focal neurological deficits were independent predictors of in-hospital mortality in HIV-infected children (Gumbo et al. 2002). Poor prognostic factors associated with failure of amphotericin B therapy or relapse after therapy include an initial positive CSF India ink test result, high CSF opening pressure, low CSF leukocyte count (<20 cells/mm^3), cryptococci isolated from extraneural sites, absent anticryptococcal antibody, initial CSF or serum cryptococcal antigen titre of 1:32 or more, post-treatment titres of 1:8 or more, corticosteroid therapy, lymphoreticular malignancy, and a CSF glucose concentration that remained abnormal during 4 weeks or more of therapy (Graybill et al. 2000, Perfect 2004). Predictors of failure to sterilize CSF in patients with AIDS include very high CSF antigen titres (≥1:1024), low serum albumin concentration, low CD4 cell count (<5 cells/mL), and increased intracranial pressure in excess of 250mmH$_2$O (Perfect 2004).

Candida meningitis has a mortality of 10%–20%; permanent neurological or cognitive deficits may remain in survivors. Poor prognostic factors include late diagnosis (more than 2 weeks after onset of symptoms), CSF glucose concentrations less than 35mg/dL, and development of raised intracranial pressure and focal neurological deficits (Perfect 2004).

Histoplasma meningitis has a mortality of 20%–40% and a high relapse rate of about 50% (Pereira et al. 2008). Coccidioidal meningitis has a poor survival rate (~50%) and extremely high risk of relapse; patients frequently require lifelong suppressive therapy. Childhood CNS aspergillosis had a very high fatality rate of 83% in cases reported before 1990; however, it has halved to about 40% in cases reported after 1990 (Dotis et al. 2007). In patients with disseminated aspergillosis with CNS involvement mortality is almost 100%.

Prevention

Both fluconazole and itraconazole can prevent cryptococcal meningitis cases in HIV-infected adults, but survival benefit is seen in patients with very low CD 4 count (100 cells/mL) or those living in an area with high incidence of cryptococcal meningitis. Azole prophylaxis is therefore recommended in children with low CD 4 count, living in endemic areas, and who are not on or are in the early stages of HAART (highly active antiretroviral treatment) (Thurey and Molyneux 2008). A cryptococcal vaccine has been developed but is not routinely used. Prophylactic use of azoles to prevent histoplasmosis and coccidioidomycosis in HIV-infected patients is being evaluated.

REFERENCES

Amador JT, Guillen Martin S, Prieto Tato L (2011) [Why might micafungin be the drug of choice in paediatric patients?] *Enferm Infecc Microbiol Clin* 29 (Suppl 2): 23–8.
Bariola JR, Perry P, Pappas PG, et al. (2010) Blastomycosis of the central nervous system: a multicenter review of diagnosis and treatment in the modern era. *Clin Infect Dis* 50: 797–804.

Blyth CC, Hale K, Palasanthiran P, et al. (2010) Antifungal therapy in infants and children with proven, probable or suspected invasive fungal infections. *Cochrane Database Syst Rev* 2: CD006343.

Caudle KE, Inger AG, Butler DR, Rogers PD (2012) Echinocandin use in the neonatal intensive care unit. *Ann Pharmacother* 46: 108–16.

Chen TL, Chen HP, Fung CP, et al. (2004) Clinical characteristics, treatment and prognostic factors of candidal meningitis in a teaching hospital in Taiwan. *Scand J Infect Dis* 36: 124–30.

Dotis J, Iosifidis E, Roilides E (2007) Central nervous system aspergillosis in children: a systematic review of reported cases. *Int J Infect Dis* 11: 381–93.

Fernandez M, Moylett EH, Noyola DE, Baker CJ (2000) Candidal meningitis in neonates: a 10 year review. *Clin Infect Dis* 31: 458–463.

Franzot SP, Salkin IF, Casadevall A (1999) *Cryptococcus neoformans* var. *grubii*: separate varietal status for Cryptococcus neoformans serotype A isolates. *J Clin Microbiol* 37: 838–40.

Graybill JR, Sobel J, Saag M, et al. (2000) Diagnosis and management of increased intracranial pressure in patients with AIDS and cryptococcal meningitis. *Clin Infect Dis* 30: 47–54.

Gumbo T, Kadzirange G, Mielke J, et al. (2002) *Cryptococcus neoformans* meningoencephalitis in African children with acquired immunodeficiency syndrome. *Pediatr Infect Dis J* 21: 54–6.

Hamilton JF, Bartkowski HB, Rock JP (2003) Management of CNS mucormycosis in the pediatric patient. *Pediatr Neurosurg* 38: 212–5.

Hong XY, Chou YC, Lazareff JA (2008) Brain stem candidiasis mimicking cerebellopontine angle tumor. *Surg Neurol* 70: 87–91.

Jain KK, Gupta RK, Mittal SK, Kumar S (2007) Imaging features of central nervous system fungal infections. *Neurol India* 55: 241–50.

Katragkou A, Roilides E (2011) Best practice in treating infants and children with proven probable or suspected invasive fungal infections. *Curr Opin Infect Dis* 24: 225–9.

Katragkou A, Dotis J, Kotsiou M, et al. (2007) *Scedosporium apiospermum* infection after near-drowning. *Mycoses* 50: 412–21.

Likasitwattanakul S, Poneprasert B, Sirisanthana V (2004) Cryptococcosis in HIV-infected children. *Southeast Asian J Trop Med Public Health* 35: 935–9.

Lindsley MD, Mekha N, Baggett HC, et al. (2011) Evaluation of a newly developed lateral flow immunoassay for the diagnosis of cryptococcosis. *Clin Infect Dis* 53: 321–5.

Luthra G, Parihar A, Nath K, et al. (2007) Comparative evaluation of fungal, tubercular, and pyogenic brain abscesses with conventional and diffusion MR imaging and proton MR spectroscopy. *AJNR Am J Neuroradiol* 28: 1332–8.

Marr KA, Boeckh M, Carter RA, et al. (2004) Combination antifungal therapy for invasive aspergillosis. *Clin Infect Dis* 39: 797–802.

Mohindra S, Mukherjee KK, Chhabra R, et al. (2008) Invasive intracranial aspergillosis: the management dilemmas. *Surg Neurol* 69: 496–505.

Murthy JMK (2007) Fungal infections of the central nervous system: the clinical syndromes. *Neurol India* 55: 221–5.

Mussini C, Pezzotti P, Miró JM, et al. (2004) Discontinuation of maintenance therapy for cryptococcal meningitis in patients with AIDS treated with highly active antiretroviral therapy: an international observational study. *Clin Infect Dis* 38: 565–71.

Pappas PG, Kauffman CA, Andes D, et al. (2009) Clinical practice guidelines for the management of candidiasis: 2009 update by the Infectious Diseases Society of America. *Clin Infect Dis* 48: 503–35.

Park BJ, Wannemuehler KA, Marston BJ, et al. (2009) Estimation of the current global burden of cryptococcal meningitis among persons living with HIV/AIDS. *AIDS* 23: 525–30.

Pereira GH, Pádua SS, Park MV, et al. (2008) Chronic meningitis by histoplasmosis: report of a child with acute myeloid leukemia. *Braz J Infect Dis* 12: 555–7.

Perfect JR (2004) Fungal meningitis. In: Scheld WM, Whitley RJ, Marra CM, eds. *Infections of the Central Nervous System. 3rd edn.* Philadelphia: Lippincott Williams & Wilkins, pp. 691–712.

Perfect JR, Cox GM, Lee JY, et al. (2001) The impact of culture isolation of *Aspergillus* species: a hospital-based survey of aspergillosis. *Clin Infect Dis* 33: 1824–33.

Perfect JR, Dismukes WE, Dromer F, et al. (2010) Clinical practice guidelines for the management of cryptococcal disease: 2010 update by the Infectious Diseases Society of America. *Clin Infect Dis* 50: 291–322.

Redmond A, Dancer C, Woods ML (2007) Fungal infections of the central nervous system: a review of fungal pathogens and treatment. *Neurol India* 55: 251–9.

Saini J, Gupta AK, Jolapara MB, et al. (2010) Imaging findings in intracranial aspergillus infection in immunocompetent patients. *World Neurosurg* 74: 661–70. doi: 10.1016/j.wneu.2010.06.017.

Schwartz S, Reisman A, Troke PF (2011) The efficacy of voriconazole in the treatment of 192 fungal central nervous system infections: a retrospective analysis. *Infection* 39: 201–10.

Shih CC, Chen YC, Chang SC, et al. (2000) Cryptococcal meningitis in non-HIV infected patients. *QJM* 93: 245–51.

Singhi SC, Mathew JL, Jindal A (2011) Clinical pearls in respiratory diseases. *Indian J Pediatr* 78: 603–8. doi: 10.1007/s12098-010-0270-3.

Skiada A, Lanternier F, Groll AH, et al. (2013) Diagnosis and treatment of mucormycosis in patients with hematological malignancies: guidelines from the 3rd European Conference on Infections in Leukemia (ECIL 3). *Haematologica* 98: 492–504. doi: 10.3324/haematol.2012.065110.

Spellberg B, Walsh TJ, Kontoyiannis DP, et al. (2009) Recent advances in the management of mucormycosis: from bench to bedside. *Clin Infect Dis* 48: 1743–51.

Sundaram C, Mahadevan A, Laxmi V, et al. (2005) Cerebral zygomycosis. *Mycoses* 48: 396–407.

Susever S, Yegenoglu Y (2011) Evaluation of the significance of molecular methods in the diagnosis of invasive fungal infections: comparison with conventional methods. *Mikrobiyol Bul* 45: 325–35.

Teive H, Carsten AL, Iwamoto FM, et al. (2008) Fungal encephalitis following bone marrow transplantation: clinical findings and prognosis. *J Postgrad Med* 54: 203–5.

Thurey J, Molyneux E (2008) Evidence behind the WHO guidelines: Hospital Care for Children: the usefulness of azole prophylaxis against cryptococcal meningitis in HIV-positive children. *J Trop Pediatr* 54: 361–3.

Traunmüller F, Popovic M, Konz KH, et al. (2011) Efficacy and safety of current drug therapies for invasive aspergillosis. *Pharmacology* 88: 213–24.

Walsh TJ, Anaissie EJ, Denning DW, et al. (2008) Treatment of aspergillosis: clinical practice guidelines of the Infectious Diseases Society of America. *Clin Infect Dis* 46: 327–60.

Walsh TJ, Driscoll T, Milligan PA, et al. (2010) Pharmacokinetics, safety, and tolerability of voriconazole in immunocompromised children. *Antimicrob Agents Chemother* 54: 4116–23.

Wheat LJ (2003) Rapid diagnosis of invasive aspergillosis by antigen detection. *Transpl Infect Dis* 5: 158–66.

Zaoutis TE, Roilides E, Chiou CC, et al. (2007) Zygomycosis in children: a systematic review and analysis of reported cases. *Pediatr Infect Dis J* 26: 723–7.

16
PARASITIC INFECTIONS

Richard Idro and Charles R Newton

Parasitic infections or infestations (referred to hereafter as infections) are a leading cause of central nervous system (CNS) morbidity worldwide, particularly in resource-poor areas and tropical countries. They may occur with ingestion of contaminated water or food, via penetration of the skin by parasite larval forms, or by direct inoculation of parasites by an infested insect's bite. CNS disease is often secondary, the primary sites being elsewhere, particularly in the gastrointestinal system or peripheral blood. In this chapter, common parasitic infections that cause CNS disease in children are considered. Infections such as CNS toxoplasmosis in neonates and immuno-compromised persons are described in Chapter 5.

Malaria

AETIOLOGY, EPIDEMIOLOGY AND LIFE CYCLE

Malaria is a leading cause of ill health in tropical countries. In 2008, there were an estimated 243 million clinical cases worldwide and 863 000 deaths (WHO 2009). Four *Plasmodium* species – *P. vivax*, *P. ovale*, *P. malariae* and *P. falciparum* – cause human disease; one monkey species, *P. knowelsi*, may also cause malaria (White et al. 2014). *P. falciparum* is responsible for most cases of severe disease and the largest number of malaria-related deaths worldwide, although *P. vivax* is also known to cause severe malaria. Children living in sub-Saharan Africa bear the brunt of the disease. Repeated infections over several years induce partial immunological protection so that severe disease is uncommon among adults in endemic areas. Non-immune travellers to endemic countries and pregnant women remain susceptible.

Malaria is transmitted by species of female *Anopheles* mosquitoes. The parasite develops in the gut and salivary glands of the mosquito. The mosquito injects sporozoites into human blood while feeding. Sporozoites rapidly enter liver hepatocytes to start the exo-erythrocytic cycle, which culminates in hepatocyte rupture, release of merozoites back into the blood, and their entry into erythrocytes. It is this erythrocytic stage that is responsible for the symptoms and complications of malaria.

PATHOGENESIS

P. falciparum is unique in that later erythrocytic stages of the parasite sequester within deep vascular beds in organs, especially the brain. Sequestration results from cytoadherence of parasitized erythrocytes to the host endothelial lining via parasite-derived proteins exposed on erythrocyte surface. A group of parasite antigens including the *P. falciparum* erythrocyte membrane protein-1 mediate this binding to host receptors, of which intercellular adhesion molecule-1 (ICAM-1), whose expression is upregulated by the parasites, is the most important. The sequestered parasite mass is further increased when adherent erythrocytes agglutinate with other parasitized erythrocytes, form rosettes with non-parasitized erythrocytes or use platelet-mediated clumping to bind to each other. Sequestration may impair perfusion, which is aggravated by the decreased ability of parasitized cells to deform and pass through the microvasculature (Rogerson et al. 2004). In addition, local and systemic cytokine and chemokine expression plays a complex role in pathogenesis with both protective and harmful effects (Clark 2009). Microparticles from the blood and endothelial cells also contribute.

CLINICAL PRESENTATION

Children with malaria usually have a history of fever, although the absence of fever does not exclude the diagnosis. Children often have high temperatures (>38°C), which may be continuous or irregular without a definite pattern. Vomiting and, to a lesser extent, diarrhoea are common, and may contribute to dehydration or electrolyte depletion.

Neurological involvement is observed in nearly 50% of children with falciparum malaria requiring hospital care (Idro et al. 2007), but is rare in infections with other species. Neurological manifestations of falciparum malaria include headache, irritability, restlessness or agitation, seizures, prostration, drowsiness or coma. Cerebral malaria is the most severe neurological manifestation. It is a clinical syndrome characterized by coma in which (1) the child is unable to localize a painful stimulus at least 1 hour after the last seizure; (2) asexual forms of *P. falciparum* are seen on smears of peripheral blood; and (3) other causes of encephalopathy (e.g. meningitis, encephalitis or hypoglycaemia) have been excluded (WHO 2000). However, this strict definition is reserved for research purposes, and any child in an endemic area with *P. falciparum* and disturbed consciousness should be treated for cerebral malaria. Seizures occur in over 80% of children with cerebral malaria, and are very common with falciparum, and to a lesser extent vivax malaria. Seizures commonly precipitate the coma. The cause of seizures is unclear; they are not simply febrile seizures since many occur in afebrile periods, and are often complicated: many recur during the same acute illness and may be focal or prolonged (Waruiru et al. 1996). Most do not appear to be related to electrolyte abnormalities or hypoglycaemia.

Brainstem signs including dysconjugate eye movement and decorticate or decerebrate posturing are observed. Meningism may be present, such that cerebral malaria cannot be differentiated clinically from bacterial meningitis (Idro et al. 2005). Direct CNS involvement of *P. falciparum* is difficult to define since there are no pathognomonic pathological features except a distinctive retinopathy (best seen by indirect ophthalmoscopy) that includes retinal haemorrhages, retinal whitening, blood-vessel colour changes and less frequently papilloedema (Fig. 16.1). These features may be caused by parasite sequestration in the brain and may help differentiate cerebral malaria from other causes of encephalopathy (Kariuki et al. 2014). They resolve over 1–4 weeks (Lewallen et al. 2000).

The liver and spleen are often enlarged, and spontaneous bleeding from the gastrointestinal tract may occur, especially in adults with multiorgan failure.

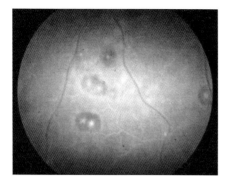

Fig. 16.1. Retina in a 3-year-old child with cerebral malaria showing haemorrhages, white exudates and changes in the colour of the vessels. (Reproduced by courtesy of Nick Beare.) A colour version of this figure is available in the plate section at the end of the book.

Other complications such as anaemia, hypoglycaemia and metabolic acidosis may occur concurrently or separately. Metabolic acidosis manifests with deep breathing, and is often associated with hyperlactataemia caused by hypovolaemia, inadequate tissue perfusion, anaemia and increased lactate production from the anaerobic parasites. Children with dehydration often have transient impairment of renal function, but, unlike in adults, overt renal failure is rare. Multiple complications in a child are associated with poor prognosis.

LABORATORY FEATURES

In endemic areas, malaria should be suspected in any child with fever. In non-endemic areas, it should be considered in a child who has visited or even transiently landed at an airport in an endemic area within the last 3 months and develops fever, headache or change in cognitive status. A diagnosis of malaria in symptomatic individuals is made on peripheral blood smears or rapid diagnostic tests. The parasite count in falciparum malaria varies considerably, ranging from a barely detectable parasitaemia to more than 20% of erythrocytes infected. The lack of detectable parasitaemia especially in non-immune travellers does not exclude the diagnosis, since parasites may be sequestered within deep vascular beds or chemoprophylaxis may have suppressed peripheral parasitaemia. In such cases, blood smears should be examined every 6–8 hours for 48 hours before excluding the infection. Rapid diagnostic tests such as the immunochromatographic test for *P. falciparum* histidine-rich protein 2 and lactate dehydrogenase are more sensitive. Parasite mRNA or DNA testing is more sensitive than microscopy, but is expensive, more laborious and does not estimate parasite load.

Anaemia, usually with evidence of haemolysis (raised unconjugated bilirubinaemia and low haptoglobin), is a consquence of the infection. Thrombocytopenia is common, usually not severe enough to cause spontaneous bleeding. Fibrin degradation products are raised, but frank disseminated intravascular coagulation is uncommon. Hypoglycaemia and lactic acidosis are the major metabolic complications. Hypoxaemia is associated with pulmonary oedema. Renal impairment is common. Hyponatraemia is mainly caused by salt depletion, but some cases may be due to inappropriate antidiuretic hormone secretion. Hypophos-

TABLE 16.1
Parenteral antimalarial treatment for severe falciparum malaria

Drug	Route	Loading dose	Maintenance dose
Artesunate	IV/IM	2.4mg/kg, repeated after 8 hours	2.4mg/kg once daily, either until the patient can take orally when this is replaced with a full course of first-line artemether-based combination therapy, or artesunate is continued for a maximum of 7d
Artemether	IM	3.2mg/kg	1.6mg/kg/d until able to take orally or for a minimum of 5d
Quinine dihydrochloride	IV	20mg salt/kg over 2–4h	10mg salt/kg every 8–12h until able to take orally
Quinine dihydrochloride	IM	20mg salt/kg (dilute IV formulation to 60mg/mL) given in two injection sites	10mg salt/kg every 8–12h until able to take orally
Quinidine gluconate	IV	15mg base/kg (24mg/kg salt) in normal saline over 4h; *or* 6.25mg base/kg (10mg salt/kg) over 2h	7.5mg base/kg (12mg salt/kg) infused over 4h, every 8–12h with ECG monitoring; then 0.0125mg base/kg/min (0.02mg salt/kg/min) as a continuous infusion for 24h

phataemia is a feature of severe malaria and may be exacerbated by glucose therapy.

In cerebral malaria, brain swelling is observed on neuroimaging, with abnormal T2 signal intensities and diffusion-weighted abnormalities in the cortical, deep grey and white matter structures on MRI (Potchen et al. 2012). The encephalogram recording is characterized by slow and high-amplitude waves, and ictal discharges may be seen even in some children with no clinical convulsions (Gwer et al. 2012). The cerebrospinal fluid (CSF) is usually acellular, and other diagnoses such as encephalitis should be considered if pleocytosis is found, although cerebral malaria cannot be excluded. CSF lactate concentrations are raised, but total protein and glucose concentrations are usually normal. Blood cultures may detect concurrent bacteraemia, particularly caused by gram-negative organisms.

MANAGEMENT

Antimalarial therapy
The cinchona alkaloids (quinine and its diastereomer quinidine) or the artemesinin compounds (artesunate, artemether and arteether) are the first-line antimalaria drugs for the treatment of severe malaria (Table 16.1) (White et al. 2014). The artemesinin compounds are fast acting and, unlike the cinchona alkaloids, act against all blood stages, reducing the time to parasite clearance and fever resolution. Artesunate is the favoured drug, since it can

be administered intravenously or intramuscularly, is associated with less neurotoxicity in animal models, and has reduced mortality in African children with severe malaria (Dondorp et al. 2010). In children with non-severe CNS manifestations, e.g. seizures, the first-line oral artemisinin-based combination therapy may be used.

Quinine is more widely available. An initial loading dose of 20mg/kg is recommended in cerebral malaria to rapidly achieve high therapeutic levels but should be avoided in children who have received cinchonoids or mefloquine within the previous 24 hours. Side-effects are common, particularly cinchonism (tinnitus, hearing impairment, nausea, restlessness and blurred vision). In addition, serious cardiovascular adverse events including hypotension and cardiac arrhythmias may also occur especially if the drugs are administered rapidly. The Q–T interval should be monitored during the infusion. Since quinine for intravenous administration is unavailable in the USA, quinidine is used (Table 16.1).

In addition to the artemisinin-based combination drugs, other antimalarial drugs (atova-quone-proguanil, sulphonamides) can be used with the cinchinoids to shorten the course of therapy or for the treatment of non-severe falciparum malaria. The spread of resistance to the sulphonamides (sulphadoxine, sulphalene and trimethoprim) have limited their usefulness. The biguanides (proguanil and chlorproguanil) are useful prophylactic drugs. Halofantrine is an effective drug, but has significant cardiovascular toxicity. The antibiotics, clindamycin and tetracycline, are effective against the blood stages, but should not be used as primary antimalarial drugs.

SUPPORTIVE TREATMENT

Supportive treatment is important in children with severe malaria, since most deaths occur within 24 hours of admission, before antimalarials have had time to work. Correction of hypoxaemia, hypoglycaemia, shock and metabolic acidosis and control of seizures are a priority (Idro et al. 2006).

Patients should be monitored closely; blood glucose should be measured every 6 hours, and parasitaemia and haematocrit every 12 hours; and electrolytes, blood gases and renal function tests should be conducted at least daily during the acute stages. Fluid balance is critical in severe malaria, as many children are hypovolaemic (Maitland et al. 2005), but overaggressive fluid therapy can precipitate pulmonary oedema and aggravate intracranial hypertension, and has been associated with increased mortality (Maitland et al. 2011). Recurrences of hypoglycaemia may be prevented by continuous infusion of glucose-containing fluids until consciousness is regained. Renal function should be carefully monitored especially in non-immune patients because acute renal failure is a common cause of death. Patients with pulmonary oedema or respiratory distress syndrome require supplemental oxygen and positive pressure ventilation, as well as diuretics or haemofiltration to correct fluid overload.

Single seizures must be treated promptly with a benzodiazepine, and status epilepticus with phenobarbital or phenytoin. Prevention of seizures in children with cerebral malaria using phenobarbital is associated with increased mortality especially in unventilated children also given three or more doses of benzodiazepines (Crawley et al. 2000), and phosphenytoin does not appear to prevent seizures (Gwer et al. 2013). Because brain swelling is relatively common in children with deep coma, lumbar puncture should either be delayed or brain swelling excluded on CT before the procedure is conducted. Mannitol may reduce intracranial pressure but does not prevent progression in those with severe intracranial hypertension (Okoromah et al. 2011). Of note, treatment with steroids is associated with an increased incidence of gastrointestinal bleeding without any beneficial effect on outcome (Krishna 2012, Warrell et al. 1982).

Hyperpyrexia should be treated with standard modalities for lowering temperature including paracetamol although this may increase parasite clearance time. Blood transfusion should be considered when the haematocrit falls toward 20% or the child has evidence of cardiovascular compromise. However, in African children, transfusion is recommended at a lower haematocrit (WHO 2000). The role of exchange transfusions is controversial; it has been recommended in patients with parasitaemia in excess of 10% and in patients deteriorating despite conventional treatment. Vitamin K and cryoprecipitate should be administered if a patient has a bleeding diathesis.

Secondary bacterial infections should always be suspected. Blood, urine and CSF should be sent for culture, and repeated examinations of the chest should be performed because aspiration or hypostatic pneumonia may develop in comatose patients. Broad-spectrum antimicrobial treatment should be started as soon as a complicating infection is suspected.

OUTCOME

CNS involvement in childhood malaria is associated with an increased risk of death, 4.4% versus 1.3% (Idro et al. 2007). Mortality in the picture defined as 'cerebral malaria' (see above) is even higher, at 10%–20%, with patients usually dying within the first 48 hours of hospitalization (Newton and Krishna 1998). About two-thirds of childhood malaria deaths are due to cardiorespiratory arrest associated with metabolic derangements and the remaining third to respiratory arrest, most with features of raised intracranial pressure.

Among surviving children, neurological deficits are common and severe, and include motor impairment, central hypotonia, ataxia, cortical blindness and epileptic seizures, while some patients are left in a vegetative state. Up to 25% of children have neurocognitive deficits following cerebral malaria (Carter et al. 2005). Long-term impairment of a wide range of cognitive functions has been documented, particularly in memory, attention, executive functions and language (Idro et al. 2005). The risk of subsequent epilepsy increases with time after exposure (Carter et al. 2004, Birbeck et al. 2010), and long-term behaviour problems including hyperactivity and conduct difficulties are increasingly described (Idro et al. 2010).

In Malawian children who survived cerebral malaria (Kampondeni et al. 2013), MRI detected periventricular T2 signal changes (53%), atrophy (47%), subcortical T2 signal changes (18%), and focal cortical defects (16%) (Fig. 16.2). Acute focal seizures were associated with atrophy, papilloedema with subcortical T2 signal changes, and peripheral retinal whitening and a higher admission white blood cell count with periventricular T2 signal changes. These findings suggest that seizures, increased intracranial pressure and microvascular ischaemia contribute to clinically relevant brain injury following cerebral malaria.

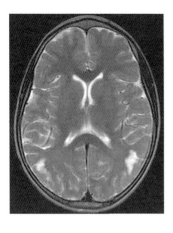

Fig. 16.2. T2-weighted MRI showing focal cortical changes in a male Malawian child who survived cerebral malaria. (Reproduced by courtesy of Sam Kampodeni and Gretchen Birbeck.)

Schistosomiasis

AETIOLOGY AND EPIDEMIOLOGY

Schistosomiasis, also known as bilharzia, is caused by trematodes that are endemic in 70 countries and infect over 200 million people. The disease is caused by *Schistosomia haematobium* and *S. mansoni* in Africa and the Middle East, *S. japonicum* in the Far East, and *S. mekongi* and *S. intercalatum* in southeast Asia and central west Africa (Gray et al. 2010).

Humans are the definitive host, and snails the intermediate host. Adult worms live in the human abdominal venous circulation where they release hundreds of eggs responsible for most schistosome pathology. The eggs can penetrate the intestinal and bladder walls into stool or urine, causing tissue injury and blood loss, and if excreted in the open, get washed into fresh water sources. These rapidly hatch into miracidia, a short-lived stage that seeks and penetrates a snail, the intermediary host. Inside the snail, the parasites multiply asexually and are then released into a water body as a larval form, the cercaria. Humans are infected when they make contact with infested water and the cercaria penetrate the skin. Within weeks, the worms mature inside the abdominal venous circulation and produce eggs into stool or urine to continue the cycle.

The prevalence of *S. mansoni* in the CNS varies from 0.3% to 30% of infected individuals, mainly in the spinal cord; with *S. japonica* brain involvement is more frequent.

PATHOGENESIS

Neurological complications generally occur in the later stages of schistosomiasis and are caused by a granuloma reaction around eggs or adult forms in the CNS (Carod Artal 2012). Schistosome eggs are thought to deposit in the spinal cord through one of two mechanisms. First, an increase in intra-abdominal pressure may cause retrograde venous flow through the Batson venous plexus, a valve-free venous system connecting intra-abdominal and spinal veins and draining the lower spinal cord. As the intra-abdominal pressure is relieved, venous blood may flow back and leave the schistosome eggs in the spinal cord. Second, abnormally migrating adult worms may deposit eggs directly inside the vessels. The interval between infestation and development of symptoms varies from days to 6 years. Vascular lesions are responsible for the neurological sequelae. Subsequent extension of the lesion depends on the degree of infestation and the host's immunological response. Vascular obstruction in the spinal cord is secondary to the formation of a granuloma. An intense inflammatory reaction with a degree of ischaemic necrosis is observed even in some cases where eggs are not found in the nervous system (Pittella 1997). Clinical signs of acute cerebral schistosomiasis suggest cerebral vasculitis (Sarazin et al. 2004). Schistosome eggs or micro-emboli from the heart may be responsible for the vasculitis, mediated partly by eosinophil toxicity.

CLINICAL FEATURES

Cerebral schistosomiasis
Acute schistosomiasis (also known as invasive schistosomiasis or Katayama fever), most often caused by *S. japonicum* infection, may be complicated by life-threatening neurological involvement manifesting with encephalitis and focal neurological deficits 2–6 weeks after exposure. There is fever, disorientation, irritability and confusion, psychomotor slowing, insomnia, depressed consciousness and focal motor weakness. Splinter haemorrhages (a sign of vasculitis) may be detected. The C-reactive protein is elevated, and inverted ST waves may be seen on electrocardiogram leads V3–V5.

Spinal-cord schistosomiasis
Up to 75%–80% of spinal-cord schistosomiasis is asymptomatic. Three types of clinical disease are observed: (1) myelitic form, the most frequent clinical manifestation occurring in about 60% of cases; (2) the pseudotumour or granulomatous form, which is more common in children than in adults; and (3) a radicular or myeloradicular form (Ferrari et al. 2004). The more common presentation of the granulomatous disease form in childhood is thought to be related to the immunological reaction of the younger host.

The onset of symptoms may be acute or subacute. Patients are fully conscious but report pain in the lower limbs that may limit walking. Lower-limb weakness and sphincter involvement develops, with the child having more difficulty in walking. The urinary sphincters are more commonly involved than the anal sphincters, so urinary incontinence and retention often precedes faecal incontinence. The most frequently affected spinal-cord levels are of the lower thoracic and sacrolumbar regions, the conus medullaris and the cauda equina (Araujo et al. 2006).

Upper and lower motor neuron signs may be observed, depending on the spinal level, and paraparesis is often asymmetrical. Most patients with spinal-cord schistosomiasis do not have clinical evidence of hepatosplenic involvement, and diagnosis is often made after spinal-cord damage has already occurred. A few patients, however, may have fever and abdominal discomfort, pain or diarrhoea before onset of spinal-cord signs.

INVESTIGATIONS

In both the cerebral and spinal forms of the disease there is marked eosinophilia and the serum tests positive for anti-schistosomal antibodies, but this only proves exposure. CSF enzyme-linked immunosorbent assay (ELISA) and immunoblot titres may be more elevated than serum. The CSF may show a lymphocytic pleocytosis (from 4 to >200 cells/mm^3) and eosinophilia, elevated protein (0.5 to >4.0g/L) particularly of the gammaglobulin component, and low or normal glucose level. A combination of elevated CSF gammaglobulin and *Schistosoma* eggs in a faecal smear confirms diagnosis. However, absence of eggs in stool does not exclude diagnosis since stool examination is positive in only 50% of cases. Repeated stool examinations may therefore be required. Rectal biopsy is more sensitive and should be performed when stool examinations are negative. In cerebral disease, the ECG may be abnormal and troponin levels elevated, but echocardiography is normal.

Brain MRI may show multiple infarcts in the cortex and white matter in border-zone areas in cerebral schistosomiasis. Spinal MRI helps confirm the level of the lesion in spinal-cord schistosomiasis: an enlarged conus medullaris is seen on T1-weighted images; T2-weighted images show signal hyperintensity or a heterogeneous pattern of enhancement with contrast material (Paz et al. 2002, Saleem et al. 2005). Studies from China have found specific arborized lesions on T1-weighted images characterized by multiple enhancing punctate nodules around a central linear enhancement (Liu et al. 2008). These lesions were associated with the granuloma formation around schistosomal eggs surrounded by inflammation and venous congestion.

TREATMENT

Acute cerebral schistosomiasis should initially be treated with corticosteroids, methylprednisolone or prednisone. Praziquantel is given after neurological recovery has started, since it can precipitate acute neurological deterioration. Corticosteroids attenuate the neurological and cardiac toxicity of eosinophils and the hypersensitivity reaction to parasite toxins (Jaureguiberry et al. 2007). In both cerebral and spinal-cord schistosomiasis, praziquantel can be administered as two 20–35mg/kg doses or as a single dose of 40mg/kg. Oxaminiquine 15–30mg/kg may also be used. Laminectomy and intra-operative biopsy is indicated if other diagnoses are considered, and spinal-cord decompression may be needed for some patients with pseudotumoural forms (Paz et al. 2002).

PROGNOSIS

In a review of 45 patients with spinal schistosomiasis, neurological function was unchanged with treatment in 11, and one patient died. The remaining patients achieved either partial or total improvement (Paz et al. 2002). Recovery is observable within 48 hours of treatment (Ferrari et al. 2004). The outcome of treatment is dependent on the degree of neural injury at the time treatment is initiated. Most patients improve, with full functional recovery described in a third, but those with the pseudotumoral form have a worse prognosis than those with the myelitic and myeloradicular forms.

Toxocariasis

AETIOLOGY AND EPIDEMIOLOGY

Toxocariasis is caused by dog and cat intestinal nematodes, *Toxocara canis* and *T. catis* respectively. Most transmission is vertical; transplacental in the dog fetus or transmammary (during lactation) in young cats. Adult animals may acquire infection by ingesting the parasite's embryonated eggs. Human beings are incidental hosts; transmission mostly occurs though hand-to-mouth contact with *Toxocara* egg-contaminated soil and consumption of contaminated raw vegetables. The parasites cannot fully mature in the human host; instead, the immature and invasive larval forms first penetrate the intestinal wall, after which they migrate to the liver, lungs, CNS and other organs, where they can reside for months or years, until they are overcome by the body's immune system and die (Hotez and Wilkins 2009). People living in areas with high dog and cat populations especially in resource-poor settings have the highest positive seroprevalence rates. Children are particularly prone since they are exposed to the eggs in playgrounds where the soil is contaminated with dog faeces.

CLINICAL FEATURES

The clinical manifestations include visceral larva migrans, ocular larva migrans, covert toxocariasis and 'common' toxocariasis. Visceral and ocular larva migrans are rare. Instead, toxocariasis manifests with only some of the clinical features of visceral larva migrans (especially wheezing and pulmonary infiltrates), and in adults, weakness, pruritus, rash, breathing difficulty and abdominal pain (Magnaval et al. 1994).

Visceral larva migrans

Visceral larva migrans most commonly occurs in young children and manifests with hepatitis and pneumonitis as the larvae migrate through the liver and lungs. The child may have fever, abdominal pain, hepatomegaly, limb pains, decreased appetite, nausea, vomiting, pharyngitis, cervical lymphadenopathy, cough, wheezing, headache, restlessness, sleep and behaviour disorders, lethargy, eosinophilia and, on radiography, pulmonary infiltrates.

Ocular larva migrans

Ocular larva migrans is more frequent in the older child or adolescent, is usually unilateral, and can result from migration of even a single larva into the eye. The resulting inflammatory reaction manifests as either a granuloma or a granulomatous larval track in the retina or endophthalmitis (Good et al. 2004). The most common symptom is visual loss, with onset over a period of days to weeks. There may be uveitis, endophthalmitis, papillitis or inflammatory masses (snow-banks) in the peripheral vitreous (Tran et al. 1999). These signs may fluctuate over years. Ocular infection, however, may be subclinical and only detected during a routine eye examination.

Central nervous system toxocariasis

CNS involvement is relatively rare. The clinical signs are non-specific: the presence of

Toxocara larvae in the CNS can result in seizures from meningo-encephalitis, cerebritis or acute disseminated encephalitis (Marx et al. 2007). Long-standing infections have been associated with epilepsy, intellectual disability and developmental delay (Nelson et al. 1996, Marx et al. 2007). Since pica is a risk factor for both toxocariasis and lead ingestion, lead toxicity needs to be excluded as a potential cause of some of these cognitive deficits.

DIAGNOSIS
Like most helminthic infections, visceral toxocariasis is associated with peripheral blood eosinophilia (Saporito et al. 2008). Total serum IgE concentration may also be high. However, eosinophilia is not common in ocular disease, probably due to the low larval burden, and may also be absent on covert disease. Stool examination is not helpful.

Diagnosis is based on testing for antibodies against *Toxocara* excretory–secretory antigens from the infective-stage larvae by ELISA or enzyme immunoassay. Enzyme immunoassay detects *T. canis* and *T. catis* infections. The sensitivity and specificity of both tests at a titre of 1:32 are 78% and 92%, respectively (Glickman et al. 1978), but they do not distinguish between exposure or active disease. The serum test, however, is less sensitive for the diagnosis of ocular larva migrans; therefore, vitreous fluid may be used. A mobile larva may also be observed directly under the retina. Tests based on polymerase chain reaction are also available.

TREATMENT
There is controversy as to whether the infection should be treated. Thus, only patients with features consistent with toxocariasis, a high eosinophil count and positive serological test, i.e. active disease, are considered for treatment. Serum total IgE over 500 IU/mL provides further evidence of recent infection. The detection of the eosinophil cationic protein released by activated eosinophils may also be helpful (Magnaval et al. 2001).

Effective drugs include albendazole, mebendazole, thiabendazole and diethylcarbamazine. Albendazole (10mg/kg/d for 5 days) is the treatment of choice since it has better penetration into the CSF and is less toxic. Mebendazole (20–25mg/kg/d for 3 weeks) or thiabendazole (25–50mg/kg/d for 3–7 days) can also be used. Corticosteroids (prednisolone 1mg/kg/d) for 1 month or more may reduce inflammation and ocular damage in ocular larva migrans. Laser photocoagulation may be used if the larva is directly visible. Ocular granulomas can be treated with cryopexy. Pars plana vitrectomy is used to remove the epiretinal as well as the subretinal component of a *Toxocara* retinal granuloma. However, if the use of oral and/or topical corticosteroids does not result in full recovery, specific antihelminthic treatment should be considered.

Trichinosis

AETIOLOGY, TRANSMISSION AND EPIDEMIOLOGY
Trichinosis is acquired by eating undercooked pork or wild game meat infected with larvae of a species of the nematode *Trichinella*. Three species cause human disease: *T. spiralis*, *T.*

nativa and *T. brotiva*, with *T. spiralis* being the most pathogenic. Infection occurs when *Trichinella* larvae, encysted in the animal's muscle tissue, are ingested. The cyst wall breaks down in gastric juice, and the larvae are released into the intestine where they develop. Female adult worms produce larvae over several years that migrate through the intestinal wall into the bloodstream and invade many organs including the lungs, eyes, brain, and muscle tissue including the heart and diaphragm.

CLINICAL FEATURES

The clinical course of *Trichinella* infection ranges from no symptoms to severe and even fatal disease. Infestation occurs in two phases: an intestinal (or enteral) phase, and a muscular or systemic phase. Infestations with low intensities can remain asymptomatic, but parasite burdens higher than a few hundred larvae can initially cause gastroenteritis (Pozio and Darwin Murrell 2006). Early symptoms include nausea, vomiting, fatigue, fever, cough, abdominal discomfort and diarrhoea. Headache, joint and muscle pains, itchy skin or constipation may follow. Muscle pain is most pronounced especially with breathing or chewing, or while using large muscles. These symptoms subside within a few months, although fatigue and diarrhoea may last several months. Infection may be detected only years later when calcium deposits are detected around dead cysts on radiography or CT.

CNS disease occurs mainly with heavier infection. Children may experience seizures with an encephalitis-like illness, eye swelling with eyelid oedema, blindness, and coordination difficulties (Ozdemir et al. 2005). Acutely, the patient may be disoriented and drowsy, and focal neurological deficits including hemiparesis may be observed.

Pneumonia or pneumonitis may manifest with breathing difficulties, while heart-muscle involvement is associated with arrhythmias, myocarditis and/or cardiac failure. Such severe infestations are more difficult to treat and may result in death.

INVESTIGATION

Raised creatine kinase from muscle is suggestive. ELISA is sensitive, and increasing *Trichinella* antibody titres on indirect immunofluorescence is diagnostic. CSF may be normal. Moderate cerebral dysfunction may be seen on the electroencephalogram (EEG). On CT or MRI, multifocal small lesions located in the cerebral cortex and white matter are seen (Gelal et al. 2005). Encysted *Trichinella* larvae may be seen in muscle biopsy.

TREATMENT

The infestation is self-limiting and most individuals have no symptoms. Treatment of early infections is with mebendazole (200–400mg three times a day for 3 days, followed by 400–500mg three times a day for 10 days) or albendazole (400mg twice daily for 8–14 days). There is no specific treatment for trichinosis once the larvae have invaded the muscles. The cysts can remain viable for years. Analgesics may be used to relieve muscle pains. More severe infections may be difficult to treat, although in patients with CNS disease, treatment with mebendazole and prednisolone may produce favourable results. Control relies on prevention.

OUTCOME

After infection, patients may have persistent symptoms, particularly muscular, ocular, cardiac, headaches and other neurological complaints as well as tiredness and weakness (Feldmeier et al. 1991). Some children have persistent infections with continuing immunological response.

Onchocerciasis

Onchocerciasis is caused by *Onchocerca volvulus*, a nematode that is found in the tropical regions of Africa and Latin America. It causes river blindness, the second most common infective cause of blindness in the world.

O. volvulus is transmitted by blackflies of *Simulium* species, which live near fast-flowing rivers. The flies carry immature larval forms that, when injected in the human, form nodules in the subcutaneous tissue, where they mature to adult worms. After mating, the female adult worm can release up to 1000 microfilariae a day into the bloodstream.

River blindness may be partly a consequence of an inflammatory reaction to antigens of the *O. volvulus* endosymbiotic bacterium, *Wolbachia pipientis*, which are released when the worms die, causing a severe inflammatory response in the retina that produces blindness. Nodules in the subcutaneous tissue and severe itching with cutaneous marks from scratching are clinical characteristics.

Onchocerciasis appears to be associated with epilepsy in adults (Pion et al. 2009), and also in children according to a recent study from central Ghana and southern Tanzania (Ngugi et al. 2013). A significant proportion of the subcutaneous nodules found in patients living in onchocerciasis-endemic areas of Uganda were found to be caused by *Taenia solium*, questioning the attribution of epilepsy to onchocerciasis in areas where both conditions occur (Katabarwa and Lakwo 2008). However, there is a report on reduced seizure frequency following mass ivermectin treatment for onchocerciasis in an endemic area in Uganda (Kipp et al. 1992), but it is unclear whether this reduction is sustained, translates into a reduction in epilepsy, or is caused by possible antiepileptic properties of ivermectin itself.

The cause of epilepsy in onchocerciasis is unclear. Other clinical manifestations, e.g. blindness, are thought to be caused by the inflammatory responses to dead or dying microfilariae (>100 000 microfilariae die every day in a heavily infected person) and/or coinfection with *W. pipientis*. The immune responses are predominantly antibody mediated, but cellular components are also important. Other proposed mechanisms of epileptogenesis due to onchocerciasis include entry of the adult worm into the CNS, and the generation of autoantibodies. There are no pathological studies that have reported adult worms within the CNS, and there are no neuroimaging studies that have demonstrated lesions associated with adult worms. Microfilariae have been seen in the CSF of untreated patients with onchocerciasis and after the onset of treatment (Marin et al. 2006), but no studies have examined the association of microfilariae in the CSF with epilepsy. Autoantibodies to the retinal photoreceptors have been found in the inner retina of patients with onchocerciasis, but the relationship with retinal damage is not clear. There have been no reports on the association between autoantibodies and epilepsy in onchocerciasis.

Nodding syndrome

Nodding syndrome was first described in Southern Tanzania in the 1960s, and has subsequently been reported in localized areas in Liberia, South Sudan and Northern Uganda, but is rarely seen outside these areas. It is characterized by head nodding, often precipitated by seeing or eating food, or by cold air on the face or cold weather (Sejvar et al. 2013). The head nodding represents atonic seizures, often occurring in association with other seizure types, especially myoclonic seizures, absences and generalized tonic–clonic seizures. In a Ugandan study, the median age at onset was 6 years (range 4–10) (Idro et al. 2013). The syndrome is associated with malnutrition (stunting and wasting), lip changes and muscle wasting. There is progressive cognitive impairment, with psychiatric manifestations such as disorientation, aggression, depression and disordered perception. The EEG is abnormal, suggesting symptomatic generalized epilepsy in most cases. On MRI, there is cortical and cerebellar atrophy (Sejvar et al. 2013).

The cause of nodding syndrome is not clear, but an association with onchocerciasis and/or vitamin B6 deficiency is found in some areas. If the seizures are not controlled with antiepileptic drugs, then there is a decline characterized by progressive wasting and cognitive impairment. Death may occur, mostly from seizure-related events.

Trypanosomiasis

AETIOLOGY AND EPIDEMIOLOGY

Trypanosomes are unicellular protozoa, and those that cause human trypanosomiasis are *Trypanosoma cruzi* (American trypanosomiasis), *T. brucei gambiensi* (west African trypanosomiasis) (97%) and *T. brucei rhodensiensi* (southeast African type).

African trypanosomiasis or sleeping sickness is transmitted by the tsetse fly (*Glossina* spp.) (Kennedy 2013). The disease is exclusive to sub-Saharan Africa, with over 60 million people at risk (Kennedy 2013). The reduction of the reservoirs of infection (e.g. cattle), control of tsetse flies, and early diagnosis and treatment have improved control.

American trypanosomiasis, also called Chagas disease, is transmitted by reduvid bugs and affects approximately 8 million people in Latin American countries (Viotti et al. 2009).

AFRICAN TRYPANOSOMIASIS

Pathogenesis

The inoculated parasites initially multiply in the human lymphatic system before being released into blood circulation and spreading to other organs. The disease therefore progresses through two stages: a haemolymphatic stage, and later, a meningoencephalitic stage. The parasites escape the host immune response by varying the surface glycoprotein coat.

In the brain, trypanosomes are first restricted to periventricular areas and the choroid plexus, outside of the blood–brain barrier, and to the dorsal root ganglia in the spinal cord, appearing as perivascular cuffing on histology (Kristensson et al. 2010). They eventually cross the blood–brain barrier at postcapillary venules, where they induce cytokine response.

The trypanosomes cause secretion of several prostaglandins and interact with the host's immune system to release proinflammatory cytokines. The involvement of the CNS leads to an irreversible demyelinating process. Several neuronal functions and endogenous biological rhythms are altered, the most prominent being the circadian rhythm and the 24 hour sleep–wake cycle. A number of neural pathways, including the suprachiasmatic nucleus and its connections, may be involved through altered effects of cytokines on synaptic functions to cause the changes characteristic of the disease (Kristensson et al. 2010).

Clinical features
T. b. rhodensiense presents more acutely with symptoms developing within days or weeks, whereas in *T. b. gambiense* infection the disease is chronic and may last several years without any major signs or symptoms.

The bite of the tsetse fly and site of parasite inoculation erupts into an inflamed swelling and within weeks the patient experiences fever, lymphadenopathy (Winterbottom sign), aching muscles and joints, headache and irritability. After migration into the CNS, the parasites cause several neurological changes including alterations in behaviour, psychiatric disorders, seizures, coma and ultimately death. The biological clock is altered so that the patient sleeps during the day and is awake at night; confusion, slurred speech, seizures, and difficulties in walking and talking may occur. These problems can develop over months to years depending on aetiology and, if not treated, are fatal.

Diagnosis
Diagnosis requires confirmation of parasite presence in any body fluid, usually blood or the lymphatic system. Early diagnosis is hampered by the lack of specific signs or symptoms in the earlier stages of the disease and the lack of sensitive parasitological tests. Serological tests available today are useful only to screen for *T. b. gambiense* and establish suspicion of infection. Confirmation requires the performance of parasitological tests to demonstrate trypanosomes in the patient. The parasites can be found in most body fluids. However, the number of parasites can be very low, especially in *T. b. gambiense* infection. Thus a negative parasitological result in the presence of a positive serological test does not necessarily indicate absence of infection, and tests may have to be repeated over time to achieve diagnosis. In acute CNS disease, MRI is not diagnostic but is useful to discriminate between acute encephalitis induced by the parasites and post-treatment reactive encephalopathy, a severe and often fatal complication of treatment, particularly with arsenic treatment (Kager et al. 2009).

Treatment
Untreated, African trypanosomiasis is fatal. Reliable distinction between early-stage and late-stage disease, after trypanosomes have traversed the blood–brain barrier, is important for deciding type and duration of treatment (Lejon and Buscher 2005). Accordingly, examination of CSF is essential in diagnosis, selection of drugs for treatment and post-treatment follow-up (Kennedy 2013).

Four drugs are used for the treatment of African trypanosomiasis: pentamidine, suramin, melarsoprol and eflornithine. All are associated with significant toxicity. Pentamidine and suramin are used in the early stage of *T. b. gambiense* and *T. b. rhodesiense* infections, and melarsoprol for the late stage of both forms of the disease. Treatment with melarsoprol, however, may be followed by a severe post-treatment reactive encephalopathy which can be fatal (Kennedy 2006). A combination therapy with eflornithine and nifurtimox, a drug used to treat American trypanosomiasis, reduces the duration of eflornithine monotherapy in treating African trypanosomiasis. More recently, there have been increased efforts for new antitrypanosomal drugs, and the diamidine compounds have shown promising prospects (Kennedy 2013).

AMERICAN TRYPANOSOMIASIS

Pathogenesis
T. cruzi escapes host immune response through intracellular localization. Seven to fourteen days after an infectious bite, the trypanosomes localize in lymph nodes where they divide and aggregate to form pseudocysts, which release parasites on rupture. The parasites invade the bloodstream and lymphatic circulation, lodging in skeletal and heart muscle, gut and phagocytic cells causing inflammatory lesions. The amastigotes elicit an immune response that causes cell and neuron destruction and fibrosis, blockage of the heart's conductive system, arrhythmias, heart failure and aperistalsis of the gastrointestinal system.

Clinical features
Chagas disease may be asymptomatic or characterized by an acute phase in which a swelling (inoculation chagoma or Romana sign) may develop on the skin at the site of parasite penetration. Patients may have fever, lymph-node enlargement and hepatosplenomegaly. Acute disease may be completed by anaemia, muscle pain and neurological manifestations. Acute CNS disease presents as meningoencephalitis especially in children aged 2 years or under, and is potentially fatal if it coexists with concurrent myocarditis and cardiac insufficiency (Cordova et al. 2010). *T. cruzi* can cross the placenta, and fetal infection from chronically infected pregnant mothers can occur, with possibly fatal outcome.

Chronic disease occurs mostly in adults, probably following infection in childhood, and consists of neurological disorder, megacolon, mega-oesophagus and myocarditis. It may be mild and sometimes asymptomatic, or may be associated with significant neural injury resulting in cessation of gut smooth-muscle contractions, cardiac arrhythmias, chronic encephalopathy, and sensory and motor deficits. In 10% of patients, neuritis may diminish reflexes and sensation (Cordova et al. 2010). Immune suppression, as in HIV infection or with drug therapy in organ transplantation, may reactivate *T. cruzi* infection. In these patients, meningoencephalitis and brain abscesses may occur, and mortality is high despite specific treatment (Py 2011).

Treatment
Currently, benznidazole and nifurtimox are the only specific treatments available for American

trypanosomiasis, but these are not as effective against amastigotes in the indeterminate and chronic stages of the disease (Perez-Molina et al. 2009). Treatment is for 30–60 days. Concurrent treatment for the cardiac complications including arrhythmias, ventricular dysfunction and thromboembolism is essential as these are associated with increased mortality (Dubner et al. 2008).

Cystic echinococcosis

AETIOLOGY AND EPIDEMIOLOGY

Cystic echinococcosis is a larval disease of the tapeworm, *Echinococcus*. *E. granulosus* occurs worldwide, typically in rural areas of Africa, the Middle East, southern Europe, Russia, China, Australia and South America. Other species such as *E. multilocularis* present only in the northern hemisphere, and *E. vogeli* in Central and South America. These are responsible for polycystic echinococcosis. The epidemiology, clinical features, diagnosis and treatment of *E. granulosus* differ from the other species. The life cycle involves a definitive host, usually a dog, and intermediate hosts such as sheep, goats and swine. The adult tapeworm lives in the canine intestine and excretes eggs in faeces, contaminating the environment and leading to infection of the intermediate hosts. The hatched larvae can penetrate the intestinal wall and become widely distributed in the body, developing into hydatid cysts. Dogs become infected by ingesting the protoscolices in intermediate hosts. Human infection is usually accidental, through contact with canine faeces (Altinors et al. 2000).

CLINICAL FEATURES

E. granulosus hydatid cysts grow very slowly; thus infected persons often remain asymptomatic for many years. Symptoms are usually caused by mass effect or less commonly by bacterial superinfection and allergic symptoms, especially if a cyst ruptures. Depending on the location of the cyst, patients may have abdominal pain, jaundice and a palpable mass, cough and dyspnoea. Loss of appetite, weight loss and generalized weakness are common. Bone pain and spontaneous fractures have been reported (Altinors et al. 2000).

Hydatid cysts may be intracranial and intraspinal (Altinors et al. 2000). Cerebral cysts are rare, occurring mostly in the white matter of children. Symptoms depend on location, size and number of the cysts (Ozek 1994). Headache and motor weakness are the most common initial symptoms, and a round cystic lesion may be seen on CT (Tuzun et al. 2004). The cysts may rupture into the subarachnoid space leading to widespread dissemination and an anaphylactic reaction. Some children have atypical CNS manifestations such as cerebrovascular occlusive disease and disorders of movement. Neuroimaging is important for diagnosis and correct localization of the cysts (Turgut 2002).

Spinal hydatid cysts occur mainly in the extradural space, sometimes extending intradurally. Symptoms arise from compression. Early symptoms include back, leg or radicular pain in most patients; some may report difficulty in walking. Later, about one-half present with paraparesis that may be asymmetrical.

A positive Casoni skin test is diagnostic of hydatid disease but a negative test does not exclude diagnosis. The test can be negative in solitary cerebral hydatid cyst. Serological ELISA and indirect haemagglutination tests are more sensitive and positive in 85% of patients. Radiological findings depend upon the type of infestation. Solitary cysts with scolices are diagnostic (Reddy 2009).

TREATMENT

Complete surgical excision is the treatment of choice. It is preceded by radiological evaluation and preoperative therapy with albendazole, especially in patients with multiple cerebral cysts where the risk of cyst rupture is very high or if the cyst is in the brainstem. In the latter case, 3% saline may also be injected into the cyst to kill viable scolices before excision (Turgut 2002, Reddy 2009). Surgical excision with the Dowling–Orlando technique is recommended. Complications of CNS cyst excision include intra-operative cyst rupture with an anaphylactic reaction, haemorrhage, pneumocephalus, subdural effusion and development of a porencephalic cyst (Tuzun et al. 2010). Prognostic factors include the location and rupture of the cyst and dissemination of its content. Although cysts are resectable, recurrence remains a major problem with spinal hydatid cysts, at 30%–100% (Kalkan et al. 2007). The therapeutic benefit of methylprednisolone is unclear.

Long-term chemotherapy with albendazole or mebendazole may also be administered to inoperable patients. Albendazole (15mg/kg/d 12 hourly for 28 days not exceeding 800mg/d) is the drug of choice. The regimen may be repeated as needed for 1–3 months. Response to therapy is best monitored by serial imaging studies.

In all cases, preventive programmes should break the parasite life cycle and also educate the farmers in endemic areas.

Paragonimiasis

AETIOLOGY

Paragonimiasis is caused by lung flukes of the genus *Paragonimus*. It is most common in East Asia but is also found in the Americas and in Africa. Human infections are most commonly caused by *P. westermani*, by eating inadequately cooked crab or crayfish infected with metacercariae. The parasite's unembryonated eggs are excreted in sputum or may be swallowed and passed in stool. They become embryonated in the environment and hatch into miracidia which seek their first intermediate host, a snail in which they develop into cercariae. The cercariae invade the second intermediate host, a crab or crayfish, in which they encyst and become metacercariae and infect mammals. The metacercariae excyst in the duodenum and penetrate through the intestinal wall into the peritoneal cavity, then through the diaphragm into the lungs, where they develop into adults; they may also reach the brain and striated muscles (Blair et al. 1999).

CLINICAL FEATURES AND DIAGNOSIS

In endemic areas, acute paragonimiasis should be suspected in children presenting with fever, cough, diarrhoea, abdominal pain, urticaria, hepatosplenomegaly and eosinophilia.

The cough may be productive with blood-stained sputum or frank haemoptysis. Pleural effusion can be present. Extrapulmonary disease may manifest with cholecystitis or CNS symptoms. Parasite localization in the brain is associated with headache, focal or generalized convulsive seizures, hemianopsia, focal motor weakness, sensory disorders, gait disturbances and coma (Xu et al. 2012, Chen et al. 2013). Haemorrhagic stroke and meningitis have also been described. On MRI, parasite nodules and haemorrhagic lesions, some of which have surrounding oedema, are seen as conglomerates of multiple ring-like enhancements. Rarely, there is a 'tunnel sign', which is a track left by a migrating adult worm. On CT, large calcified nodules of chronic infection are visible (Kaw and Sitoh 2001). Cystic lesions may be seen in the cerebral cortex on biopsy specimens. Diagnosis is based on microscopic demonstration of eggs in stool or sputum, but these are not present until 2–3 months after infection. The eggs may also be found in pleural effusion or biopsy material. CNS paragonimiasis may be misdiagnosed as tuberculosis.

TREATMENT
Praziquantel is the drug of choice to treat paragonimiasis. Bithionol is an alternative drug. Brain lesions causing significant focal symptoms may also be surgically excised (Miyazaki 1975).

Amoebic brain infections
Amoebic CNS infections include amoebic abscess and meningoencephalitis.

AMOEBIC BRAIN ABSCESS
Amoebic brain abscess is a rare complication of *Entamoeba histolytica*. The amoebic trophozoites bore and penetrate the intestinal wall, enter the bloodstream and spread to extra-intestinal sites where the trophozoites form abscesses, usually in the liver but occasionally in the lungs, spleen and brain. A common outcome of extra-intestinal spread is amoebic liver abscess, although on rare occasions, amoebic lung, bone, splenic and brain abscesses may develop.

E. histolytica primarily causes amoebic dysentery, a disease characterized by fatigue, abdominal pain, bloody diarrhoea and weight loss. The most common initial presentations of amoebic brain abscess are headache and an altered mental state. Patients develop fever, confusion, vomiting, disorientation and progressive weakness. Depending on the location of the abscess, focal deficits such as hemiplegia and impaired sensation develop, and cranial nerve palsies are frequently observed (Ohnishi et al. 1994, Shah et al. 1994). In addition, some patients have signs of meningism. However, some have no history of dysentery.

The CSF is abnormal in the majority of patients. The erythrocyte sedimentation rate is elevated and there is neutrophilia. On brain CT, patients may have ring-like enhancing lesions predominantly in the white matter with surrounding oedema and, often, a midline shift. Liver abscesses may be visualized on abdominal ultrasound. Diagnosis can be established on light microscopy of an unstained wet preparation of the abscess showing motile amoebic trophozoites with four nuclei, and can also be facilitated by serology including indirect haemagglutination antibody (IHA) test, latex agglutination test, countercurrent immunoelectrophoresis, indirect immunofluorescence, radioimmunoassay or ELISA. A negative IHA, ELISA and indirect immunofluorescence make the diagnosis of invasive amoebiasis unlikely. For histology, tissue is best obtained from the periphery of the lesion. Permanent Wright stain, Feulgen reaction and immunofluorescent-labelled antibodies directed against the amoebae in tissue may be used, or amoebae isolated and cultured (Ohnishi et al. 1994, Shah et al. 1994).

Treatment is with intravenous or oral metronidazole and dehydroemetine. Surgical decompression and drainage of the abscess with removal of necrotic and infected material may be required for the control of intracranial pressure (Ohnishi et al. 1994, Sundaram et al. 2004).

PRIMARY AMOEBIC MENINGOENCEPHALITIS

Primary amoebic meningoencephalitis is a rare but often fatal CNS infection caused by *Naegleria fowleri*, *Acanthamoeba* spp. or *Bulamuthia mandillaris*.

Most *N. fowleri* infection occurs in healthy young boys exposed to infection in recreational waters, lakes and ponds in warm-weather locations (Yoder et al. 2010). Symptoms are similar to bacterial and viral meningitis. Patients complain of fever, reduced appetite, severe headache, occasional vomiting and a stiff neck. There is rapid progression of the infection with agitation, seizures and development of altered consciousness or coma. Death may result in 3–7 days. On autopsy, there is acute haemorrhagic necrosis of the olfactory bulb and cerebral cortex. Diagnosis is established on microscopy with the presence of *N. fowleri* trophozoites on a fresh wet preparation of CSF centrifuge sediment, Giemsa–Wright stained films or indirect fluorescent antibody tests, and by polymerase chain reaction. Treatment should be in an intensive care setting using intravenous and intrathecal amphotericin B or fluconazole, azithromycin, rifampicin and metronidazole (CDC 2008).

Acanthamoeba spp. are free-living amoebae that cause granulomatous encephalitis especially in debilitated and immunocompromised hosts probably with depressed cell-mediated immunity. The pathogenesis is poorly understood (Khan 2010) but most likely includes induction of proinflammatory responses, invasion of the blood–brain barrier and connective tissue, and neuronal injury leading to brain dysfunction particularly in the midbrain, basal areas of the temporal and occipital lobes, and posterior fossa structures. The routes of entry include the olfactory neuroepithelium or the lower respiratory tract, followed by haematogenous spread. Skin lesions (ulcers and nodules) may provide direct entry into the bloodstream. The clinical course is insidious, usually similar to a brain abscess, but may mimic bacterial meningitis or tuberculous meningitis. Patients complain of headache and low-grade fever, and present with seizures, neuropsychiatric symptoms, keratitis, focal neurological signs, hemiparesis and coma, progressing to death.

The CSF pressure is elevated, cells (lymphocytes and plasma cells) are increased, glucose is low, and the protein levels are high. CT is non-specific. Acanthamoebic trophozoites and cysts can be found in the haemorrhagic and necrotic cerebral tissues in autopsy specimens. Severe angiitis and fibrinoid necrosis of the vascular wall with perivascular cuffing by lymphocytes and plasma cells may also be seen (Lu et al. 1999). Rapid diagnosis is critical for early treatment. Microscopic examination and culture of CSF, biopsy specimens and corneal scrapings, and real-time polymerase chain reaction assays are used for diagnosis (da Rocha-Azevedo et al. 2009). Treatment is with antimicrobial combinations of azoles (clotrimazole, miconazole, ketoconazole, fluconazole, itraconazole), pentamidine isethionate, 5-fluorocytosine and sulphadiazine. Rarely, excision of the brain lesion(s) may be possible (Aichelburg et al. 2008).

Bulamuthia mandillaris is similar to *Acanthamoeba* spp. in that it causes a granulomatous amoebic encephalitis, but it causes disease in immune-competent as well as immune-compromised children. It is found in the soil, and most cases have been reported from North, Central and South America and Australia (Hill et al. 2011). To date there are a few case reports in which the children present with fever, headaches, seizures, hemiparesis and coma. It can cause mycotic aneurysms giving rise to strokes. Treatment is similar to *Acanthamoeba* infections.

Summary

Parasite infections and infestations of the CNS are common in the world, but their distribution depends upon local ecological conditions and wealth of the populations. CNS symptoms and signs in children who have travelled, been in contact with animals or come from resource-poor areas should arouse suspicion.

REFERENCES

Aichelburg AC, Walochnik J, Assadian O, et al. (2008) Successful treatment of disseminated *Acanthamoeba* sp. infection with miltefosine. *Emerg Infect Dis* 14: 1743–6.

Altinors N, Bavbek M, Caner HH, Erdogan B (2000) Central nervous system hydatidosis in Turkey: a cooperative study and literature survey analysis of 458 cases. *J Neurosurg* 93: 1–8.

Araujo KC, Rosa e Silva Cd, Barbosa CS, Ferrari TC (2006) Clinical–epidemiological profile of children with schistosomal myeloradiculopathy attended at the Instituto Materno-Infantil de Pernambuco. *Mem Inst Oswaldo Cruz* 101 Suppl 1: 149–56.

Birbeck GL, Molyneux ME, Kaplan PW, et al. (2010) Blantyre Malaria Project Epilepsy Study (BMPES) of neurological outcomes in retinopathy-positive paediatric cerebral malaria survivors: a prospective cohort study. *Lancet Neurol* 9: 1173–81.

Blair D, Xu ZB, Agatsuma T (1999) Paragonimiasis and the genus *Paragonimus*. *Adv Parasitol* 42: 113–222.

Carod Artal FJ (2012) Cerebral and spinal schistosomiasis. *Curr Neurol Neurosci Rep* 12: 666–74.

Carter JA, Neville BG, White S, et al. (2004) Increased prevalence of epilepsy associated with severe falciparum malaria in children. *Epilepsia* 45: 978–81.

Carter JA, Mung'Ala-Odera V, Neville BG, et al. (2005) Persistent neurocognitive impairments associated with severe falciparum malaria in Kenyan children. *J Neurol Neurosurg Psychiatry* 76: 476–81.

CDC (2008) Primary amebic meningoencephalitis — Arizona, Florida, and Texas, 2007. *MMWR Wkly Rep* 57: 573–7.

Chen J, Chen Z, Lin J, et al. (2013) Cerebral paragonimiasis: a retrospective analysis of 89 cases. *Clin Neurol Neurosurg* 115: 546–51.

Clark IA (2009) Along a TNF-paved road from dead parasites in red cells to cerebral malaria, and beyond. *Parasitology* 19: 1–12.

Cordova E, Maiolo E, Corti M, Orduna T (2010) Neurological manifestations of Chagas' disease. *Neurol Res* 32: 238–44.

Crawley J, Waruiru C, Mithwani S, et al. (2000) Effect of phenobarbital on seizure frequency and mortality in childhood cerebral malaria: a randomised, controlled intervention study. *Lancet* 355: 701–6.

da Rocha-Azevedo B, Tanowitz HB, Marciano-Cabral F (2009) Diagnosis of infections caused by pathogenic free-living amoebae. *Interdiscip Perspect Infect Dis* 2009: 251406. doi: 10.1155/2009/251406.

Dondorp AM, Fanello CI, Hendriksen IC, et al. (2010) Artesunate versus quinine in the treatment of severe falciparum malaria in African children (AQUAMAT): an open-label, randomised trial. *Lancet* 376: 1647–57.

Dubner S, Schapachnik E, Riera AR, Valero E (2008) Chagas disease: state-of-the-art of diagnosis and management. *Cardiol J* 15: 493–504.

Feldmeier H, Bienzle U, Jansen Rosseck R, et al. (1991) Sequelae after infection with Trichinella spiralis: a prospective cohort study. *Wien Klin Wochenschr* 103: 111–6.

Ferrari TC, Moreira PR, Cunha AS (2004) Spinal cord schistosomiasis: a prospective study of 63 cases emphasizing clinical and therapeutic aspects. *J Clin Neurosci* 11: 246–53.

Gelal F, Kumral E, Vidinli BD, et al. (2005) Diffusion-weighted and conventional MR imaging in neurotrichinosis. *Acta Radiol* 46: 196–9.

Glickman L, Schantz P, Dombroske R, Cypess R (1978) Evaluation of serodiagnostic tests for visceral larva migrans. *Am J Trop Med Hyg* 27: 492–8.

Good B, Holland CV, Taylor MR, et al. (2004) Ocular toxocariasis in schoolchildren. *Clin Infect Dis* 39: 1738.

Gray DJ, McManus DP, Li Y, et al. (2010) Schistosomiasis elimination: lessons from the past guide the future. *Lancet Infect Dis* 10: 733–6.

Gwer S, Idro R, Fegan G, et al. (2012) Continuous EEG monitoring in Kenyan children with non-traumatic coma. *Arch Dis Child* 97: 343–9.

Gwer SA, Idro RI, Fegan G, et al. (2013) Fosphenytoin for seizure prevention in childhood coma in Africa: a randomized clinical trial. *J Crit Care* 28: 1086–92.

Hill CP, Damodaran O, Walsh P, et al. (2011) Balamuthia amebic meningoencephalitis and mycotic aneurysms in an infant. *Pediatr Neurol* 45: 45–8.

Hotez PJ, Wilkins PP (2009) Toxocariasis: America's most common neglected infection of poverty and a helminthiasis of global importance? *PLoS Negl Trop Dis* 3: e400.

Idro R, Jenkins NE, Newton CR (2005) Pathogenesis, clinical features, and neurological outcome of cerebral malaria. *Lancet Neurol* 4: 827–40.

Idro R, Aketch S, Gwer S, et al. (2006) Research priorities in the management of severe *Plasmodium falciparum* malaria in children. *Ann Trop Med Parasitol* 100: 95–108.

Idro R, Ndiritu M, Ogutu B, et al. (2007) Burden, features, and outcome of neurological involvement in acute falciparum malaria in Kenyan children. *JAMA* 297: 2232–40.

Idro R, Kakooza-Mwesige A, Balyejjussa S, et al. (2010) Severe neurological sequelae and behaviour problems after cerebral malaria in Ugandan children. *BMC Res Notes* 3: 104.

Idro R, Opoka RO, Aanyu HT, et al. (2013) Nodding syndrome in Ugandan children—clinical features, brain imaging and complications: a case series. *BMJ Open* 3(5): e002540. doi: 10.1136/bmjopen-2012-002540.

Jaureguiberry S, Ansart S, Perez L, et al. (2007) Acute neuroschistosomiasis: two cases associated with cerebral vasculitis. *Am J Trop Med Hyg* 76: 964–6.

Kager PA, Schipper HG, Stam J, Majoie CB (2009) Magnetic resonance imaging findings in human African trypanosomiasis: a four-year follow-up study in a patient and review of the literature. *Am J Trop Med Hyg* 80: 947–52.

Kalkan E, Cengiz SL, Cicek O, et al. (2007) Primary spinal intradural extramedullary hydatid cyst in a child. *J Spinal Cord Med* 30: 297–300.

Kampondeni SD, Potchen MJ, Beare NA, et al. (2013) MRI findings in a cohort of brain injured survivors of pediatric cerebral malaria. *Am J Trop Med Hyg* 88: 542–6.

Kariuki SM, Gitau E, Gwer S, et al. (2014) Value of *Plasmodium falciparum* histidine-rich protein 2 level and malaria retinopathy in distinguishing cerebral malaria from other acute encephalopathies in Kenyan children. *J Infect Dis* 209: 600–9. doi: 10.1093/infdis/jit500.

Katabarwa M, Lakwo T, Habumogisha P, et al. (2008) Could neurocysticercosis be the cause of "onchocerciasis-associated" epileptic seizures? *Am J Trop Med Hyg* 78: 400–1.

Kaw GJ, Sitoh YY (2001) Clinics in diagnostic imaging (58). Chronic cerebral paragonimiasis. *Singapore Med J* 42: 89–91.

Kennedy PG (2006) Diagnostic and neuropathogenesis issues in human African trypanosomiasis. *Int J Parasitol* 36: 505–12.

Kennedy PGE (2013) Clinical features, diagnosis, and treatment of human African trypanosomiasis (sleeping sickness). *Lancet Neurol* 12: 186–94.

Khan NA (2010) Novel in vitro and in vivo models to study central nervous system infections due to *Acanthamoeba* spp. *Exp Parasitol* 126: 69–72.

Kipp W, Burnham G, Kamugisha J (1992) Improvement in seizures after ivermectin. *Lancet* 340: 789–90.

Krishna S (2012) Adjunctive management of malaria. *Curr Opin Infect Dis* 25: 484–8.

Kristensson K, Nygard M, Bertini G, Bentivoglio M (2010) African trypanosome infections of the nervous system: parasite entry and effects on sleep and synaptic functions. *Prog Neurobiol* 91: 152–71.

Lejon V, Buscher P (2005) Cerebrospinal fluid in human African trypanosomiasis: a key to diagnosis, therapeutic decision and post-treatment follow-up. *Trop Med Int Health* 10: 395–403.

Lewallen S, White VA, Whitten RO, et al. (2000) Clinical–histopathological correlation of the abnormal retinal vessels in cerebral malaria. *Arch Ophthalmol* 118: 924–8.

Liu H, Lim CC, Feng X, et al. (2008) MRI in cerebral schistosomiasis: characteristic nodular enhancement in 33 patients. *AJR Am J Roentgenol* 191: 582–8.

Lu D, Luo L, Xu Q, Li C (1999) [A clinico-pathological study of granulomatous amoebic encephalitis.] *Zhonghua Bing Li Xue Za Zhi* 28: 169–73.

Magnaval JF, Michault A, Calon N, Charlet JP (1994) Epidemiology of human toxocariasis in La Réunion. *Trans R Soc Trop Med Hyg* 88: 531–3.

Magnaval JF, Berry A, Fabre R, Morassin B (2001) Eosinophil cationic protein as a possible marker of active human Toxocara infection. *Allergy* 56: 1096–9.

Maitland K, Nadel S, Pollard AJ, et al. (2005) Management of severe malaria in children: proposed guidelines for the United Kingdom. *BMJ* 331: 337–43.

Maitland K, Kiguli S, Opoka RO, et al. (2011) Mortality after fluid bolus in African children with severe infection. *N Engl J Med* 364: 2483–95.

Marin B, Boussinesq M, Druet-Cabanac M, et al. (2006) Onchocerciasis-related epilepsy? Prospects at a time of uncertainty. *Trends Parasitol* 22: 17–20.

Marx C, Lin J, Masruha MR, et al. (2007) Toxocariasis of the CNS simulating acute disseminated encephalomyelitis. *Neurology* 69: 806–7.

Miyazaki I (1975) Cerebral paragonimiasis. *Contemp Neurol Ser* 12: 109–32.

Nelson S, Greene T, Ernhart CB (1996) Toxocara canis infection in preschool age children: risk factors and the cognitive development of preschool children. *Neurotoxicol Teratol* 18: 167–74.

Newton CR, Krishna S (1998) Severe falciparum malaria in children: current understanding of pathophysiology and supportive treatment. *Pharmacol Ther* 79: 1–53.

Ngugi AK, Bottomley C, Kleinschmidt I, et al. (2013) Prevalence of active convulsive epilepsy in sub-Saharan Africa and associated risk factors: cross-sectional and case–control studies. *Lancet Neurol* 12: 253–63.

Ohnishi K, Murata M, Kojima H, et al. (1994) Brain abscess due to infection with *Entamoeba histolytica*. *Am J Trop Med Hyg* 51: 180–2.

Okoromah CA, Afolabi BB, Wall EC (2011) Mannitol and other osmotic diuretics as adjuncts for treating cerebral malaria. *Cochrane Database Syst Rev* (4): CD004615.

Ozdemir D, Ozkan H, Akkoc N, et al. (2005) Acute trichinellosis in children compared with adults. *Pediatr Infect Dis J* 24: 897–900.

Ozek MM (1994) Complications of central nervous system hydatid disease. *Pediatr Neurosurg* 20: 84–91.

Paz JA, Valente M, Casella EB, Marques-Dias MJ (2002) Spinal cord schistosomiasis in children: analysis of seven cases. *Arq Neuropsiquiatr* 60: 224–30.

Perez-Molina JA, Perez-Ayala A, Moreno S, et al. (2009) Use of benznidazole to treat chronic Chagas' disease: a systematic review with a meta-analysis. *J Antimicrob Chemother* 64: 1139–47.

Pion SD, Kaiser C, Boutros-toni F, et al. (2009) Epilepsy in onchocerciasis endemic areas: systematic review and meta-analysis of population-based surveys. *PLoS Negl Trop Dis* 3: e461.

Pittella JE (1997) Neuroschistosomiasis. *Brain Pathol* 7: 649–62.

Potchen MJ, Kampondeni SD, Seydel KB, et al. (2012) Acute brain MRI findings in 120 Malawian children with cerebral malaria: new insights into an ancient disease. *AJNR Am J Neuroradiol* 33: 1740–6.

Pozio E, Darwin Murrell K (2006) Systematics and epidemiology of trichinella. *Adv Parasitol* 63: 367–439.

Py MO (2011) Neurologic manifestations of Chagas disease. *Curr Neurol Neurosci Rep* 11: 536–42. doi: 10.1007/s11910-011-0225-8.

Reddy DR (2009) Managing cerebral and cranial hydatid disease. *Neurol India* 57: 116–8.

Rogerson SJ, Grau GE, Hunt NH (2004) The microcirculation in severe malaria. *Microcirculation* 11: 559–76.

Saleem S, Belal AI, el-Ghandour NM (2005) Spinal cord schistosomiasis: MR imaging appearance with surgical and pathologic correlation. *AJNR Am J Neuroradiol* 26: 1646–54.

Saporito L, Scarlata F, Colomba C, et al. (2008) Human toxocariasis: a report of nine cases. *Acta Paediatr* 97: 1301–2.

Sarazin M, Caumes E, Cohen A, Amarenco P (2004) Multiple microembolic borderzone brain infarctions and endomyocardial fibrosis in idiopathic hypereosinophilic syndrome and in *Schistosoma mansoni* infestation. *J Neurol Neurosurg Psychiatry* 75: 305–7.

Sejvar JJ, Kakooza AM, Foltz JL, et al. (2013) Clinical, neurological, and electrophysiological features of nodding syndrome in Kitgum, Uganda: an observational case series. *Lancet Neurol* 12: 166–74.

Shah AA, Shaikh H, Karim M (1994) Amoebic brain abscess: a rare but serious complication of *Entamoeba histolytica* infection. *J Neurol Neurosurg Psychiatry* 57: 240–1.

Sundaram C, Prasad BC, Bhaskar G, et al. (2004) Brain abscess due to *Entamoeba histolytica*. *J Assoc Physicians India* 52: 251–2.

Tran VT, Lumbroso L, LeHoang P, Herbort CP (1999) Ultrasound biomicroscopy in peripheral retinovitreal toxocariasis. *Am J Ophthalmol* 127: 607–9.

Turgut M (2002) Hydatidosis of central nervous system and its coverings in the pediatric and adolescent age groups in Turkey during the last century: a critical review of 137 cases. *Childs Nerv Syst* 18: 670–83.

Tuzun Y, Kadioglu HH, Izci Y, et al. (2004) The clinical, radiological and surgical aspects of cerebral hydatid cysts in children. *Pediatr Neurosurg* 40: 155–60.

Tuzun Y, Solmaz I, Sengul G, Izci Y (2010) The complications of cerebral hydatid cyst surgery in children. *Childs Nerv Syst* 26: 47–51.

Viotti R, Vigliano C, Lococo B, et al. (2009) Side effects of benznidazole as treatment in chronic Chagas disease: fears and realities. *Expert Rev Anti Infect Ther* 7: 157–63.

Warrell DA, Looareesuwan S, Warrell MJ, et al. (1982) Dexamethasone proves deleterious in cerebral malaria. A double-blind trial in 100 comatose patients. N Engl J Med 306: 313–9.

Waruiru CM, Newton CR, Forster D, et al. (1996) Epileptic seizures and malaria in Kenyan children. *Trans R Soc Trop Med Hyg* 90: 152–5.

White NJ, Pukrittayakamee S, Hien TT, et al. (2014) Malaria. *Lancet* 383: 723–5. doi: 10.1016/S0140-6736(13)60024-0.

WHO (2000) Severe falciparum malaria. *Trans R Soc Trop Med Hyg* 94 Suppl 1: S1–90.

WHO (2009) *World Malaria Report 2009*. Geneva: World Health Organization (online: http://www.who.int/malaria/world_malaria_report_2009/en/index.html).

Xu HZ, Tang LF, Zheng XP, Chen ZM (2012) Paragonimiasis in Chinese children: 58 cases analysis. *Iran J Pediatr* 22: 505–11.

Yoder JS, Eddy BA, Visvesvara GS, et al. (2010) The epidemiology of primary amoebic meningoencephalitis in the USA, 1962–2008. *Epidemiol Infect* 138: 968–75.

17
NEUROCYSTICERCOSIS

Pratibha Singhi

Neurocysticercosis (NCC), caused by infection of the central nervous system (CNS) with encysted larvae of *Taenia solium*, is a common parasitic disease of the human nervous system and a major cause of epilepsy and neurological disease worldwide. It has varied manifestations, and it is therefore important for physicians to be aware of the disease, its diagnosis and management.

Epidemiology

NCC is endemic in large parts of Asia, Latin America and southeast Africa. The exact prevalence of NCC is difficult to determine as neuroimaging is required for confirmation of diagnosis. NCC is highly prevalent in pig-rearing communities and is linked with low economic development; the burden is highest in south Asia followed by sub-Saharan Africa (WHO 2003). In endemic regions, NCC is a very common cause of acquired epilepsy. In Latin America, NCC accounts for about one-third of all patients with epilepsy (Villarán et al. 2009). In a rural community of north India, 25% of patients with seizure disorder had active NCC and 10% had remote symptomatic seizures related to calcified granuloma (Goel et al. 2011). In sub-Saharan Africa it is estimated that NCC is responsible for 30%–50% of acquired epilepsy (Winkler 2012). In a systematic review, the pooled estimate for the proportion of NCC among people with epilepsy was 29% (Ndimubanzi et al. 2010). There are no community-based studies specifically addressing children, but the pooled estimates are similar for children and adults. A point prevalence of 4.5/1000 for NCC was reported from north India (Raina et al. 2012). Hospital-based studies in Peru and north India have shown that the proportion of children with partial seizures who have NCC is over 50% (Gaffo et al. 2004, Singhi and Singhi 2004). NCC results in huge economic losses in resource-poor countries where it is endemic.

NCC is also being increasingly reported from many resource-rich countries, mainly because of the increasing numbers of immigrants from, and travel to, endemic areas. It is estimated that between 1320 and 5050 new cases of NCC occur every year in the USA (Serpa and White 2012). A population-based active surveillance in Oregon, USA, found an annual incidence of 0.5 cases per 100 000 general population and 5.8 cases per 100 000 Hispanics (O'Neal et al. 2011).

Life cycle of the parasite

Humans are the definitive host for the adult tapeworm. They acquire intestinal *T. solium* (taeniasis) from pigs by ingestion of uncooked/undercooked pork infested with live *T. solium* cysticerci. These cysticerci release larvae, which develop into adult worms that live in the intestine. The female worm sheds thousands of extremely contagious eggs, which are passed in the human faeces contaminating the soil, particularly in areas with poor sanitation and open defecation. Pigs are the intermediate host and are infected by grazing on such contaminated soil or by coprophagia. In the pigs' intestines the eggs hatch into larvae that invade the mucosa, reaching various tissues where they mature into cysticerci over a period of 3 weeks to 2 months. The life cycle of the parasite is completed when humans consume undercooked pork containing the cysts.

Humans get neurocysticercosis by ingestion of *T. solium* eggs, via intake of contaminated food, through infected food handlers, or by autoingestion of ova through the faeco-oral route in tapeworm carriers. In the human intestine the eggs hatch to release larvae that penetrate the intestinal mucosa, and migrate throughout the body to produce cysticercosis. Although the cysts may lodge in any tissue, most mature cysts are found in the CNS, skeletal muscle, subcutaneous tissue and the eyes.

Pathogenesis

In the brain, most cysts locate at the grey–white matter junction. Generally, cysticerci live asymptomatically within host tissues for prolonged periods (years) because of various protective mechanisms. Although there is no reliable animal model of NCC, murine models using the cestode *Mesocestoides corti* suggest that the parasite releases glycoconjugates at the time of penetration into the CNS and then continuously. This leads to a suppressive and immunoregulatory environment that protects the parasite from host inflammatory responses. Once the parasite dies, this balance ends and an inflammatory reaction starts (Alvarez et al. 2008). Both Th1- and Th2-type mechanisms (Kashyap et al. 2011) and Toll-like receptors (Verma et al. 2010) are involved in the immune response in symptomatic NCC.

In the brain parenchyma the cyst evolves through four stages. The *vesicular cyst* (metacestode) is viable, filled with clear fluid, and has a thin semitransparent wall with an eccentric opaque 4–5mm scolex. There is no evident inflammation around it and it is usually asymptomatic. After some time an inflammatory response is elicited, the larva undergoes hyaline degeneration, and the clear cyst fluid is replaced with opaque gelatinous material. This is termed the *colloidal stage*. This is followed by the *granular nodular stage* in which the cyst contracts and the walls are replaced by focal lymphoid nodules and necrosis. Most cysts then calcify – the *nodular calcified stage* (Escobar 1983). Some cysts may resolve completely without calcification.

Degenerating cysts are termed 'active', whereas vesicular (viable) and calcified cysts are termed 'inactive' by some experts. There is increasing evidence that not all cysticercus granulomas represent degenerating old cysts, and that many may represent fresh infections wherein the parasite has been rapidly destroyed by the host's immune system (Garcia et al. 2010).

Clinical manifestations

The exact proportion of people with NCC who remain asymptomatic is not known. In community-based studies, asymptomatic NCC was found in 15% and 9% of adults in north India (Prasad et al. 2011) and Mexico (Fleury et al. 2003) respectively.

The clinical presentation of NCC is very diverse and depends on the location, number and viability of the cysts. Parenchymal NCC usually presents with seizures and is generally benign, whereas extraparenchymal NCC usually presents with hydrocephalus and is generally severe and difficult to treat. However, both types may be seen in a single patient. Extraparenchymal NCC is uncommon, particularly in children.

PARENCHYMAL NEUROCYSTICERCOSIS

Parenchymal NCC is common in both adults and children. Most symptomatic cases of childhood NCC are seen after 5 years of age, although some are seen even in infants and toddlers (Del Brutto 2013). The most common presentation is with sudden-onset seizures in an otherwise healthy child. In a series of 500 children from India who had NCC, seizures were reported in 95% (Singhi et al. 2000). Other studies show similar figures of 70%–90% (Carabin et al. 2011). Most children (84%–87%) present with partial, particularly complex partial, seizures; about a quarter have simple partial seizures. The seizures are short, less than 5 minutes in most cases; status epilepticus has been reported in 2%–32% of patients. Often there is a single seizure. Clustering of seizures, commonly reported in adults, is less common in children. It is presumed that degeneration of the cysts and the associated inflammatory response evokes seizures; however, in Latin America, some patients with seizures are found on neuroimaging to have vesicular cysts, whereas in the Indian subcontinent, symptomatic NCC is seen when the cysts start degenerating. Seizures can also be seen with calcified cysts. Regional differences in the clinical presentation of NCC may indicate genetic differences in the host or the parasite.

Headache and vomiting occur in about a third of cases, often in association with seizures (Baranwal et al. 1998, Singhi et al. 2000). Chronic tension-type headaches and migraine, reported in adults, are rarely seen in children. Papilloedema has been reported in 2%–7% of children. Signs of raised intracranial pressure (ICP) are less common in children than in adults. Neurological deficits are reported in 16% of adults, but are uncommon (4%–6%) in children. Transient hemiparesis, monoparesis and oculomotor abnormalities may be seen; cerebrovascular disease is reported in 4%–12% of adults (Marquez and Arauz 2012) but is rare in children. Ptosis due to midbrain NCC (Singhi et al. 2008) and movement disorder due to basal ganglia NCC (Karnik et al. 2011) are reported.

CYSTICERCAL ENCEPHALITIS

An acute encephalitic presentation with severe acute raised ICP is occasionally seen in young children and adolescents with massive cyst burden and diffuse cerebral oedema. These patients are difficult to treat and have a poor prognosis.

EXTRAPARENCHYMAL NEUROCYSTICERCOSIS

Extraparenchymal NCC presents as obstructive hydrocephalus when ventricular or subarachnoid cysts block the CSF flow, usually in the fourth ventricle; associated inflammation may worsen the obstruction. Cysts in the sylvian fissure can involve the middle cerebral artery, or they may lodge in the basal areas and cause chronic arachnoiditis or meningitis. Some subarachnoid cysts may enlarge considerably without scolices, become racemose and cause mass effects, hydrocephalus and infarcts. Rarely, symptoms and signs of spinal dysfunction including radicular pain, paraesthesia, sphincteric disturbances and paraplegia may be seen when cysts locate in the leptomeningeal space, or within the cord. A high frequency (61%) of spinal cysts was reported in adults with intracranial subarachnoid NCC (Callacondo et al. 2012). Cysts can also lodge anywhere in the eyes including the extra-ocular muscles, subretinal space, vitreous humor, subconjunctiva or anterior chamber. Symptoms occur accordingly and include limitation of eye movements, visual deficits and even sudden blindness.

Several unusual presentations of NCC such as behavioural changes and psychiatric manifestations, dorsal midbrain syndrome, papillitis, cerebral haemorrhage, dystonia and neurocognitive deficits have been reported, but are rare in children.

Diagnosis

The mainstay of diagnosis is neuroimaging; other indicators such as epidemiology, serology and a history of travel to endemic areas can corroborate the diagnosis.

COMPUTERIZED TOMOGRAPHY (CT)

Parenchymal neurocysticercosis

In the Indian subcontinent the usual CT finding is a single small (<20mm) low-density lesion with ring or disc enhancement and an eccentric scolex that appears as a bright high-density nodule and is pathognomonic of NCC. This is termed a single small enhancing CT lesion or a single cysticercal granuloma (Fig. 17.1) and represents a degenerating cyst. In most cases there is perilesional oedema, which is usually mild to moderate, occasionally severe. Some children may have two or more lesions; multiple NCC with numerous cysts of varying stages may give the so-called 'starry sky' appearance that is typical of NCC (Fig. 17.2). In Latin America and Africa the proportion of cases with multiple lesions is much higher than in India.

Calcified cysts are usually punctate or a few millimetres in size, single or multiple, generally without any surrounding oedema. Oedema may at times be seen around calcified lesions in children with active seizures and is thought to represent inflammation secondary to host response to newly released/recognized parasite antigen (Nash 2012). Vesicular cysts generally appear as small round lesions with CSF-density cystic fluid; the wall is isodense to the brain parenchyma. They are non-enhancing or mildly enhancing and are not surrounded by oedema. Viable lesions are very rarely seen in India, whereas they are commonly seen in Latin America and China.

Extraparenchymal neurocysticercosis

Extraparenchymal NCC features of arachnoiditis and chronic meningitis such as enhance-

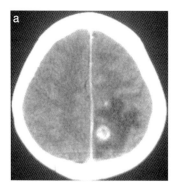
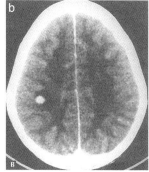

Fig. 17.1. Single small enhancing lesion in a child. (a) CT showing ring enhancement with scolex and perilesional oedema. (b) CT showing disc enhancement.

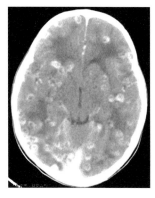

Fig. 17.2. CT showing multiple neurocysticercosis lesions in a child.

ment of tentorium and basal cisterns, hydrocephalus and occasionally infarcts may be seen in cases of subarachnoid NCC. Intraventricular cysts may cause obstruction and hydrocephalus; racemose cysts may be seen as cystic hypodense lesions in the sylvian fissure or cerebellopontine angle.

MAGNETIC RESONANCE IMAGING (MRI)
MRI is more sensitive than CT for visualization of scolex and extraparenchymal cysts. The scolex is seen as a nodule that is isointense or hyperintense relative to white matter, and is best seen on proton density-weighted images. On T2-weighted images, the perilesional oedema appears bright, and because of the high-intensity cystic fluid, the scolex may not be seen. The MRI characteristics change as the cyst evolves. On T2 images the cystic contents change from hyperintense to hypointense and the cyst wall changes from hypointense to hyperintense. Gadolinium-enhanced MRI shows ring enhancement of the lesion, followed by disc enhancement.

Calcified lesions appear hypointense on all MRI sequences and may at times be missed. Vesicular cysts appear as round lesions, either isointense or slightly hyperintense to the CSF.

MRI is ideal in defining NCC lesions and differentiating them from other similar-looking lesions. However, in many resource-poor countries patients often cannot afford MRI, and CT is generally sufficient for making a diagnosis. MRI may be required in cases where the scolex is not seen and in extraparenchymal NCC.

SEROLOGICAL TESTS

Several serodiagnostic tests are available; they have variable sensitivity and specificity depending on the antigen and the technique used. Low positivity of 17%–25% has been reported for single lesions. The seropositivity depends on the parasite load and may also vary because of differences between the genotypes of *T. solium* (Asian versus African/Latin American).

The enzyme-linked immunoelectro-transfer blot (EITB) assay using purified glycoprotein antigens from *T. solium* cysticerci is reported to be highly specific and nearly 100% sensitive for patients with either multiple active parenchymal cysts or extraparenchymal NCC (Tsang et al. 1989). However, it is less sensitive for patients with single cysts or calcification. The EITB assay is more sensitive than the enzyme-linked immunosorbent assay (ELISA), especially in serum (Proaño-Narvaez et al. 2002). A comparative study of antigen-detecting ELISA and antibody-detecting dot-blot assay in children found that both were more sensitive in patients with multiple brain lesions (100%) than in those with a single lesion (87%) (Mandal et al. 2006). Antibody-detecting tests have similar sensitivity in serum and CSF, whereas the antigen-detecting ELISA has better sensitivity in CSF as compared to serum. The use of excretory–secretory antigens (Sahu et al. 2009), synthetic peptides and newer modalities such as 'nanobodies' (single-domain antibody fragments consisting of heavy chain only) is being evaluated (Esquivel-Velázquez et al. 2011). The ideal immunodiagnostic test for single-lesion NCC is still awaited. A positive test supports the diagnosis of NCC; a negative test, however, does not exclude the diagnosis. False-positive serology can be seen in people from endemic areas.

OTHER TESTS

Biopsy of subcutaneous nodules for presence of parasite and radiography of skeletal muscles to detect calcified cysts corroborate the diagnosis in some adults but are hardly ever useful in children. Stool examination for tapeworms, although indicative of taeniasis, is rarely helpful in the diagnosis of NCC. Peripheral eosinophilia is seen in about a third of cases.

Cerebrospinal fluid

CSF examination is not helpful in cases of parenchymal NCC, as it is usually normal. In patients with NCC meningitis, CSF may show mild elevation of protein, hypoglycorrhachia, and pleocytosis that may be lymphocytic, monocytic or polymorphonuclear. Other laboratory tests are usually normal in NCC.

Diagnostic criteria for neurocysticercosis incorporating clinical, radiological, immuno-logical and epidemiological data of patients have been proposed and revisited (Del Brutto 2012). However, they have not been validated in different parts of the world. The presenta-tion of NCC is pleomorphic, and it needs to be considered in the differential diagnosis of several neurological disorders, particularly seizures.

Differential diagnosis

In endemic countries, NCC is usually the first diagnosis considered in an otherwise healthy, afebrile child who presents with sudden-onset partial seizures. NCC is also considered in the differential diagnosis of children with headache, vomiting and other neurological symptoms and signs.

PARENCHYMAL NEUROCYSTICERCOSIS

If the scolex is clearly identified on neuroimaging, it is diagnostic of NCC; if not, the most important differential diagnosis of single small enhancing CT lesion includes a tuberculoma, particularly in countries where tuberculosis is endemic. Presence of raised ICP, progressive focal neurodeficit, size of CT lesion greater than 20mm, lobulated irregular shape, and marked oedema causing midline shift are some of the criteria in favour of a tuberculoma (Rajshekhar et al. 1993). The site of the lesion(s) may also be helpful, as tubercular lesions are usually seen at the base of the brain whereas NCC lesion(s) are often seen at the grey–white matter junction. In endemic countries, tuberculosis needs to be excluded in all cases by a good history, examination and other tests such as Mantoux test, and chest radiography. Sophisticated neuroimaging techniques are being investigated for use in cases where the scolex is not well seen and it is difficult to make the diagnosis of NCC with certainty. These include diffusion-weighted MRI, 3D constructive interference in steady state (CISS), and proton magnetic resonance spectroscopy (MRS). Presence of a lactate peak and choline/creatine ratio greater than 1 on MRS is suggestive of a tuberculoma (Pretell et al. 2005).

The other differential diagnoses of enhancing lesions include microabscess, toxoplas-mosis, fungal lesions, low-grade astrocytoma and cystic cerebral metastasis (Singhi and Baranwal 2001).

EXTRAPARENCHYMAL NEUROCYSTICERCOSIS

Meningitis and hydrocephalus due to NCC need to be differentiated from tubercular, fun-gal and other causes of chronic meningitis, and of acquired hydrocephalus. Fast imaging employing steady-state acquisition (FIESTA) and susceptibility-weighted angiography (SWAN) sequences have been reported to better delineate NCC in the CSF spaces (Neyaz et al. 2012).

Treatment

The management of a child with NCC involves (1) symptomatic/supportive therapy, and (2) definitive medical/surgical treatment for cysts.

Children with acute manifestations of NCC such as status epilepticus and raised ICP require urgent stabilization and appropriate management of the underlying problem.

Antiepileptic therapy
Seizures due to single-lesion NCC are usually well controlled with a single antiepileptic drug (AED), usually carbamazepine. The optimal duration of AED therapy is a matter of debate. Although the general practice has been to use AEDs for a 2 years seizure-free interval, shorter durations of AEDs may be sufficient. Seizure recurrence after AED therapy for 1 year versus 2 years seizure-free interval was not significantly different and correlated significantly with an abnormal CT (persistence or calcification of lesion) and an abnormal EEG at the time of AED withdrawal (Singhi et al. 2003b). Thus AEDs may be withdrawn after a 1 year seizure-free interval in cases where the lesion has disappeared and the EEG has normalized; longer durations may be needed for those with persistent or calcified lesions.

Corticosteroids
Oral corticosteroids are generally administered for a few days starting a day or two before anticysticercal therapy so as to reduce the perilesional oedema and prevent any adverse reactions that may occur due to the host inflammatory reaction. Usually oral prednisolone 1–2mg/kg is used; IV dexamethasone (0.1/mg/kg/d) is used in some cases, particularly when there are features of raised ICP. In children with numerous disseminated lesions and extensive cerebral oedema, steroids may be required for several weeks.

DEFINITIVE THERAPY

Cysticidal therapy
Both praziquantel and albendazole destroy viable cysts. However, their use in patients with enhancing lesions has been debated as these lesions are considered to represent degenerating cysts and spontaneous resolution occurs in some cases.

In a double-blind, placebo-controlled trial in 63 children with single-lesion NCC, the use of albendazole within 3 months of onset of seizures was associated with a significantly increased and faster disappearance of lesions after 1 month (41%) as compared to placebo (16%), and after 3 months (albendazole 65% vs placebo 38%) (Baranwal et al. 1998). These findings have been substantiated by other trials (Carpio et al. 2008, Thussu et al. 2008). Other studies did not find beneficial effect of albendazole therapy (Padma et al. 2004, Das et al. 2007), although there were some methodological issues.

Cysticidal drugs were found to improve seizure control in adults with epilepsy associated with vesicular lesions as well as with enhancing lesions (Garcia et al. 2004). Other studies have not found any significant improvement in seizure control (Das et al. 2007, Carpio et al. 2008).

A meta-analysis of studies between 1979 and 2005 found that cysticidal therapy was associated with a significantly higher rate of complete resolution of vesicular cystic lesions than in patients not receiving cysticidal therapy (44% vs 19%), and a trend toward increased resolution of enhancing lesions that became statistically significant when an outlier trial was excluded from the analysis (69% vs 55%). The risk for seizure recurrence was also lower after cysticidal therapy (Del Brutto et al. 2006). Another meta-analysis found rates of seizure remission and disappearance of lesions to be slightly better in children treated with albendazole as compared to controls (Mazumdar et al. 2007). A recent Cochrane review reported increased disappearance of lesions but no difference in seizure control with cysticidal therapy in adults with viable lesions. In children with nonviable lesions, seizure recurrence was lower with albendazole therapy (Abba et al. 2010). A recent meta-analysis concluded that anthelmintic treatment was associated with increased rates of both seizure control and resolution of lesions in patients with single lesions (Otte et al. 2013). Based on evidence, the American Academy of Neurology guidelines recommend the use of albendazole and corticosteroids for adults and children with parenchymal NCC, both to reduce the number of active lesions on neuroimaging and to reduce long-term seizure frequency (Baird et al. 2013).

Although the efficacy rates of praziquantel and albendazole are similar, albendazole is preferred as it is less expensive, better tolerated, and has better penetration into the subarachnoid space. Co-administration of steroids increases the bioavailability of albendazole but decreases that of praziquantel. Co-administration of phenytoin or carbamazepine does not affect the bioavailability of albendazole but decreases that of praziquantel. Albendazole is used in a dose of 15mg/kg/d in two or three divided doses, usually for 28 days (Garcia et al. 2002); shorter durations of 8–14 days have also been used. A 1 week albendazole therapy was found to be equally effective as 4 weeks therapy in children with one to three enhancing lesions (Singhi et al. 2003a). Side-effects of albendazole such as urticaria and rashes are extremely rare.

Praziquantel is used in a dose of 50mg/kg/d for a period of 15 days. A 1 day therapy (three 25mg/kg doses) was found to be as effective as 7 days treatment with albendazole (Pretell et al. 2000); however, it was not found to be effective for multiple lesions (Pretell et al. 2001). Side-effects of praziquantel include abdominal pain, dizziness, headache and allergic reactions but are uncommon.

A combination therapy of albendazole and praziquantel in children with single-lesion NCC was associated with a higher resolution of lesions as compared to albendazole alone, but the difference was not statistically significant (Kaur et al. 2009). Combined albendazole and praziquantel therapy is associated with increased albendazole sulphoxide plasma concentrations and may contribute to increased cysticidal efficacy (Garcia et al. 2011). Larger trials are needed to study the role of combination therapy in NCC.

Corticosteroids have also been found to be helpful in cyst resolution in some studies both in children and in adults (Singhi et al. 2004, Kishore and Misra 2007). However, larger trials are needed (Nash et al. 2011). A recent meta-analysis of 13 studies concluded that although corticosteroids can reduce the rate of seizure recurrence and hasten the resolution of lesions on neuroimaging, quantifying this effect remains problematic due to methodological issues (Cuello-García et al. 2013).

Cysticidal therapy should not be used in patients with markedly elevated ICP, nor in ophthalmic NCC, as the host inflammatory response may lead to worsening; steroids alone are recommended. Cysticidal therapy has no effect on calcified lesions. An individualized approach is recommended for the treatment of different types of NCC (Nash et al. 2006).

SURGICAL MANAGEMENT
Patients with obstructive hydrocephalus need endoscopic removal of cysts from the ventricles and shunt placement. Simultaneous administration of steroids and albendazole is recommended to reduce the rate of re-obstruction (Sinha and Sharma 2012).

Repeat CT is usually done after 3–6 months in all children on treatment to determine whether the lesions have resolved. In cases with persistent lesions, a repeat course of cysticidal therapy is usually given.

Prognosis

Single-lesion NCC, particularly a degenerating lesion, has a good prognosis: seizures are usually well controlled, and the lesion disappears within 6 months in more than 60% of cases. Recurrence of seizures in children with single lesions varies from 10% to 20% (Baranwal et al. 2001). Multiple cystic lesions and calcified lesions often have frequent seizure recurrences. A correlation between calcified NCC and hippocampal sclerosis is thought to exist in adults (Rathore et al. 2012). The prognosis is poorer in cysticercus encephalitis and extraparenchymal NCC.

Prevention

NCC can be prevented by ensuring proper hygiene and sanitation, and enforcing strict animal husbandry and meat-inspection procedures. Mass deworming of the population with niclosamide or praziquantel and mass vaccination of pigs with newer effective vaccines such as TSOL18, along with treatment of pigs with oxfendazole, have been recommended (Willingham et al. 2008). Community interventions have been found to reduce the rate of epilepsy in hyperendemic areas provided they are carried out properly (Medina et al. 2011).

Conclusion

Neurocysticercosis is the most common cause of acquired seizures in children in some areas. As neurocysticercosis may have variable neurological manifestations, it should be considered in the differential diagnosis of a number of neurological conditions. Treatment with cysticidal drugs is associated with increased and faster resolution of lesions and is usually well tolerated; however, it needs to be individualized. Children with single or few lesions have a good outcome, whereas those with multiple lesions often develop epilepsy. Public sanitation and hygiene are of utmost importance in prevention.

REFERENCES

Abba K, Ramaratnam S, Ranganathan LN (2010) Anthelmintics for people with neurocysticercosis. *Cochrane Database Syst Rev* 3: CD000215. doi: 10.1002/14651858.CD000215.pub4.
Alvarez JI, Rivera J, Teale JM (2008) Differential release and phagocytosis of tegument glycoconjugates in

neurocysticercosis: implications for immune evasion strategies. *PLoS Negl Trop Dis* 2: e218.

Baird RA, Wiebe S, Zunt JR, et al. (2013) Evidence-based guideline: treatment of parenchymal neurocys-ticercosis: report of the Guideline Development Subcommittee of the American Academy of Neurology. *Neurology* 80: 1424–9.

Baranwal AK, Singhi PD, Khandelwal N, Singhi SC (1998) Albendazole therapy in children with focal seizures and single small enhancing computerized tomographic lesions: a randomized, placebo-con-trolled, double blind trial. *Pediatr Infect Dis J* 17: 696–700.

Baranwal AK, Singhi P, Singhi S, Khandelwal N (2001) Seizure recurrence in children with focal seizures and single small enhancing computed tomographic lesions. Prognostic factors on long-term follow-up. *J Child Neurol* 16: 443–5.

Callacondo D, Garcia HH, Gonzales I, et al. (2012) High frequency of spinal involvement in patients with basal subarachnoid neurocysticercosis. *Neurology* 78: 1394–400.

Carabin H, Ndimubanzi PC, Budke CM, et al. (2011) Clinical manifestations associated with neurocysticer-cosis: a systematic review. *PLoS Negl Trop Dis* 5: e1152.

Carpio A, Kelvin EA, Bagiella E, et al. (2008) Effects of albendazole treatment on neurocysticercosis: a ran-domised controlled trial. *J Neurol Neurosurg Psychiatry* 79: 1050–5.

Cuello-García CA, Roldán-Benítez YM, Pérez-Gaxiola G, Villarreal-Careaga J (2013) Corticosteroids for neurocysticercosis: a systematic review and meta-analysis of randomized controlled trials. *Int J Infect Dis* 17: e583–92.

Das K, Mandal GP, Banerjee M, et al. (2007) Role of antiparasitic therapy for seizures and resolution of lesions in neurocysticercosis patients: an 8 year randomised study. *J Clin Neurosci* 14: 1172–7.

Del Brutto OH (2012) Diagnostic criteria for neurocysticercosis, revisited. *Pathog Glob Health* 106: 299–304.

Del Brutto OH (2013) Neurocysticercosis in infants and toddlers: report of seven cases and review of pub-lished patients. *Pediatr Neurol* 48: 432–5.

Del Brutto OH, Roos KL, Coffey CS, García HH (2006) Meta-analysis: cysticidal drugs for neurocysticer-cosis: albendazole and praziquantel. *Ann Intern Med* 145: 43–51.

Escobar A (1983) The pathology of neurocysticercosis. In: Palacios E, Rodriguez-Carbajal KJ, Taveras J, eds. *Cysticercosis of the Central Nervous System.* Springfield, IL: Charles C Thomas, pp. 27–54.

Esquivel-Velázquez M, Ostoa-Saloma P, Morales-Montor J, et al. (2011) Immunodiagnosis of neurocysticer-cosis: ways to focus on the challenge. *J Biomed Biotechnol* 2011: 516042. doi: 10.1155/2011/516042.

Fleury A, Gomez T, Alvarez I, et al. (2003) High prevalence of calcified silent neurocysticercosis in a rural village of Mexico. *Neuroepidemiology* 22: 139–45.

Gaffo AL, Guillén-Pinto D, Campos-Olazábal P, Burneo JG (2004) [Cysticercosis as the main cause of partial seizures in children in Peru.] *Rev Neurol* 39: 924–6.

Garcia HH, Evans CA, Nash TE, et al. (2002) Current consensus guidelines for treatment of neurocysticer-cosis. *Clin Microbiol Rev* 15: 747–56.

Garcia HH, Pretell EJ, Gilman RH, et al. (2004) A trial of antiparasitic treatment to reduce the rate of seizures due to cerebral cysticercosis. *N Engl J Med* 350: 249–58.

Garcia HH, Gonzalez AE, Rodriguez S, et al. (2010) Neurocysticercosis. Unraveling the nature of the single cysticercal granuloma. *Neurology* 75: 654–8.

Garcia HH, Lescano AG, Lanchote VL, et al. (2011) Pharmacokinetics of combined treatment with prazi-quantel and albendazole in neurocysticercosis. *Br J Clin Pharmacol* 72: 77–84.

Goel D, Dhanai JS, Agarwal A, et al. (2011) Neurocysticercosis and its impact on crude prevalence rate of epilepsy in an Indian community. *Neurol India* 59: 37–40.

Karnik PS, Tullu MS, David JJ, Ghildiyal RG (2011) Neurocysticercosis-induced hemiballismus in a child. *J Child Neurol* 26: 904–6. doi: 10.1177/0883073810393966.

Kashyap B, Das S, Jain S, et al. (2011) Correlation between the clinico radiological heterogeneity and the immune-inflammatory profiles in pediatric patients with neurocysticercosis from a tertiary referral centre. *J Trop Pediatr* 58: 320–3.

Kaur S, Singhi P, Singhi S, Khandelwal N (2009) Combination therapy of praziquantel and albandazole ver-sus albandazole alone in children with single lesion NCC—a randomized placebo controlled double blind trial. *Ped Infect Dis J* 28: 403–6.

Kishore D, Misra S (2007) Short course of oral prednisolone on disappearance of lesion and seizure recur-rence in patients of solitary cysticercal granuloma with single small enhancing CT lesion: an open label randomized prospective study. *J Assoc Physicians India* 55: 419–24.

Mandal J, Singhi PD, Khandelwal N, Malla N (2006) Evaluation of ELISA and dot blots for the serodiagnosis of neurocysticercosis, in children found to have single or multiple enhancing lesions in computerized tomographic scans of the brain. *Ann Trop Med Parasitol* 100: 39–48.

Marquez JM, Arauz A (2012) Cerebrovascular complications of neurocysticercosis. *Neurologist* 18: 17–22.

Mazumdar M, Pandharipande P, Poduri A (2007) Does albendazole affect seizure remission and computed tomography response in children with neurocysticercosis? A systematic review and meta-analysis. *J Child Neurol* 22: 135–42.

Medina MT, Aguilar-Estrada RL, Alvarez A, et al. (2011) Reduction in rate of epilepsy from neurocysticercosis by community interventions: the Salamá, Honduras study. *Epilepsia* 52: 1177–85.

Nash T (2012) Edema surrounding calcified intracranial cysticerci: clinical manifestations, natural history and treatment. *Pathog Glob Health* 106: 275–9.

Nash TE, Singh G, White AC, et al. (2006) Treatment of neurocysticercosis: current status and future research needs. *Neurology* 67: 1120–7.

Nash TE, Del Brutto OH, Butman JA, et al. (2004) Calcific neurocysticercosis and epileptogenesis. *Neurology* 62: 1934–8.

Nash TE, Mahanty S, Garcia HH; Cysticercosis Group in Peru (2011) Corticosteroid use in neurocysticercosis. *Expert Rev Neurother* 118: 1175–83.

Ndimubanzi PC, Carabin H, Budke CM, et al. (2010) A systematic review of the frequency of neurocysticercosis with a focus on people with epilepsy. *PLoS Negl Trop Dis* 411: e870.

Neyaz Z, Patwari SS, Paliwal VK (2012) Role of FIESTA and SWAN sequences in diagnosis of intraventricular neurocysticercosis. *Neurol India* 60: 646–7.

O'Neal S, Noh J, Wilkins P, et al. (2011) *Taenia solium* tapeworm infection, Oregon, 2006–2009. *Emerg Infect Dis* 17: 1030–6.

Otte WM, Singla M, Sander JW, Singh G (2013) Drug therapy for solitary cysticercus granuloma: a systematic review and meta-analysis. *Neurology* 80: 152–62.

Padma MV, Behari M, Misra NK, Ahuja N (1994) Albendazole in single CT ring lesions in epilepsy. *Neurology* 44: 1344–6.

Prasad KN, Verma A, Srivastava S, et al. (2011) An epidemiological study of asymptomatic neurocysticercosis in a pig farming community in northern India. *Trans R Soc Trop Med Hyg* 105: 531–6.

Pretell EJ, Garcia HH, Custodio N, et al. (2000) Short regimen of praziquantel in the treatment of single brain enhancing lesions. *Clin Neurol Neurosurg* 102: 215–8.

Pretell EJ, Garcia HH, Gilman RH, et al. (2001) Failure of one-day praziquantel treatment in patients with multiple neurocysticercosis lesions. *Clin Neurol Neurosurg* 103: 175–7.

Pretell EJ, Martinot C Jr, Garcia HH, et al. (2005) Differential diagnosis between cerebral tuberculosis and neurocysticercosis by magnetic resonance spectroscopy. *J Comput Assist Tomogr* 29: 112–4.

Proaño-Narvaez JV, Meza-Lucas A, Mata-Ruiz O, et al. (2002) Laboratory diagnosis of human neurocysticercosis: double-blind comparison of enzyme-linked immunosorbent assay and electroimmunotransfer blot assay. *J Clin Microbiol* 40: 2115–8.

Raina SK, Razdan S, Pandita KK, et al. (2012) Active epilepsy as indicator of neurocysticercosis in rural northwest India. *Epilepsy Res Treat* 2012: 802747. doi: 10.1590/s0004-282x2011000200004.

Rajshekhar V, Haran RP, Prakash S, Chandy MJ (1993) Differentiating solitary small cysticercus granulomas and tuberculomas in patients with epilepsy—clinical and computerized tomographic criteria. *J Neurosurg* 78: 402–7.

Rathore C, Thomas B, Kesavadas C, Radhakrishnan K (2012) Calcified neurocysticercosis and hippocampal sclerosis: potential dual pathology? *Epilepsia* 53: e60–2.

Sahu PS, Parija SC, Narayan SK, Kumar D (2009) Evaluation of an IgG-ELISA strategy using *Taenia solium* metacestode somatic and excretory-secretory antigens for diagnosis of neurocysticercosis revealing biological stage of the larvae. Acta Trop 110: 38–45.

Serpa JA, White AC Jr (2012) Neurocysticercosis in the United States. *Pathog Glob Health* 106: 256–60. doi: 10.1179/2047773212Y.0000000028.

Singhi P, Singhi S (2004) Neurocysticercosis in children. *J Child Neurol* 19: 482–92.

Singhi P, Ray M, Singhi S, Khandelwal N (2000) Clinical spectrum of 500 children with neurocysticercosis and response to albendazole therapy. *J Child Neurol* 15: 207–13.

Singhi P, Devi Dayal, Khandelwal N (2003a) One week versus four weeks of albendazole therapy for neurocysticercosis in children: a randomized placebo controlled double blind trial. *Pediatr Infect Dis J* 22: 268–72.

Singhi P, Dinakaran, Khandelwal NK (2003b) One year versus two years of antiepileptic therapy for SSECTL. *J Trop Pediatr* 5: 274–8.

Singhi P, Jain V, Khandelwal N (2004) Corticosteroids versus albendazole for treatment of single small enhancing CT lesions in children with NCC. *J Child Neurol* 19: 323–7.

Singhi P, Mahajan V, Khandelwal N (2008) Sudden-onset ptosis caused by midbrain neurocysticercosis in two children. *J Child Neurol* 23: 334–7.

Singhi PD, Baranwal AK (2001) Single small enhancing computed tomographic lesion in Indian children— I: Evolution of current concepts. *J Trop Pediatr* 47: 204–7.

Sinha S, Sharma BS (2012) Intraventricular neurocysticercosis: a review of current status and management issues. *Br J Neurosurg* 26: 305–9.

Thussu A, Chattopadhyay A, Sawhney IM, Khandelwal N (2008) Albendazole therapy for single small enhancing CT lesions (SSECTL) in the brain in epilepsy. *J Neurol Neurosurg Psychiatry* 79: 238–9.

Tsang VC, Brand JA, Boyer AE (1989) An enzyme-linked immunoelectro-transfer blot assay and glycoprotein antigens for diagnosing human cysticercosis (*Taenia solium*). *J Infect Dis* 159: 50–9.

Verma A, Prasad KN, Gupta RK, et al. (2010) Toll-like receptor 4 polymorphism and its association with symptomatic neurocysticercosis. *J Infect Dis* 202: 1219–25.

Villarán MV, Montano SM, Gonzalvez G, et al. (2009) Epilepsy and neurocysticercosis: an incidence study in a Peruvian rural population. *Neuroepidemiology* 33: 25–31.

WHO (2003) Control of neurocysticercosis. Report by the Secretariat, Fifty-sixth World Health Assembly. Document A56/10. Geneva: World Health Organization (online: http://apps.who.int/iris/bitstream/ 10665/78210/1/ea5610.pdf?ua=1).

Willingham AL 3rd, Harrison LJ, Fèvre EM, et al. (2008) Inaugural meeting of the Cysticercosis Working Group in Europe. *Emerg Infect Dis* 14: e2.

Winkler AS (2012) Neurocysticercosis in sub-Saharan Africa: a review of prevalence, clinical characteristics, diagnosis, and management. *Pathog Glob Health* 106: 261–74.

18
SPIROCHAETAL INFECTIONS

Charles R Newton

Spirochaetes are a group of gram-negative bacteria characterized by elongated and spiral-shaped organisms, measuring 5–250µm with flagellae running lengthwise. They belong to a single order, Spirochaetales, which includes pathogenic *Borrelia* and *Leptospira* species and *Treponema pallidum*. This chapter discusses borreliosis and leptospirosis; syphilis is covered in the chapter on congenital infections.

Neuroborreliosis

Lyme disease (borreliosis) is caused by *Borrelia* species, which are transmitted by *Ixodes* species ticks that are distributed through North America, Europe and Asia. Mammals such as deer act as the main reservoirs (Pachner and Steiner 2007).

Neuroborreliosis is the second most common complication of *Borrelia* spp. infection in Europe after cutaneous involvement, while in North America cutaneous and joint involvement are more common (Pachner and Steiner 2007). Neuroborreliosis is caused by *B. afzelii*, *B. garinii* and *B. burgdorferi* sensu stricto in Europe, but predominantly by *B. burgdorferi* sensu stricto in North America. In Europe, the isolation of *B. garinii* from cerebrospinal fluid (CSF) is reported in adults with radiculitis (painful radiculitis or meningoradiculoneuritis), whereas infections with *B. afzelii* have less specific symptoms such as dizziness or memory disturbances.

PATHOGENESIS

Borrelia spp. enter humans through the skin during tick bites, during which they may cause erythema migrans. They spread through the blood to the peripheral and central nervous system (CNS) and other organs. The *Borrelia* spirochaetes evade the human immune system in the blood and other parts of the body by reducing immunogenic surface proteins, active immune suppression by downregulating the human immune response and neutralizing its effector mechanisms, and invading the extracellular matrix with the help of flagella and proteins, thus hiding from leukocytes (Rupprecht et al. 2008). Outer surface protein A (OspA) is a key molecule for evading detection in the tick and humans.

The spirochaetes probably adhere to endothelium with upregulation of endothelial proteins, but it is unclear how they cross the blood–brain barrier: either through or between the endothelial cells. They may also be transported by peripheral nerves and possibly the lymph system. In the brain and peripheral nerves, the spirochaetes are detected by local immune cells, but escape destruction by immune modulation (Rupprecht et al. 2008).

The neurological complications arise from direct cytotoxicity, neurotoxic mediators and/or autoimmune reactions. The spirochaetes adhere to neuronal and glial cells causing necrosis, and OspA induces apoptosis of these cells. The *Borrelia* spp. induce production of nitric oxid, quinolinic acid, interleukin-6 and tumour necrosis factor, all of which are toxic to neurons. Antibodies to the flagellum of the spirochaetes may also damage neuronal cells through complement-mediated membrane attack complex deposits and macrophage infiltrates.

CLINICAL FEATURES

The clinical features of neuroborreliosis depend upon age, region, endemicity and species (Pachner and Steiner 2007). Facial nerve palsy and subacute aseptic meningitis are the most common neurological manifestations in children. Other manifestations include other cranial nerve palsies, ocular involvement, benign intracranial hypertension, cerebellar ataxia, hemiparesis, acute transverse myelitis, and painful radiculitis (Garin-Bujadoux–Bannwarth syndrome) (Tuerlinckx and Glupczynski 2010).

Facial nerve palsy

Borreliosis is the most common cause of facial nerve palsy in endemic areas, accounting for 33%–65% of all cases. Facial nerve palsy is more frequent in Europe than in North America or endemic areas (Tuerlinckx and Glupczynski 2010). It is most common in children aged 4–9 years, with a higher incidence in summer and autumn. Facial nerve palsy is often associated with anorexia, fatigue, headache and meningism. CSF abnormalities (pleiocytosis, elevated protein concentration and/or intrathecal production of antibodies) are found in 68%–99% of children with facial nerve palsy, even in the absence of other clinical signs. Lumbar puncture is not indicated in all cases of facial nerve palsy but should be considered in any child with severe or prolonged headache, or signs of meningism.

Radiculitis

Radiculitis presents with a lancinating pain that radiates down a dermatomal distribution. It may be associated with symmetrical or asymmetrical sensory abnormalities, such as numbness or tingling, and motor weakness. Lyme meningoradiculoneuritis (Garin-Bujadoux–Bannwarth syndrome) includes painful asymmetrical sensory and motor dysfunctions and lymphocytes in the CSF.

Meningitis

Borrelia meninigitis is less frequent in children than in adults. In up to 40% of patients it is preceded by erythema migrans, which presents about 2–10 weeks before the onset of meningitic symptoms. Headaches are the most common feature; neck stiffness and photophobia are less common. Systemic symptoms, e.g. fever, myalgia and arthralgia, occur in a third. Asymptomatic pleocytosis is common. The meningitic symptoms usually last 1–2 months but can persist for up to a year, and patients can have recurrent episodes.

The main differential diagnosis is that of viral meningitis or aseptic meningitis. *Borrelia* meningitis is suggested by a long duration of symptoms, cranial nerve palsy (particularly facial nerve palsy), a low percentage of CSF neutrophils or a high percentage of CSF mononuclear cells. A diagnosis is unlikely if the proportion of CSF neutrophils is greater than 10% (negative predictive value: 99%–100%) (Avery et al. 2006). A 'rule of 7s' has been suggested – i.e. headache lasting less than 7 days, no VIIth nerve palsy and less than 70% of mononuclear cells in the CSF – to exclude *Borrelia* meningitis. Other authors have suggested adding low CSF protein levels to increase specificity (Tuerlinckx and Glupczynski 2010).

DIAGNOSIS

The diagnosis of neuroborreliosis is usually based on a characteristic clinical picture, exposure to ticks in an endemic area, and a positive antibody response to *B. burgdorferi*. In North America, an enzyme-linked immunosorbent assay (ELISA) is performed, and those with equivocal or positive results are then tested with a Western blot (Aguero-Rosenfeld et al. 2005). In Europe, because strains causing borreliosis are more heterogeneous, the European Society of Clinical Microbiology and Infectious Diseases study group recommends a two-step test procedure with the detection of intrathecal antibodies being the mainstay of laboratory diagnosis. Specific intrathecal antibodies were found in over 70% of children (Christen et al. 1993), although the sensitivity of intrathecal anti-*Borrelia* antibodies is lower in children presenting with a short duration of symptoms at the time of the lumbar puncture. In one study of 146 children with a definite diagnosis of borreliosis, the authors reported a positive antibody index in 80% of children with symptoms lasting for 7 days or longer, versus 51% of children with symptoms for up to 7 days (Tveitnes et al. 2009). Other tests such as the C6 ELISA may be more specific, since C6 is a synthetic peptide based on a conserved immunodominant peptide across all species (Steere et al. 2008). The sensitivity and specificity of the C6 ELISA test were 100% and 96% compared with 100% and 99%, respectively, for the two-step approach in patients with disseminated infection (Steere et al. 2008). The diagnostic sensitivity of polymerase chain reaction (PCR) or culture of *Borrelia* in the CSF is low (10%–50%), higher in those with a short duration of illness (Pachner and Steiner 2007).

TREATMENT

For facial nerve palsy, older children can be treated with oral doxycycline (2mg/kg twice daily, maximum 200–400mg/dose) without the need of a lumbar puncture. Younger children (<8 years) should be given either oral ampicillin (25mg/kg three times a day, max. 500mg/dose) or cefuroxime (15mg/kg twice a day, max. 500mg/dose). Treatment should last for 14 days.

In meningitis and radiculitis, IV ceftriaxone (50–75mg/kg/d every 24 hours, max 2g) is the drug of choice, but cefotaxime (50mg/kg every 6–8 hours, max. 6g/d) or benzyl penicillin (50 000U/kg every 4 hours) can be used. Some authorities have suggested that these complications can be treated with oral doxycycline (2mg/kg twice a day, max. 200–400mg/dose) in children aged over 8 years. Treatment should be for at least 14 days and may be continued to 28 days.

OUTCOME

The clinical outcome of neuroborreliosis is more favourable in children than in adults. In a Swedish study, 73% of children appeared to recover fully (Berglund et al. 2002). Persistent facial nerve palsy occurred in 13%, while other motor or sensory deficits were found in another 14%. There was little effect on daily activities or school performance. Long-term neuropsychological disorders appear to be very uncommon in children recovering from neuroborreliosis (Tuerlinckx and Glupczynski 2010).

PREVENTION

Borreliosis is prevented by avoiding tick bites. This includes not entering endemic areas, particularly during summer months, wearing protective clothing (long trousers and shirts), using insect repellents, e.g. DEET (N,N-diethyl-meta-toluamide), and removing ticks as soon as possible.

Leptospirosis

Leptospirosis is found throughout the world, but the greatest burden is in Africa, the western Pacific, Americas and southeast Asia. It is most common in tropical and rural areas, and epidemics occur after flooding (Hartskeerl et al. 2011). In resource-rich countries, it is often associated with swimming in contaminated water.

The spirochaete, *Leptospira interrogans*, is the pathogenic form in humans. This species consists of 23 serogroups, which contain over 200 serovars (serotypes) (Palaniappan et al. 2007). Three serogroups – *canicola*, *icterohaemorrhagiae* and *pomona* – are associated with CNS complications. Most infections are transmitted via the urine of animals, most commonly rats, cats, dogs, pigs and cattle. Thus it is more common in rural than in urban areas. Contaminated water is the primary source of the infection. The spirochaetes invade the body through cuts and the mucosa of the nose, mouth and eyes. The incubation period is 1–2 weeks, after which there is an initial leptospiraemic phase lasting 3–7 days followed by an immune-mediated phase lasting 1–4 weeks.

In the central and peripheral nervous system, there is endothelial damage and vasculitis. There are exudates, and meningeal congestion of the brain and spinal cord, with haemorrhages and oedema. Microscopically, there is perivascular infiltration of small and medium-sized blood vessels, and patchy demyelination.

CLINICAL FEATURES

Most cases are asymptomatic. In children it typically presents as a febrile illness with nausea, vomiting, myalgia, headache, bleeding (particularly epistaxis) and confusion. On examination there is often conjunctival injection, jaundice and hepatomegaly. Respiratory difficulty may be caused by pulmonary or cardiac complications, which are associated with a high mortality.

The CNS involvement includes a wide range of manifestations. Although 50%–90% of patients may have CSF pleocytosis, only half of these patients are symptomatic. CNS manifestations may occur without the features of the typical febrile illness (Panicker et al. 2001),

TABLE 18.1
Differential diagnosis in leptospirosis

Central nervous system	Peripheral nervous system
Aseptic meningitis	Polyradiculitis including Guillain–Barré syndrome
Encephalitis	Mononeuritis and neuralgias; facial palsy
Cerebellitis	Autonomic lability
Intracranial haemorrhage	Polymyositis
Stroke	
Movement disorder	
Myelitis	

and thus leptospirosis should be considered in the differential diagnosis of the neurological syndromes listed in Table 18.1.

The most common manifestation is aseptic meningitis. During the leptospiraemic phase, signs of meningeal irritation are uncommon, but leptospirae can be isolated from the CSF. The immune phase is characterized by headache, vomiting and meningeal irritation. The meninges are most commonly affected, and there is evidence of parenchymal involvement, giving rise to a meningoencephalitis. The opening CSF pressure may be raised, with a lymphocytic pleocytosis, increased protein and normal glucose.

Stroke secondary to vasculitis is rarely seen in children, but cerebral haemorrhage may occur. Leptospirosis may also cause an acute disseminated encephalomyelitis as part of the immune-mediated stage (Lelis et al. 2009). Facial nerve palsy, unilateral or bilateral, is also described.

DIAGNOSIS

Diagnosis is confirmed by serological tests. The microscopic agglutination test (MAT) is considered the criterion standard test, but only detects the antibodies 5–7 days after the infection (Toyokawa et al. 2011). The sensitivity and specificity of MAT are 92% and 95% respectively; other serological tests are not as sensitive. The organism can be isolated from urine, but culture is labour intensive, takes days to weeks to grow, and thus is often insensitive. PCR-based techniques have been developed but the commonly used 16S rRNA gene sequence is not sufficiently polymorphic for accurate identification of the serovars. Newer molecular techniques are being developed but are not in use for the clinical diagnosis.

There are no pathognomonic features on neuroimaging. Cerebral oedema may be seen in the acute stages, and demyelination during the second phase (Panicker et al. 2001, Mathew et al. 2006).

TREATMENT

Treatment is controversial, since there is little evidence that antibiotics influence the outcome (Brett-Major and Coldren 2012). Benzyl penicillin (25 000–50 000U/kg/d IV or IM, divided into 6-hourly doses) or ampicillin (100–400mg/kg/d IV or IM divided into 6-hourly doses) may reduce the duration of the illness if administered during the first 4 days of illness.

However, it does influence the immune-mediated phase. Tetracyclines have been used (load with 4.4mg/kg/d orally or IV, divided into 12-hourly doses, then 2.2–4.4mg/kg/d orally or IV given daily or divided into twice-daily doses for 7 days). Corticosteroids (methylpred-nisolone 30mg/kg/d or dexamethasone) may reduce the duration and severity of illness, but randomized clinical trials have not been conducted.

OUTCOME

Prognosis depends on the clinical manifestations: impaired consciousness and seizures are associated with worse outcome. Meningitis usually resolves by 3–6 weeks, although chronic meningitis may develop. Encephalomyelitis has a high mortality (up to 25%), but if the patient survives, it will resolve over a few months. Mononeuritis resolves within 2 months and polyradiculitis within 8 weeks. There appear to be few neurological sequelae, except deafness and uveitis, although detailed studies have not been conducted.

PREVENTION

Leptospirosis is prevented in children by not allowing them to have contact with contaminated water. This is often difficult in poor areas, but rat-infested areas should be avoided.

REFERENCES

Aguero-Rosenfeld ME, Wang G, Schwartz I, Wormser GP (2005) Diagnosis of lyme borreliosis. *Clin Microbiol Rev* 18: 484–509.
Avery RA, Frank G, Glutting J, Eppes SC (2006) Prediction of Lyme meningitis in children from a Lyme disease-endemic region: a logistic-regression model using history, physical, and laboratory findings. *Pediatrics* 117: e1–e7.
Berglund J, Stjernberg L, Ornstein K, et al. (2002) 5-y follow-up study of patients with neuroborreliosis. *Scand J Infect Dis* 34: 421–5.
Brett-Major DM, Coldren R (2012) Antibiotics for leptospirosis. *Cochrane Database Syst Rev* (2): CD008264.
Christen HJ, Hanefeld F, Eiffert H, Thomssen R (1993) Epidemiology and clinical manifestations of Lyme borreliosis in childhood. A prospective multicentre study with special regard to neuroborreliosis. *Acta Paediatr Suppl* 386: 1–75.
Hartskeerl RA, Collares-Pereira M, Ellis WA (2011) Emergence, control and re-emerging leptospirosis: dynamics of infection in the changing world. *Clin Microbiol Infect* 17: 494–501.
Lelis SS, Fonseca LF, Xavier CC, et al. (2009) Acute disseminated encephalomyelitis after leptospirosis. *Pediatr Neurol* 40: 471–3.
Mathew T, Satishchandra P, Mahadevan A, et al. (2006) Neuroleptospirosis – revisited: experience from a tertiary care neurological centre from south India. *Indian J Med Res* 124: 155–62.
Pachner AR, Steiner I (2007) Lyme neuroborreliosis: infection, immunity, and inflammation. *Lancet Neurol* 6: 544–52.
Palaniappan RU, Ramanujam S, Chang YF (2007) Leptospirosis: pathogenesis, immunity, and diagnosis. *Curr Opin Infect Dis* 20: 284–92.
Panicker JN, Mammachan R, Jayakumar RV (2001) Primary neuroleptospirosis. *Postgrad Med J* 77: 589–90.
Rupprecht TA, Koedel U, Fingerle V, Pfister HW (2008) The pathogenesis of Lyme neuroborreliosis: from infection to inflammation. *Mol Med* 14: 205–12.
Steere AC, McHugh G, Damle N, Sikand VK (2008) Prospective study of serologic tests for Lyme disease. *Clin Infect Dis* 47: 188–95.
Toyokawa T, Ohnishi M, Koizumi N (2011) Diagnosis of acute leptospirosis. *Expert Rev Anti Infect Ther* 9: 111–21.
Tuerlinckx D, Glupczynski Y (2010) Lyme neuroborreliosis in children. *Expert Rev Anti Infect Ther* 8: 455–63.
Tveitnes D, Oymar K, Natas O (2009) Laboratory data in children with Lyme neuroborreliosis, relation to clinical presentation and duration of symptoms. *Scand J Infect Dis* 41: 355–62.

19
MYCOPLASMAL INFECTIONS

Ari Bitnun and Susan E Richardson

Mycoplasma spp. and *Ureaplasma* spp. are members of the class *Mollicutes*, the smallest self-replicating prokaryotic organisms capable of cell-free existence (Waites and Talkington 2004). More than 200 species have been identified, of which approximately 15 have been associated with human mucous membrane colonization, and three, *M. pneumoniae*, *M. hominis* and *U. urealyticum/U. parvum*, have been associated with central nervous system (CNS) disease in otherwise healthy individuals. Rare cases of CNS disease attributable to other *Mycoplasma* species have been reported, primarily in immunocompromised children.

Mycoplasmas are primarily extracellular pathogens that adhere closely to epithelial cells of the respiratory or genitourinary tract. A highly specialized organelle that contains a network of adhesin proteins (P1, P30, P40, P90, HMW1, HMW2 and HMW3) mediates adherence (Atkinson et al. 2008). Owing to the lack of a cell wall, they are pleomorphic in shape and cannot be classified as either cocci or bacilli, are highly susceptible to adverse environmental conditions such as heat or drying, and are resistant to β-lactam and glycopeptide antibiotics. They lack the ability to synthesize peptidoglycan, are dependent on host-cell nutrients for their survival, and are fastidious to grow in artificial media.

Mycoplasma pneumoniae

EPIDEMIOLOGY
M. pneumoniae is primarily a respiratory-tract pathogen that can infect both the upper and lower respiratory tracts. It is a leading cause of community-acquired pneumonia, accounting for approximately 10% of cases in children less than 5 years of age, 20%–40% in children 5–15 years of age, and almost 50% in college students and military recruits. Epidemics occur every 3–7 years superimposed on a low-level, constant, endemicity.

CNS complications develop in up to 0.1% of individuals with *M. pneumoniae* infection (Tsiodras et al. 2005). However, among patients hospitalized with serologically confirmed *M. pneumoniae* infection, the prevalence of such complications may be as high as 10% (Ponka 1980). Clusters of cases with neurological complications have been observed during epidemics of respiratory disease due to *M. pneumoniae* (Walter et al. 2008).

Young children are disproportionately more affected. Among 560 patients hospitalized with serologically confirmed *M. pneumoniae* infections from several centres in Finland, 15 of 27 with neurological complications were under 10 years old (Ponka 1980). Children account for approximately 70% of patients with *M. pneumoniae* CNS disease in whom the organism is detected in brain tissue or cerebrospinal fluid (CSF) by culture, polymerase chain reaction (PCR) or other direct detection techniques (Bitnun and Richardson 2010). *M. pneumoniae* is one of the leading identifiable causes of acute encephalitis among children in North America and Europe, contributing to 5%–13% of cases (Koskiniemi et al. 1991, Bitnun et al. 2001, Christie et al. 2007a). A prevalence of 7% was observed in Canadian children using more stringent microbiological criteria for *M. pneumoniae* infection (Bitnun et al. 2001).

PATHOGENESIS

M. pneumoniae-induced neurological disease has been linked with three broad pathophysiological mechanisms: (1) direct infection with local tissue injury related to either the organism itself or the immune response to it; (2) autoimmunity; and (3) vascular occlusion (Atkinson et al. 2008, Waites et al. 2008, Narita 2009).

Direct infection of the brain parenchyma has been demonstrated in three fatal encephalitis cases involving generally healthy adults whose neurological symptoms were preceded by a respiratory illness. In these three cases the diagnosis was based on isolation of *M. pneumoniae* in culture from brain tissue, detection of *M. pneumoniae* by nucleic acid hybridization in temporobasal brain tissue, or demonstration of *Mycoplasma* antigens within macrophages in perivascular infiltrates in the cerebral hemispheres, medulla oblongata and spinal cord (Bitnun and Richardson 2010). Polyclonal antimycoplasmal antibody has been detected in multiple cell types within the brain parenchyma in a child with encephalitis (Powers and Johnson 2012). *M. pneumoniae* has also been cultured from or detected by PCR in the CSF of approximately 50 patients, 70% of whom were children, and 80% of whom had meningitis, meningoencephalitis or encephalitis (Bitnun and Richardson 2010). The pathophysiological mechanisms of CNS injury following direct infection of the brain parenchyma are largely unknown. Elevated CSF levels of intrathecally produced interleukins IL-6 and IL-8, but not interferon-γ, tumour necrosis factor alpha (TNF-α), transforming growth factor-β1 or IL-18, suggest a prominent pathophysiological role for cytokines that differs from that seen with bacterial or viral meningitis, in which interferon-γ and TNF-α are elevated (Narita 2009). Replication of organism within the CNS and production of injurious metabolic by-products such as hydrogen peroxide, superoxide radicals and highly reactive hydroxyl radicals has also been implicated.

The type and extent of the host immune response appears to influence the risk of systemic dissemination (Narita 2009). The risk of disseminated disease due to *Mycoplasma* is elevated in patients with hypogammaglobulinaemia. A robust immune response appears to result in more severe respiratory illness, but a lower risk of extrapulmonary dissemination (Waites and Talkington 2004).

Antigenic mimicry is thought to play a central role in the pathogenesis of *M. pneumoniae*-associated 'postinfectious' neurological syndromes such as acute disseminated encephalomyelitis (ADEM), transverse myelitis and Guillain–Barré syndrome (Waites and Talkington 2004, Atkinson et al. 2008, Narita 2009). The specific *M. pneumoniae* epitopes and human brain-tissue antigens involved in autoimmunity remain largely unknown. Antiganglioside antibodies have been demonstrated in sera of patients with *M. pneumoniae*-associated postinfectious encephalitis, Bickerstaff brainstem encephalitis and Guillain–Barré syndrome, and glycolipid epitopes of *M. pneumoniae* have been shown to cross-react with brain tissue as well as several gangliosides (Narita 2009, Bitnun and Richardson 2010). However, such autoantibodies have also been detected in the sera in approximately 25%–50% of individuals with *M. pneumoniae* infections restricted to the respiratory tract and in 3%–5% of healthy controls (Nishimura et al. 1996, Ang et al. 2002). In another study, 50% of patients with *M. pneumoniae*-associated encephalitis and neuro-imaging evidence of demyelination had antiganglioside antibodies in the CSF (Christie et al. 2007b). This observation is consistent with the hypothesis that neuronal injury may only occur if antiganglioside antibodies can traverse the blood–brain barrier or be synthesized intrathecally.

Stroke secondary to occlusion of major cerebral arteries or their tributaries is described in association with *M. pneumoniae* infection in both children and adults who had a respiratory illness preceding it by 3–21 days (mean 10.5 days) (Narita 2009, Bitnun and Richardson 2010). In some cases a procoagulable state is implicated, and in others, a cytokine-mediated systemic or focal vasculitic process. Biopsy-proven cutaneous leukocytoclastic vasculitis with multiple periventricular T2-weighed hyperintense lesions on MRI and angiographic evidence of focal cerebral vasculitis have been demonstrated in stroke victims with serologically confirmed *M. pneumoniae* infection (Perez and Montes 2002).

CLINICAL MANIFESTATIONS

Neurological complications associated with *M. pneumoniae* infection include meningitis, encephalitis, ADEM, postinfectious haemorrhagic leukoencephalitis (Hurst disease), acute bilateral striatal necrosis, Bickerstaff brainstem encephalitis, transverse myelitis, Guillain–Barré syndrome, polyradiculitis, opsoclonus–myoclonus syndrome and stroke (Waites and Talkington 2004, Winchell et al. 2008, Powers and Johnson 2012). A summary of selected salient clinical manifestations and investigative features of *M. pneumoniae*-associated neurological syndromes is provided in Table 19.1.

A respiratory prodrome occurs in the majority of older children and adults with *M. pneumoniae* neurological disease. In children under 5 years of age, respiratory symptoms may be absent or extremely mild (Bitnun and Richardson 2010). A short interval of 7 days or less between the respiratory symptoms and onset of neurological symptoms is common in disease entities attributable to direct invasion of the CNS, such as meningitis or acute encephalitis. Detection of the organism by PCR or culture in blood, CSF or brain tissue is typical of such patients. An interval of 1–3 weeks or longer is characteristic of postinfectious immune-mediated disorders such as ADEM, transverse myelitis and Guillain–Barré syndrome. In these patients, the organism is only rarely detected in CSF or brain tissue, but can often be demonstrated in respiratory tract samples (Narita 2009, Bitnun and Richardson 2010).

TABLE 19.1

Selected clinical and investigative findings in *M. pneumoniae*-associated clinical neurological syndromes

Clinical neurological entity	Proposed pathogenesis	Selected clinical and investigative findings
Meningitis	Direct infection	• More common in adults; benign clinical course • Onset usually within 7 days of respiratory symptom onset • Lymphocytic pleocytosis (usually <200 cells/μL) • *M. pneumoniae* may be detected in the CSF by PCR
Acute encephalitis	Direct infection or immune-mediated	• More common in children; common manifestations include encephalopathy, fever, focal or generalized seizures, ataxia; neurological sequelae in 40%–60% of patients • Detection of organism in CSF or blood usually associated with neurological symptom onset within 7 days of respiratory symptom onset (or in absence of such symptoms); detection of organism in the respiratory tract, but not in the CSF or blood, usually associated with a respiratory prodrome of more than 7 days • Lymphocytic pleocytosis (usually <200 cells/μL), mildly elevated CSF protein • MRI: normal or non-specific abnormalities such as brain oedema, inflammatory lesions • *M. pneumoniae* may be detected in the CSF by PCR
Acute disseminated encephalomyelitis	Immune-mediated	• Polysymptomatic with encephalopathy, focal neurological deficits; neurological sequelae observed in 40%–60% of patients • Onset usually 1–4 weeks after respiratory illness • Elevated CSF protein; lymphocytic pleocytosis (usually <200 cells/μL) • Antigalactocerebroside antibody may be present in blood or CSF • MRI: focal or multifocal lesions predominantly in white matter (hyerintense on FLAIR/T2-weighted sequences; Fig. 19.1) • *M. pneumoniae* often detected in respiratory tract, only rarely in CSF
Acute haemorrhagic leukoencephalitis (Hurst disease)	Immune-mediated	• Sudden onset of fever, encephalopathy, seizures and focal neurological signs; rapidly progressive, high mortality • Onset usually within 3 weeks of respiratory symptom onset • Pleocytosis, elevated CSF red blood cells • MRI: large bihemispheric areas of demyelination; petechial haemorrhages on T2-weighted images

TABLE 19.1
[continued]

Clinical neurological entity	Proposed pathogenesis	Selected clinical and investigative findings
Bickerstaff brainstem encephalitis	Immune-mediated	• External ophthalmoplegia, ataxia, impaired consciousness; full recovery occurs in the majority of cases • Lymphocytic pleocytosis; elevated CSF protein • Anti-GQ1b IgG antibodies in two-thirds of cases • MRI: hyperintense T2-weighted lesions in brainstem, less often in basal ganglia or thalamus
Bilateral striatal necrosis	Immune-mediated	• Encephalopathy with extrapyramidal symptoms and signs (bradykinesia, tremor, rigidity); favourable outcome • Onset usually 1–4 weeks after respiratory illness • MRI: high-signal lesions in basal ganglia on T2-weighted imaging
Opsoclonus–myoclonus syndrome	Immune-mediated	• Involuntary, irregular, multidirectional but conjugate eye movements, myoclonus (neck, trunk mainly) and ataxia • Onset 1–4 weeks after respiratory illness • Neuroimaging usually normal • Lymphocytic pleocytosis; elevated CSF protein; oligoclonal bands may be present
Transverse myelitis	Immune-mediated	• Acute progressive motor disturbance, sphincter dysfunction, bilateral segmental sensory changes • Onset usually 1–4 weeks after respiratory illness • Lymphocytic pleocytosis (40%–60%); elevated CSF protein • *M. pneumoniae* often detected in respiratory tract, only rarely in CSF
Guillain–Barré syndrome	Immune-mediated	• Ascending paralysis, areflexia, sensory deficits • Onset usually 1–4 weeks after respiratory illness • Elevated CSF protein; usually no pleocytosis • Antigalactocerebroside antibody may be present in blood or CSF • *M. pneumoniae* often detected in respiratory tract, only rarely in CSF
Stroke	Vasculitis or procoagulable state	• Focal neurological deficits corresponding with brain region affected; residual deficits common • Onset typically 3–21 days after respiratory illness • Evidence of cerebral vasculitis may be seen on neuroimaging • *M. pneumoniae* often detected in respiratory tract, only rarely in CSF

CSF, cerebrospinal fluid; PCR, polymerase chain reaction; MRI, magnetic resonance imaging; FLAIR, fluid-attenuated inversion recovery.

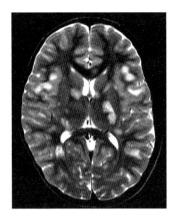

Fig. 19.1. MRI of a 10-year-old female with *Mycoplasma pneumoniae*-induced acute disseminated encephalomyelitis. On this T2-weighted axial (TR=2800, TE=90) image, multiple foci of increased signal intensity within deep grey structures and white matter are present. Upper respiratory symptoms of 2 weeks duration had resolved 1–2 weeks before the onset of encephalitis. *M. pneumoniae* was implicated on the basis of positive serology (IgM by enzyme immunoassay and acute/convalescent complement fixation titres of 1:128/1:512) and detection of the organism by polymerase chain reaction in an oropharyngeal sample. (Reproduced by permission from Bitnum et al. 2003.)

DIAGNOSIS

The clinical manifestations, routine laboratory tests (such as complete blood count and erythrocyte sedimentation rate), CSF, electroencephalography and neuroimaging findings of *M. pneumoniae*-associated CNS disease are non-specific. Clinico-radiographic evidence of atypical pneumonia is supportive. Cold haemagglutinins (autoantibodies directed against the I-antigen of human erythrocytes) are evident in 50%–60% of individuals with *M. pneumoniae* infection; however, they may also be induced by a variety of other infections or lymphoid malignancies (Jacobs 1993). The mainstays of diagnosis of *M. pneumoniae* infection are serology, culture and polymerase chain reaction (PCR). In order to enhance diagnostic accuracy in the context of CNS disease where the pretest likelihood of *M. pneumoniae* is relatively low, the combination of *M. pneumoniae* PCR and serology should be employed (Bitnun and Richardson 2010). A thorough microbiological workup that excludes alternative aetiologies is also important.

Serology

The detection of immunoglobulins IgM or IgA in acute sera, demonstration of seroconversion from negative to positive, or a four-fold rise in antimycoplasmal antibody titre between acute and convalescent sera is indicative of acute or recent infection with *M. pneumoniae* (Daxboeck et al. 2003, Atkinson et al. 2008). IgM antibody appears towards the end of the first week of illness, peaks 2–3 weeks later, and declines to undetectable levels over the course of several months. IgA antibody appears concurrently with IgM, but declines earlier (Waites and Talkington 2004). In primary infections, IgG antibody is first detectable approximately 2 weeks after the appearance of IgM. In individuals with repeated infections, an IgM response may or may not occur; in this setting, detection of IgA in acute sera or demonstration of a four-fold or greater rise in IgG titre between acute and convalescent sera can be used to establish the diagnosis (Atkinson et al. 2008).

Most serological assays used for the diagnosis of *M. pneumoniae* infection have limited specificity, probably due to the use of crude antigen. The complement fixation test (CFT), based on a methanol-chloroform lipid extract of *M. pneumoniae* that detects both IgM and IgG antibodies, has a sensitivity of 90% and a specificity of 94% in culture-positive, radiographically proven pneumonia (Kenny et al. 1990). However, cross-reactivity with *M. genitalium* and a variety of human, animal and plant epitopes is reported, and high CFT titres have been observed in a variety of non-*M. pneumoniae*-related conditions, such as acute pancreatitis and acute bacterial meningitis (Jacobs 1993). Most commercial assays have similar limitations – the poor specificity of IgM-based assays is illustrated by their detection in at least 20% of blood donors with no antecedent illness during the 30 days prior to blood sampling (Nir-Paz et al. 2006).

Culture

Culture of *M. pneumoniae* from clinical samples is complicated by its fastidious nature, complex nutritional requirements and slow growth (Waites and Talkington 2004). Even in experienced laboratories, the analytical sensitivity of culture is no more than 60% that of PCR (Waites and Talkington 2004). In the context of CNS disease, the isolation of *M. pneumoniae* from CSF or brain tissue provides reliable evidence of causality. The significance of a positive culture from a respiratory specimen is more complex because asymptomatic colonization and persistent shedding for 3 months or more after resolution of acute infection can occur despite appropriate antimicrobial therapy (Foy 1993).

Polymerase chain reaction

The principle advantages of PCR are that it is highly sensitive, does not require the organism to remain viable in clinical samples, and allows for timely diagnosis in the acute care setting prior to the development of specific antibody. A variety of PCR assays have been developed for the detection of *M. pneumoniae* in clinical samples using primers directed at genes encoding for P1 adhesin, ATPase operon, 16S RNA, tuf, and repetitive element repMp1 (Waites and Talkington 2004, Atkinson et al. 2008). Real-time PCR assays, such as those utilizing the multicopy repetitive element within the P1 adhesin gene, repMp1, or the CARDS toxin gene as targets, may offer enhanced sensitivity (Winchell et al. 2008).

Several caveats should be kept in mind when interpreting a positive *M. pneumoniae* PCR. Contamination due to a lapse in quality control must always be considered, as with any molecular assay. Confirming a positive PCR result by repeating the extraction and PCR with the same or a second primer set targeting a different gene, or repeating the specimen collection and PCR testing, could alleviate such concerns (Atkinson et al. 2008). Detection of the organism in brain tissue or CSF (if contaminated by blood) may be due to spillage of DNA of dead organism into the circulation from a damaged respiratory tract, rather than systemic spread of viable organisms. Distinguishing between asymptomatic respiratory-tract carriage, observed in 5%–13.5% of adults, prolonged respiratory shedding following infection, and truly acute infection is not possible with qualitative PCR assays. The potential role of quantitative PCR in distinguishing acute infection from asymptomatic colonization or prolonged shedding following infection has not been adequately explored.

TREATMENT

The role of antibiotic therapy in the management of *M. pneumoniae*-associated CNS complications is uncertain (Bitnun et al. 2003, Tsiodras et al. 2005). Nevertheless, given the high frequency of neurological sequelae, it is reasonable to consider antibiotic therapy on an individual basis. Unanswered questions include whether CNS penetration of the antibiotic is important, particularly when *M. pneumoniae* is detected in CSF or brain tissue, and whether eradication of the organism from the respiratory tract can limit the extent of neurological injury in immunologically mediated conditions (Narita 2009). Antibiotics with good in-vitro and in-vivo efficacy against *M. pneumoniae* include the macrolides, tetracyclines, fluoroquinolones, ketolides, streptogramins and chloramphenicol. The macrolides have the theoretical advantage of having both antimicrobial activity and anti-inflammatory properties, but their CNS penetration, with the possible exception of azithromycin, is limited (Narita 2009). For improved CSF penetration, a fluoroquinolone, tetracycline, or perhaps chloramphenicol is most appropriate. The optimal duration of antibiotic therapy is unknown, but a 2–3 week course is suggested.

Corticosteroids, intravenous immune globulin and plasma exchange have been associated with clinical improvement in *M. pneumoniae*-associated encephalitis, ADEM, transverse myelitis, Guillain–Barré syndrome and other postinfectious immunologically mediated disorders (Tsiodras et al. 2005). The evidence for these interventions is largely anecdotal, based on case reports and case series. A retrospective review of published *M. pneumoniae* encephalitis cases treated with corticosteroids found that complete or near-complete resolution of neurological manifestations occurred in 78% of patients (Carpenter et al. 2002). Without corticosteroids, resolution is seen in 35%–56% of individuals with encephalitis (Lehtokoski-Lehtiniemi and Koskiniemi 1989, Bitnun et al. 2001). On the basis of clinical experience, corticosteroids should be considered 'first-line' therapy for ADEM and transverse myelitis (Tsiodras et al. 2006). Intravenous immune globulin or plasma exchange is preferable in the setting of Guillain–Barré syndrome, and in those with ADEM or transverse myelitis who fail to respond to corticosteroids. Immunoadsorption therapy may be an option for individuals with Guillain–Barré syndrome who fail to respond to intravenous immune globulin or plasma exchange (Arakawa et al. 2005).

PROGNOSIS

The prognosis of *M. pneumoniae*-associated CNS disease is not fully elucidated, but varies by clinical syndrome. Complete recovery can be expected for those with meningitis (Daxboeck et al. 2004). *M. pneumoniae* encephalitis is a severe entity with an associated mortality of up to 10% and residual neurological sequelae in 20%–60% of survivors (Bitnun et al. 2003, Daxboeck et al. 2004, Tsiodras et al. 2005). Long-term sequelae include epilepsy, intellectual impairment, and less frequently expressive dysphasia, dysarthria, truncal ataxia, hemiparesies and quadriparesis. Among individuals with *M. pneumoniae*-associated acute transverse myelitis, 50%–60% suffer residual neurological deficits (Tsiodras et al. 2006). Focal neurological deficits are common in stroke victims.

Other *Mycoplasma* species

M. hominis and *U. urealyticum/U. parvum* account for most mycoplasmal CNS disease not attributable to *M. pneumoniae* and are the focus of this section. *U. urealyticum* and *U. parvum*, separate species within the *Ureaplasma* genus, can at present be distinguished only by serotyping or PCR; they are considered together here. All three species are commensals of the genitourinary tract. Individual case reports implicating *M. genitalium* or other mycoplasmal species have been reported, but are extremely rare.

MYCOPLASMA HOMINIS

M. hominis can be isolated from the genital tract of approximately 10%–30% of otherwise healthy women. Newborn infants acquire the infection vertically during the process of birth; 27% are colonized transiently in the respiratory or genitourinary tracts (Grattard et al. 1995). Rarely, meningitis, meningoencephalitis and intracranial or subdural abscess may ensue following haematogenous dissemination (Hata et al. 2008). Neonatal meningitis and meningoencephalitis due to *M. hominis* are indistinguishable from those due to other pathogens. The onset of symptoms ranges from days 1 to 32 of life. CSF pleocytosis is evident in most, with cell counts ranging from fewer than 5 cells/µL to as many as 32000 cells/µL. In older individuals, CNS infection results from direct inoculation of the brain or CSF following head trauma, neurosurgical procedures or haematogenous dissemination subsequent to urogenital manipulation, such as vaginal delivery or urinary catheterization. Intracranial abscesses present non-specifically with fever and focal neurological manifestations.

The key to the diagnosis of *M. hominis* CNS infections is a high index of suspicion; it should be considered when routine bacterial cultures from purulent foci or CSF are sterile in the absence of antibiotic treatment. Because the organism is extremely sensitive to environmental conditions, specimens should ideally be inoculated into appropriate transport media (such as SP4 or Shepard's 10B broth supplemented with arginine) at the bedside. PCR-based assays offer higher sensitivity and rapid turnaround, but are not widely available.

M. hominis is usually susceptible to tetracyclines, fluoroquinolones, lincosamides and chloramphenicol; it is intrinsically resistant to erythromycin and other 14- and 15-member ring macrolides (Waites et al. 2005). In the context of CNS disease, the tetracyclines (minocycline, doxycycline) and fluoroquinolones are preferred because of their superior CSF penetration. A 2–3 week course of therapy is sufficient for most cases of meningitis or meningoencephalitis. Six weeks or longer is warranted for intracranial abscesses (Hata et al. 2008).

UREAPLASMA UREALYTICUM/UREAPLASMA PARVUM

Asymptomatic colonization of the female genital tract by *U. urealyticum* or *U. parvum* is evident in 40%–80% of generally healthy sexually active women (Waites et al. 2005). Asymptomatic neonatal infection may follow ascending intrauterine infection, transplacental transmission in association with maternal bacteraemia, or infection acquired during labour and delivery. CNS disease such as meningitis and brain abscess due to *U. urealyticum/U. parvum* has been reported less frequently than with *M. hominis*. Unlike *M. hominis*, *U. urealyticum* and *U. parvum* are usually susceptible to macrolides, but relatively resistant to lincosamides (Waites et al. 2005). Infections of the CNS are most often treated with tetracyclines, fluoroquinolones or chloramphenicol.

REFERENCES

Ang CW, Tio-Gillen AP, Groen J, et al. (2002) Cross-reactive anti-galactocerebroside antibodies and *Mycoplasma pneumoniae* infections in Guillain–Barré syndrome. *J Neuroimmunol* 130: 179–83.

Arakawa H, Yuhara Y, Todokoro M, et al. (2005) Immunoadsorption therapy for a child with Guillain–Barré syndrome subsequent to *Mycoplasma* infection: a case study. *Brain Dev* 27: 431–3.

Atkinson TP, Balish MF, Waites KB (2008) Epidemiology, clinical manifestations, pathogenesis and laboratory detection of *Mycoplasma pneumoniae* infections. *FEMS Microbiol Rev* 32: 956–73.

Bitnun A, Richardson SE (2010) Mycoplasma pneumoniae: innocent bystander or a true cause of central nervous system disease? *Curr Infect Dis Rep* 12: 282–90.

Bitnun A, Ford-Jones EL, Petric M, et al. (2001) Acute childhood encephalitis and *Mycoplasma pneumoniae*. *Clin Infect Dis* 32: 1674–84.

Bitnun A, Ford-Jones E, Blaser S, et al. (2003) *Mycoplasma pneumoniae* encephalitis. *Sem Pediatr Infect Dis* 14: 96–107.

Carpenter TC (2002) Corticosteroids in the treatment of severe mycoplasma encephalitis in children. *Crit Care Med* 30: 925–7.

Christie LJ, Honarmand S, Talkington DF, et al. (2007a) Pediatric encephalitis: what is the role of *Mycoplasma pneumoniae*? *Pediatrics* 120: 305–13.

Christie LJ, Honarmand S, Yagi S, et al. (2007b) Anti-galactocerebroside testing in *Mycoplasma pneumoniae*-associated encephalitis. *J Neuroimmunol* 189: 129–31.

Daxboeck F, Krause R, Wenisch C (2003) Laboratory diagnosis of *Mycoplasma pneumoniae* infection. *Clin Microbiol Infect* 9: 263–73.

Daxboeck F, Blacky A, Seidl R, et al. (2004) Diagnosis, treatment, and prognosis of *Mycoplasma pneumoniae* childhood encephalitis: systematic review of 58 cases. *J Child Neurol* 19: 865–71.

Foy HM (1993) Infections caused by *Mycoplasma pneumoniae* and possible carrier state in different populations of patients. *Clin Infect Dis* 17 Suppl 1: S37–46.

Grattard F, Soleihac B, De Barbeyrac B, et al. (1995) Epidemiologic and molecular investigations of genital mycoplasmas from women and neonates at delivery. *Pediatr Infect Dis J* 14: 853–8.

Hata A, Honda Y, Asada K, et al. (2008) *Mycoplasma hominis* meningitis in a neonate: case report and review. *J Infect* 57: 338–43.

Jacobs E (1993) Serological diagnosis of Mycoplasma pneumoniae infections: a critical review of current procedures. *Clin Infect Dis* 17 Suppl 1: S79–82.

Kenny GE, Kaiser GG, Cooney MK, Foy HM (1990) Diagnosis of *Mycoplasma pneumoniae* pneumonia: sensitivities and specificities of serology with lipid antigen and isolation of the organism on soy peptone medium for identification of infections. *J Clin Microbiol* 28: 2087–93.

Koskiniemi M, Rautonen J, Lehtokoski-Lehtiniemi E, Vaheri A (1991) Epidemiology of encephalitis in children: a 20-year survey. *Ann Neurol* 29: 492–7.

Lehtokoski-Lehtiniemi E, Koskiniemi ML (1989) *Mycoplasma pneumoniae* encephalitis: a severe entity in children. *Pediatr Infect Dis J* 8: 651–3.

Narita M (2009) Pathogenesis of neurologic manifestations of *Mycoplasma pneumoniae* infection. *Pediatr Neurol* 41: 159–66.

Nir-Paz R, Michael-Gayego A, Ron M, Block C (2006) Evaluation of eight commercial tests for *Mycoplasma pneumoniae* antibodies in the absence of acute infection. *Clin Microbiol Infect* 12: 685–8.

Nishimura M, Saida T, Kuroki S, et al. (1996) Post-infectious encephalitis with anti-galactocerebroside antibody subsequent to *Mycoplasma pneumoniae* infection. *J Neurol Sci* 140: 91–5.

Perez C, Montes M (2002) Cutaneous leukocytoclastic vasculitis and encephalitis associated with *Mycoplasma pneumoniae* infection. *Arch Intern Med* 162: 352–4.

Ponka A (1980) Central nervous system manifestations associated with serologically verified *Mycoplasma pneumoniae* infection. *Scand J Infect Dis* 12: 175–84.

Powers JM, Johnson MD (2012) Mycoplasmal panencephalitis: a neuropathologic documentation. *Acta Neuropathol* 124: 143–8.

Tsiodras S, Kelesidis I, Kelesidis T, et al. (2005) Central nervous system manifestations of *Mycoplasma pneumoniae* infections. *J Infect* 51: 343–54.

Tsiodras S, Kelesidis T, Kelesidis I, et al. (2006) *Mycoplasma pneumoniae*-associated myelitis: a comprehensive review. *Europ J Neurol* 13: 112–24.

Waites KB, Talkington DF (2004) *Mycoplasma pneumoniae* and its role as a human pathogen. *Clin Microbiol Rev* 17: 697–728.

Waites KB, Katz B, Schelonka RL (2005) Mycoplasmas and ureaplasmas as neonatal pathogens. *Clin Microbiol Rev* 18: 757–89.

Waites KB, Balish MF, Atkinson TP (2008) New insights into the pathogenesis and detection of *Mycoplasma pneumoniae* infections. *Future Microbiol* 3: 635–48.

Walter ND, Grant GB, Bandy U, et al. (2008) Community outbreak of *Mycoplasma pneumoniae* infection: school-based cluster of neurologic disease associated with household transmission of respiratory illness. *J Infect Dis* 198: 1365–74.

Winchell JM, Thurman KA, Mitchell SL, et al. (2008) Evaluation of three real-time PCR assays for detection of *Mycoplasma pneumoniae* in an outbreak investigation. *J Clin Microbiol* 46: 3116–8.

20
RICKETTSIAL DISEASE

Timothy D Minniear and Steven C Buckingham

Rickettsiae are arthropod-borne gram-negative coccobacilli that can cause a broad range of human diseases. The agents of spotted fevers, typhus and ehrlichiosis are included within the class *Alphaproteobacteria*, all members of which are incapable of prolonged survival outside of a host cell. *Coxiella burnetii*, the causative agent of Q fever, belongs to the class *Gammaproteobacteria* and is capable of surviving in the environment.

Rickettsia: spotted fever group

EPIDEMIOLOGY
The vectors and natural hosts for the spotted fever group (SFG) rickettsiae are arachnids: ticks and mites. These rickettsiae can be found across the globe (Table 20.1). Ticks are capable of passing these organisms to other ticks through copulation, by transovarian passage, and by feeding in close proximity to other ticks. Humans are dead-end hosts for all SFG rickettsiae.

PATHOGENESIS AND CLINICAL MANIFESTATIONS
The vector primarily transmits infection via contaminated saliva during a blood meal; it takes several hours of feeding before infection is established. Once inside the host, the primary targets for all SFG rickettsiae are vascular endothelial cells, which they infect directly near the site of tick attachment or by transportation to distant endothelial cells through lymphatics or blood vessels. The ensuing endothelial necrosis and inflammatory response produce a widespread vasculitis that results in vascular leakage and intravascular coagulation and is responsible for the bulk of the manifestations in spotted fever disease (Walker et al. 2003). The rickettsia responsible for the most severe disease is *R. rickettsii*; other pathogenic rickettsiae cause similar though less severe clinical diseases.

Rickettsia rickettsii (Rocky Mountain spotted fever)
The range of clinical disease in Rocky Mountain spotted fever (RMSF) is broad. Moderate cases may resolve without medical intervention, while as many as one-third of cases are severe enough to require hospitalization (Chapman et al. 2006).

Clinical manifestations occur after an incubation period of 2 days to 2 weeks (median, 4 days) (Helmick and Bernard 1984, Buckingham et al. 2007). Typically, the initial symptoms are vague and include fever, malaise, myalgias, nausea, vomiting, abdominal pain and

TABLE 20.1
Selected pathogenic rickettsial organisms: common vectors and geographic distribution[a]

Organism	Human disease	Vector	Distribution
Rickettsia species: spotted fever group			
R. rickettsii	Rocky Mountain spotted fever	*Dermacentor variabilis* (American dog tick)	Eastern USA
		Dermacentor andersoni (wood tick)	Western USA
	Fiebre manchada	*Rhipicephalus sanguineus* (brown dog tick)	Central and South America
	Brazilian spotted fever	*Amblyomma cajennense* (cayenne tick)	South America
R. conorii	Mediterranean spotted fever	*Rhipicephalus sanguineus*	Africa, Asia, India, Mediterranean, Middle East
		Rhipicephalus simus (glossy brown tick)	Africa
		Haemaphysalis leachi (yellow dog tick)	Africa
R. africae	African tick-bite fever	*Amblyomma hebraeum* (South African bont tick)	Sub-Saharan Africa
		Amblyomma variegatum (tropical bont tick)	West Indies
R. japonica	Oriental spotted fever	*Haemaphysalis longicornis* (tick)	Japan
R. australis	Queensland tick typhus	*Ixodes holocyclus* (paralysis tick)	Australia
R. honei	Flinders Island spotted fever	*Aponomma hydrosauri* (reptilian tick)	Flinders Island
		Haemaphysalis spp. (ticks)	Australia
		Ixodes granulatus (tick)	Thailand
R. sibirica	Siberian tick typhus	*Hyalomma* spp. (ticks)	Africa, China, eastern Europe and Siberia
R. akari	Rickettsialpox	*Liponyssoides sanguineus* (mouse mite)	North America, Russia
R. felis	Flea-borne spotted fever	*Ctenocephalides felis* (cat flea)	North and Central America
Rickettsia species: typhus group			
R. typhi	Murine typhus	*Xenopsylla cheopis* (rat flea)	Subtropical and tropical zones worldwide
R. prowazekii	Epidemic typhus	*Pediculus humanus corporis* (human body louse)	North and South America, Africa, Asia

TABLE 20.1
[continued]

Organism	Human disease	Vector	Distribution
Other rickettsiae			
Ehrlichia chaffeensis	Human monocytic ehrlichiosis	*Amblyomma americanum* (Lone Star tick)	North America
Anaplasma phagocytophila	Human granulocytic anaplasmosis	*Ixodes* species (ticks)	North America, Europe
Coxiella burnetii	Q fever	Common: cattle, goats, sheep Less common: cats, dogs, rabbits, pigeons	Worldwide (except New Zealand)

[a]Raoult and Roux (1997), Raoult et al. (2000), Dumler et al. (2007).

headache. The rash generally appears 2–3 days later, although it can appear as early as the first day of illness in children (Buckingham et al. 2007). The rash is absent in 5% of paediatric cases and in up to 20% of adult cases (Helmick and Bernard 1984). Thus the lack of a rash should not dissuade the clinician from empiric treatment in an otherwise clinically compatible situation. The classic presentation of the rash is an erythematous, macular or maculopapular eruption that spreads centripetally; however, the lack of the classic progression does not rule out the diagnosis. Frequently, the rash becomes petechial; rarely, a purpuric rash similar to the purpura fulminans of meningococcal sepsis may occur. Less common clinical manifestations include peripheral or periorbital oedema, conjunctivitis, pneumonitis, pulmonary oedema, hepatomegaly and splenomegaly (Helmick and Bernard 1984, Buckingham et al. 2007). Myocarditis is found commonly on autopsies of fatal cases (Doyle et al. 2006).

Neurological symptoms in RMSF are common, can be severe, but rarely result in permanent sequelae. Local vasculitis within the brain, alone or with cerebral oedema, can induce changes in cognitive status and focal neurological deficits. Neurological symptoms range from headache to coma and can include seizures, delirium and meningitis. Significant headache is reported in 41%–70% of patients, meningismus in approximately 15%, and dizziness in 6%–17% (Haynes et al. 1970, Helmick and Bernard 1984, Kirk et al. 1990, Buckingham et al. 2007). Patients older than 15 years are more likely than children to develop neurological complications and severe disease in general (Helmick and Bernard 1984). One-third of children with confirmed RMSF have some alteration in cognitive status, and 10% will be comatose (Helmick and Bernard 1984, Buckingham et al. 2007).

A retrospective paediatric series found that 15% of children surviving severe disease were discharged with neurological deficits. Approximately 8% of children had some degree of hearing loss (Helmick and Bernard 1984), believed to result from cochlear damage due to vasculitis or direct damage to the cochlear branch of cranial nerve VIII (Dolan et al.

1986). Other neurological sequelae following severe *R. rickettsii* infection include gait disturbances, speech and swallowing problems, blindness, encephalopathy, paraesthesiae, facial palsies, proximal muscle weakness and behavioural changes (Buckingham et al. 2007).

Common laboratory abnormalities in RMSF include hyponatraemia, elevated liver enzymes and thrombocytopenia; leukocyte counts can be elevated or reduced but are usually normal. RMSF can produce aseptic meningitis with moderate cerebrospinal fluid (CSF) pleocytosis: in one study the median CSF leukocyte was 25 cells/µL (interquartile range [IQR], 3–38), the median CSF glucose was 61mg/dL (IQR, 56–70), and the median CSF protein was 0.68g/L (IQR, 35–126) in children with RNSF (Buckingham 2007). An earlier study in RMSF meningitis found a CSF leukocyte range of 11–300 cells/µL, protein range 0.41–2.00g/L, and normal glucose (Haynes et al. 1970).

Rickettsia conorii (Mediterranean spotted fever)
Mediterranean spotted fever (MSF) is caused by *R. conorii* and occurs in Africa, Europe and Asia. The pathogenesis is similar to that of RMSF, and the disease can be as severe. Common symptoms of MSF include fever, rash, headache and myalgias. A rash occurs in 94%–99% of patients, generally appearing on the third day of illness and involving the trunk and extremities (Font-Creus et al. 1985, de Sousa et al. 2008). A necrotic ulceration at the site of tick attachment, the tache noire, occurs in more than 70% of patients (Font-Creus et al. 1985), although its frequency varies depending on the infecting strain (de Sousa et al. 2008). A few patients with MSF report gastrointestinal complaints (Font-Creus et al. 1985, Cascio et al. 1998). Hepatomegaly occurs in 29%–44% of patients (Font-Creus et al. 1985, de Sousa et al. 2008); liver enzymes are elevated in more than 60%, and bilirubin is usually normal. Thrombocytopenia is common, while the leukocyte count is usually normal (de Sousa et al. 2008).

Headache occurs in approximately 70% of patients with MSF, and changes in cognitive status in 10%–38% (Font-Creus et al. 1985, de Sousa et al. 2008). Other neurological complications such as meningismus, seizures and vertigo are rare (<5%) and resolve without residual deficits (Font-Creus et al. 1985, Cascio et al. 1998, de Sousa et al. 2008). MSF is usually considered a milder disease than RMSF. However, the severity varies by strain, and the risk of death is increased by comorbidities; one study reported higher mortality (29% vs 13%) among adult patients infected with the Israeli spotted fever strain compared with other MSF strains (de Sousa et al. 2008).

Other rickettsiae
The cutaneous manifestations of rickettsialpox (caused by *R. akari* infection) are distinct from those of other SFG rickettsial infections. Rather than a tache noire at the site of tick attachment, an erythematous papule forms and transforms into a vesicle: therefore the rash of rickettsialpox is vesicular. Constitutional symptoms include fever, chills and muscle aches; regional lymphadenopathy is common. Rickettsialpox is generally mild and resolves without therapy in 1–3 weeks. Neurological complications and fatalities are not reported.

Numerous other SFG rickettsioses are described (Table 20.1), but these diseases are generally not severe and not characterized by neurological involvement. A tache noire occurs in most SFG rickettsial infections except *R. rickettsii* (Raoult and Roux 1997). *R. felis* infection rarely causes photophobia, aseptic meningitis, paraesthesiae and hearing loss (Zavala-Velazquez 2006).

DIAGNOSIS

Diagnoses of SFG rickettsial infections are based on clinical signs and symptoms. Confirmation is made by demonstrating a four-fold rise in specific antibody titres between acute and convalescent serum specimens on immunofluorescent assay (Brouqui et al. 2004, Chapman et al. 2006). A single serum titre greater than 1:64 in a clinically compatible case is sufficient for a diagnosis of probable infection (Brouqui et al. 2004). Serological tests demonstrate considerable cross-reactivity among the SFG rickettsiae. Immunohisto-chemical staining of skin biopsies (taken from where the rash is present) is sensitive, but the process is cumbersome. Because of the paucity of organism in the blood, polymerase chain reaction (PCR) testing from blood lacks sensitivity. PCR testing of tissue from a skin biopsy of the tache noire is more sensitive (Raoult et al. 2001, Chapman et al. 2006).

TREATMENT

Prompt treatment of RMSF can be lifesaving, and patients with clinically compatible disease presentations should receive therapy as soon as possible. The treatment of choice for all patients is doxycycline at 2.2mg/kg/dose (maximum 100mg) given twice a day, orally or intravenously. Therapy is continued for 3 days after defervescence. In pregnant women, doxycycline poses a risk of fetal dental and bone malformations, but this risk must be weighed against the significant risks of withholding therapy. Paediatricians should not hesitate to use doxycycline to treat children with suspected RMSF. Doxycycline does not carry the same risks of tooth staining as tetracycline, and the fear of discoloration should not outweigh the potentially catastrophic results of failing to treat RMSF. Chloramphenicol is the only alternative drug, though it is less effective than doxycycline (Holman et al. 2001).

Doxycycline is also the drug of choice for treating MSF. Children can receive doxycycline at a dose of 5mg/kg/d for 5 days; however, a 3-day course of azithromycin (10mg/kg/d) has been shown to be equally effective (Meloni and Meloni 1996). Chloramphenicol (12.5mg/kg/dose, four times a day for 7 days) is another alternative (Cascio 1998).

The other SFG rickettsiae produce milder diseases, which usually resolve spontaneously without sequelae. Doxycycline therapy, however, may shorten the duration of symptoms (Raoult et al. 2001).

PREVENTION

The prevention of tick-borne diseases depends on avoidance of tick bites and prompt removal of attached ticks. In addition to limiting time in high-risk areas such as uncultivated, overgrown fields or wooded areas, individuals can reduce their risk of tick attachment by using insect repellents containing N-N-diethyl-M-toluamide (DEET) and by spraying clothing with permethrin. Children and pets should be inspected by their guardians for ticks after spending time outdoors during seasons of tick activity. Wearing light-coloured clothing can make it easier to visualize ticks.

Attached ticks should be removed by grasping the head of the tick with tweezers and pulling with steady pressure. Ticks should not be crushed, and hands should be washed after handling ticks to prevent accidental self-inoculation. The site of attachment should be cleaned with soap and water. Other methods of tick removal (such as applying petroleum jelly or a hot match) are ineffective or even harmful and should not be used (Needham 1985).

Rickettsia: typhus group

EPIDEMIOLOGY

The typhus group rickettsiae include *R. prowazekii*, which causes epidemic typhus, and *R. typhi*, which causes endemic (murine) typhus. Endemic typhus generally occurs in subtropical and tropical zones, whereas epidemic typhus generally occurs in temperate climates. These organisms infect and are transmitted by insects (Table 20.1). Flying squirrels and humans (during epidemics) serve as the primary reservoirs for *R. prowazekii*. The common rat is the reservoir for *R. typhi*.

PATHOGENESIS AND CLINICAL MANIFESTATIONS

Typhus group rickettsiae are excreted in the faeces of the louse or flea. Mechanical trauma, such as scratching, drives the infected faeces or remains of dead lice into the body where the rickettsiae infect vascular endothelial cells. Like SFG rickettsiae, the typhus group organisms induce diffuse vasculitis with vascular leakage and widespread inflammation and coagulation (Bechah et al. 2008). Unlike other rickettsiae, *R. prowazekii* can establish life-long latency in the human host and produce recrudescent disease.

Rickettsia prowazekii (epidemic typhus)

Both epidemic typhus and murine typhus begin with a fever, headache and myalgias (Raoult and Roux 1997). The incubation period for epidemic typhus is 2 weeks, and the rash appears 4–5 days after onset of fever. Typically, the rash appears on the trunk and extremities, and spares the palms and soles. The rash can be macular or maculopapular but occasionally appears petechial (Raoult and Roux 1997). Other common symptoms include tachypnoea, abdominal pain, nausea, arthralgia and cough. Epidemic typhus can be fatal if untreated, especially in patients with underlying diseases or malnutrition (Bechah et al. 2008).

Eighty per cent of individuals infected with *R. prowazekii* experience some form of CNS abnormality ranging from drowsiness to coma. Delirium or confusion is more common than coma or seizures. Rarely, focal neurological deficits develop, and hearing loss has been reported. Common laboratory abnormalities in epidemic typhus include thrombocytopenia, elevated blood urea nitrogen and creatinine, hypoalbuminaemia, and elevated liver enzymes. Pulmonary infiltrates are often seen on chest radiographs (Bechah 2008).

Recrudescent typhus, known as Brill–Zinsser disease, is caused by *R. prowazekii* and can occur several years after the initial infection. The symptoms are similar to those of acute typhus, but the disease is usually not as severe as the original episode. Body lice can transfer infection during this recrudescence to new hosts and can quickly establish an epidemic in the appropriate setting.

Rickettsia typhi (murine or endemic typhus)

Murine typhus is a mild, non-specific disease that is rarely fatal. The incubation period is 1–2 weeks. Fever and headache, which persist for 3–7 days, are the most common symptoms (Civen and Ngo 2008). A rash occurs in fewer than half of the patients and appears later than in epidemic typhus (Raoult and Roux 1997). Confusion occurs in less than 15% of patients, and both coma and seizures are rare. Persistent, focal neurological deficits have been reported rarely. The mortality rate is less than 5%, even in the absence of antirickettsial therapy. Common laboratory abnormalities include thrombocytopenia, elevated liver enzymes and hypoalbuminaemia (Civen and Ngo 2008).

DIAGNOSIS

The diagnosis is confirmed by demonstrating a four-fold rise in convalescent serum antibody titres compared to acute titres by immunofluorescent assay. Western blot is necessary to differentiate *R. prowazekii* from *R. typhi* (Bechah et al. 2008). PCR tests for both agents of typhus have been developed, but they are not widely available (Bechah et al. 2008). In resource-poor regions, specialized diagnostic tests are often unavailable and clinicians must prescribe empiric therapy for typhus based on their clinical suspicion.

TREATMENT

Therapy is safe and well tolerated, and can save lives when given early. Therefore, presumptive treatment should not be delayed while waiting for confirmatory tests in patients with compatible presentations. Doxycycline is the treatment of choice for both epidemic and murine typhus in adults and children; chloramphenicol may be used as an alternative (Bechah et al. 2008, Civen and Ngo 2008). Five days of therapy is recommended to ensure eradication of the organism and prevent relapse. This is especially important when treating epidemic typhus in order to prevent latent disease. A single dose of doxycycline can prevent death due to epidemic typhus, but it may not prevent febrile relapses and is ineffective against other infections in the differential diagnosis, such as typhoid. Ciprofloxacin demonstrates in vitro activity against the typhus group rickettsiae; however, experts caution against its use owing to reports of fatal treatment failures. If severe complications have not evolved by the time treatment is initiated, defervescence usually occurs within 2–3 days (Bechah et al. 2008).

PREVENTION

Eliminating body lice prevents human-to-human spread of *R. prowazekii*. Washing clothes and bedding in hot water kills the lice and their eggs. Reductions in mammalian reservoirs and the use of insecticides active against fleas and lice have successfully reduced cases of epidemic typhus in the Americas. Vaccines for *R. prowazekii* have been developed, but continued marketing and development has been hindered by adverse events and the fact that effective, inexpensive treatment for typhus is widely available (Bechah et al. 2008).

Ehrlichioses

EPIDEMIOLOGY

Human monocytic ehrlichiosis (HME) and human granulocytic anaplasmosis (HGA; formerly called human granulocytic ehrlichiosis) are tick-borne infections. *Ehrlichia chaffeensis*, the cause of HME, is restricted to North America; *Anaplasma phagocytophila*, the cause of HGA, is found in both North America and Europe (Table 20.1).

PATHOGENESIS AND CLINICAL MANIFESTATIONS

As with SFG rickettsiae, humans become infected when an infected tick feeds on blood. *E. chaffeensis* is taken into the macrophage where it inhibits fusion of the lysosome and multiplies within the vacuole. *A. phagocytophila* targets granulocytic phagocytes. The pathogenesis of the ehrlichioses is not fully understood; however, immune dysregulation and widespread inflammation are likely to play important roles (Rikihisa 2006).

Ehrlichia chaffeensis (human monocytic ehrlichiosis)
The median incubation time for HME in children is 9 days, and the initial symptoms are non-specific: fever, headache, myalgia and nausea (Schutze et al. 2007). About 60% of children and 30% of adults develop a rash, usually around the fifth day of illness (Dumler et al. 2007, Schutze et al. 2007). Common laboratory findings include elevated transaminases, thrombocytopenia, leukopenia, anaemia and hyponatraemia (Dumler et al. 2007, Schutze et al. 2007).

Roughly 50% of patients with HME require hospitalization, and 17% have life-threatening complications. About one-fifth experience aseptic meningitis or meningoencephalitis. Peripheral neuropathies rarely occur (Dumler et al. 2007). In a study of children with HME, agitation or obtundation were reported in 60%. CSF evaluation in nine children demonstrated lymphocytic pleocytosis (IQR, 21–115 cells/μL), elevated protein (IQR, 0.48–1.37mg/dL) and normal glucose. Significant neurological sequelae occurred in 10% (Schutze et al. 2007).

Anaplasma phagocytophila (human granulocytic anaplasmosis)
The clinical manifestations of HGA are similar to those of HME, with a few notable distinctions. Rash appears in fewer than 10% of patients with HGA, and fewer than 10% of patients have severe disease. Meningoencephalitis occurs in approximately 1% of patients. Rarely, persistent peripheral neuropathies and facial palsies have been reported (Dumler et al. 2007).

DIAGNOSIS
The diagnosis of HME or HGA should be considered in any patient with a clinically com-

patible history, physical examination and epidemiological link. The diagnosis can be made by visualizing intracytoplasmic inclusions (morulae) in appropriate host cells on peripheral smear, but these are noted in fewer than 10% of patients. Conventionally, the diagnosis is confirmed by demonstrating a four-fold rise in antibody titres between acute and convalescent serum. Since the host cells circulate in the blood, PCR testing on whole-blood samples can be useful in the clinical setting (Dumler et al. 2007).

TREATMENT

The recommended therapy for both diseases is doxycycline, administered until 3 days after the fever has resolved; typically, this results in 5–14 days of treatment. Rifampin has been suggested as an alternative agent; however, experience with its use for ehrlichiosis is very limited (Dumler et al. 2007).

PREVENTION

There is no vaccine for *E. chaffeensis* or other ehrlichial diseases. Prevention methods are the same as for those of other tick-borne rickettsioses.

Coxiella burnetii (Q fever)

EPIDEMIOLOGY

A vast array of wild and domestic animals serve as reservoirs for *C. burnetii* (Table 20.1). Numerous species of ticks maintain the infection and transmit the organism to mammals in the zoonotic cycle. Humans generally acquire *C. burnetii* infection by inhaling or ingesting the organism following exposure to the carcasses, faeces, urine, milk or birthing products of infected animals.

PATHOGENESIS AND CLINICAL MANIFESTATIONS

C. burnetii is highly infectious; a single organism can establish infection in a human. The bacteria reside in human macrophages, where they escape destruction and multiply in phagosomes. The incubation period ranges from 1 to 3 weeks. Asymptomatic infections occur frequently.

Acute Q fever manifests as a self-limited, febrile illness with myalgia, sore throat and headache. Occasionally a maculopapular rash develops on the trunk and shoulders. The illness generally lasts between 1 and 3 weeks. Complications include pneumonia, hepatitis and encephalitis. Pneumonia occurs in approximately 50% of patients; progression to acute respiratory distress syndrome occurs rarely. Other features of acute infection include hepatitis, gastroenteritis, erythema nodosum, anaemia, central lymphadenopathy, orchitis and epididymitis (Raoult et al. 2000).

Neurological manifestations of acute Q fever are varied. Headache occurs in 40%–50% of patients (Raoult et al. 2000, Kofteridis et al. 2004). Altered cognitive status occurs in 4% of patients, and 2% have nuchal rigidity (Kofteridis et al. 2004). Significant neurological manifestations, which occur in less than 1% of patients, include aseptic meningitis, encephalitis with seizures and coma, polyradiculopathies, optic neuritis, Guillain–Barré syndrome, and the syndrome of inappropriate secretion of antidiuretic hormone (Raoult et al. 2000, Kofteridis et al. 2004).

Chronic Q fever develops in fewer than 5% of patients infected with *C. burnetii*. The most common complication of chronic Q fever is culture-negative endocarditis (Raoult et al. 2000).

DIAGNOSIS

The diagnosis of Q fever is confirmed by demonstrating a four-fold rise in specific antibody titres between acute and convalescent serum specimens using immunofluorescent assay. Serology should be repeated 6 months after disease onset; rising anti-phase-I IgG titres suggest the possibility of chronic infection. Nucleic acid amplification tests for *C. burnetii* infection are commercially available and clinically useful. Culture of the organism requires Biosafety level 3 conditions (Tissot-Dupont and Raoult 2008).

TREATMENT

For symptomatic patients of all ages, the treatment of choice for acute Q fever is doxycycline for 2–3 weeks. Alternative drugs include the fluoroquinolones and cotrimoxazole. Experts have used cotrimoxazole for treatment of Q fever in pregnant women, but it increases the risk of neonatal hyperbilirubinaemia if administered near delivery (Tissot-Dupont and Raoult 2008). Fluoroquinolones have been recommended for treatment of encephalitis because of their improved penetration of the CSF (Maltezou and Raoult 2002). To prevent the development of endocarditis, patients with valvular defects should receive hydroxychloroquine plus doxycycline for 12 months. Patients with Q fever endocarditis should receive dual therapy with doxycycline and hydroxychloroquine for at least 18–36 months (Fenollar et al. 2001, Tissot-Dupont and Raoult 2008).

PREVENTION

At-risk professionals, such as abattoir workers, veterinarians and laboratory personnel, should take measures to avoid inhalation of potentially infectious material and adhere to Biosafety protocols (US Department of Health and Human Services 2009). In Australia, an inactivated whole-cell vaccine is available for at-risk individuals (Tissot-Dupont and Raoult 2008).

REFERENCES

Bechah Y, Capo C, Mege JL, Raoult D (2008) Epidemic typhus. *Lancet Infect Dis* 8: 417–26.
Brouqui P, Bacellar F, Baranton G, et al. (2004) Guidelines for the diagnosis of tick-borne bacterial diseases in Europe. *Clin Microbiol Infect* 10: 1108–32.
Buckingham SC, Marshall GS, Schutze GE, et al. (2007) Clinical and laboratory features, hospital course, and outcome of Rocky Mountain spotted fever in children. *J Pediatr* 150: 180–4.
Cascio A, Dones P, Romano A, Titone L (1998) Clinical and laboratory findings of boutonneuse fever in Sicilian children. *Eur J Pediatr* 157: 482–6.
Chapman AS, Bakken JS, Folk SM, et al. (2006) Diagnosis and management of tickborne rickettsial diseases: Rocky Mountain spotted fever, ehrlichioses, and anaplasmosis—United States: a practical guide for physicians and other health-care and public health professionals. *MMWR Recomm Rep* 55(RR-4): 1–27.

Civen R, Ngo V (2008) Murine typhus: an unrecognized suburban vectorborne disease. *Clin Infect Dis* 46: 913–8.

de Sousa R, França A, Nòbrega SD, et al. (2008) Host- and microbe-related risk factors for pathophysiology of fatal *Rickettsia conorii* infection in Portuguese patients. *J Infect Dis* 198: 576–85.

Dolan S, Everett ED, Renner L (1986) Hearing loss in Rocky Mountain spotted fever. *Ann Intern Med* 104: 285.

Doyle A, Bhalla KS, Jones JM, Ennis DM (2006) Myocardial involvement in Rocky Mountain spotted fever: a case report and review. *Am J Med Sci* 332: 208–10.

Dumler JS, Madigan JE, Pusterla N, Bakken JS (2007) Ehrlichioses in humans: epidemiology, clinical presentation, diagnosis, and treatment. *Clin Infect Dis* 45 (Suppl 1): S45–S51.

Fenollar F, Fournier PE, Carrieri MP, et al. (2001) Risk factors and prevention of Q fever endocarditis. *Clin Infect Dis* 33: 312–6.

Font-Creus B, Bella-Cueto F, Espejo-Arenas E, et al. (1985) Mediterranean spotted fever: a cooperative study of 227 cases. *Rev Infect Dis* 7: 635–41.

Haynes RE, Sanders DY, Cramblett HG (1970) Rocky Mountain spotted fever. *J Pediatr* 76: 685–93.

Helmick CG, Bernard KW (1984) Rocky Mountain spotted fever: clinical, laboratory, and epidemiological features of 262 cases. *J Infect Dis* 150: 480–8.

Holman RC, Paddock CD, Curns AT, et al. (2001) Analysis of risk factors for fatal Rocky Mountain spotted fever: evidence for superiority of tetracyclines for therapy. *J Infect Dis* 184: 1437–44.

Kirk JL, Fine DP, Sexton DJ, Muchmore HG (1990) Rocky Mountain spotted fever. A clinical review based on 48 confirmed cases, 1943–1986. *Medicine* 69: 35–45.

Kofteridis DP, Mazokopakis EE, Tselentis Y, Gikas A (2004) Neurological complications of acute Q fever infection. *Eur J Epidemiol* 19: 1051–54.

Maltezou HC, Raoult D (2002) Q fever in children. *Lancet Infect Dis* 2: 686–91.

Meloni G, Meloni T (1996) Azithromycin vs. doxycycline for Mediterranean spotted fever. *Pediatr Infect Dis J* 15: 1042–4.

Needham GR (1985) Evaluation of five popular methods for tick removal. *Pediatrics* 75: 997–1002.

Raoult D, Roux V (1997) Rickettsioses as paradigms of new or emerging infectious diseases. *Clin Microbiol Rev* 10: 694–719.

Raoult D, Tissot-Dupont H, Foucault C, et al. (2000) Q fever 1985–1998. Clinical and epidemiologic features of 1,383 infections. *Medicine* 79: 124–5.

Raoult D, Fournier PE, Fenollar F, et al. (2001) Rickettsia africae, a tick-borne pathogen in travelers to sub-Saharan Africa. *N Engl J Med* 344: 1504–10.

Rikihisa Y (2006) Ehrlichia subversion of host innate responses. *Curr Opin Microbiol* 9: 95–101.

Schutze GE, Buckingham SC, Marshall GS, et al. (2007) Human monocytic ehrlichiosis in children. *Pediatr Infect Dis J* 26: 475–9.

Tissot-Dupont H, Raoult D (2008) Q fever. *Infect Dis Clin North Am* 22: 505–14.

US Department of Health and Human Services (2009) *Biosafety in Microbiological and Biomedical Laboratories (BMBL), 5th edn.* HHS Publication No. (CDC) 21-1112. Washington, DC: US Department of Health and Human Services (online: http://www.cdc.gov/biosafety/publications/bmbl5/BMBL.pdf).

Walker DH, Valbuena GA, Olana JP (2003) Pathogenic mechanisms of diseases caused by *Rickettsia*. *Ann NY Acad Sci* 990: 1–11.

Zavala-Velazquez J, Laviada-Molina H, Zavala-Castro J, et al. (2006) Rickettsia felis, the agent of an emerging infectious disease: report of a new case in Mexico. *Arch Med Res* 37: 419–22.

21
NEUROLOGICAL CONDITIONS CAUSED BY BACTERIAL TOXINS

Sunit Singhi and Charles R Newton

There are a few neurological conditions that are caused by toxins produced by bacteria. These bacteria are ubiquitous, but disease can be prevented by effective immunization.

Tetanus

Tetanus or 'lockjaw', described in ancient Indian literature as 'Dhanur' meaning 'arching of the body', is a disease caused by exotoxins produced by *Clostridium tetani* and characterized by muscle spasms, beginning in the jaw muscles and later becoming generalized tetanic spasms (Thwaites et al. 2006).

EPIDEMIOLOGY

Tetanus occurs worldwide and is endemic in resource-poor countries. The incidence remains under-reported. Globally, the estimated number of tetanus-related deaths in children under 5 years of age was 61 000 in 2008, of which 59 000 were attributable to neonatal tetanus (World Health Organization 2012).

    C. tetani is a gram-positive, obligate anaerobe, spore-forming bacillus. The spores are widely distributed in soil and may survive for years. They are resistant to various disinfectants and to boiling for 20 minutes. The spores usually infect the neonate through contaminated umbilical stump following non-sterile delivery or unhygienic birth and social practices. Outside the neonatal period, the common portals of entry are puncture wounds, lacerations, or even minor trauma during activities such as farming and gardening. Tetanus may complicate infections such as otitis media, skin ulcers and abscesses, and may follow burns, surgery, abortion, childbirth, body piercing or drug abuse (notably 'skin popping'). In some cases, no injury or portal of entry can be identified.

PATHOGENESIS

The spores of *C. tetani* contaminate the wounds frequently but the germination and toxin production takes place only in the absence of oxygen, in the presence of necrotic tissue, foreign bodies or active infection. *C. tetani* does not itself evoke inflammation, and the portal of entry retains a benign appearance unless co-infected with other organisms. *C. tetani* produces three types of toxins: (1) haemolysins (tetanolysin – a heat-labile, oxygen-labile haemolysin: Mitsui et al. 1980); (2) neurotoxin (tetanospasmin), released as a consequence of bacterial lysis and responsible for producing tetanus; and (3) non-spasmogenic neurotoxin, a peripherally active neurotoxin.

The neurotoxin binds to the peripheral motor neuron terminals, enters the axon, and ascends to the neuron body in the spinal cord and brainstem. It then migrates across the synapse to the presynaptic terminals, where it degrades membrane proteins of synaptic vesicles such as synaptobrevin, synaptosomal-associated protein 25 (SNAP-25) and syntaxin. This blocks the release of inhibitory neurotransmitters glycine and γ-aminobutyric acid (GABA) from the vesicles. This leads to unrestrained stimulation of motor end-plate, resulting in rigidity and spasms. Neurotoxin may also affect preganglionic sympathetic neurons and parasympathetic centres in the grey matter of the spinal cord. Loss of inhibition of preganglionic sympathetic neurons may produce sympathetic hyperactivity and high circulating catecholamine levels. Tetanospasmin blocks neurotransmitter release at the neuromuscular junction and produces weakness or paralysis; this effect is clinically evident only in cephalic tetanus.

CLINICAL MANIFESTATIONS

The incubation period is usually 1 week, but it can range from 2 days to 1 month, depending upon the amount of toxin present at the site of the wound, the immunization status of the patient, and the distance between the site of the injury and the central nervous system (CNS). The shorter the incubation period, the more severe is the disease.

Four clinical forms of the disease are described, depending upon the location and extent of the neurons involved.

Generalized tetanus

This is the most common form of tetanus. Typically, the early manifestations are difficulty in opening the mouth (trismus or lockjaw) due to increased tone of the masseters, and 'risus sardonicus' (ironic smile) due to contraction of the facial muscles causing wrinkling of the forehead and distortion of the angle of the mouth. Spasm of other muscles causes laryngospasm, dysphagia, stiffness and pain in the neck, shoulder and back muscles (opisthotonus) and rigid abdominal wall. Eventually, generalized muscle spasms appear spontaneously or following trivial stimuli such as noise, touch or nursing procedures. The spasms are immensely painful and may lead to respiratory compromise due to apnoea, hypoxia and respiratory failure. Violent spasms may cause compressive fractures of the spine, rupture of the muscles, rhabdomyolysis and renal failure. The spasms are maximal during the first two weeks of illness and decrease thereafter in frequency and intensity.

Autonomic instability develops a few days after the onset of spasms. It manifests as paroxysmal tachycardia, profuse sweating, salivation, peripheral vasoconstriction and sustained or labile hypertension. In severe forms it may cause arrhythmias, progressive and refractory hypotension, bradycardia and asystole. Gastrointestinal stasis and haemorrhage, nosocomial sepsis, multi-organ dysfunction syndrome, urinary stasis and infection may also occur (Cook et al. 2001).

Localized tetanus
Localized tetanus presents as painful spasms and stiffness of muscles adjacent to the wound site and may precede generalized tetanus. Progression to secondary generalization is an indicator of poor prognosis.

Cephalic tetanus
Cephalic tetanus is the most severe form of generalized tetanus, which results from middle-ear infections, or injuries to head, face or neck. Facial muscles are affected first, followed by muscles innervated by, in order of frequency, the VIth, IIIrd, IVth and VIIth cranial nerves. Features include retracted eyelids, gaze palsy and pharyngeal spasm. Trismus may be present but usually follows other cranial nerve deficits.

Neonatal tetanus (tetanus neonatorum)
Tetanus neonatorum is a generalized form of tetanus in neonates. It manifests 3–14 days after birth with progressive difficulty in feeding, excessive crying and irritability. This is followed by trismus, risus sardonicus and generalized spasms.

Various scoring systems (Phillips score and Ablett score) are available for assessing the severity and prognosis of tetanus (Table 21.1).

DIAGNOSIS
The diagnosis of tetanus is primarily clinical as there are no diagnostic laboratory tests. A clinical diagnosis of tetanus is made if there is an illness characterized by an acute onset of hypertonia, and/or muscle contractions and generalized muscle spasms without any other apparent causes, and the subsequent disease course is consistent with tetanus. Typically, the patient is fully conscious and there is a preceding history of an event in which the spores gained access to the body. A recent history of injury or bites, or the presence of known portals of entry (e.g. otitis media, dental abscess or an infected wound) supports the diagnosis. In patients with early signs of tetanus such as trismus or neck stiffness, a 'spatula test' may be useful. This test consists of a spatula carefully inserted into the pharynx: if the patient gags and expels the spatula, the test is negative for tetanus; if the patient bites the spatula because of the reflex spasm of the masseters, the test is considered positive. It can aid early diagnosis with 94% sensitivity and 100% specificity (Apte and Karnad 1995).

DIFFERENTIAL DIAGNOSIS
There are few differential diagnoses. Trismus caused by peritonsillar and odontogenic abscesses, and abdominal rigidity caused by local trauma or peritonitis, can be excluded by history and examination. Drug-induced dystonic reactions usually cause torticollis and oculogyric crises but do not cause spasms. Meningeal irritation caused by meningitis or meningoencephalitis can cause generalized hypertonia, neck rigidity and tonic seizures but can easily be differentiated by the presence of impaired cognition. Hypocalcaemic tetany is typically associated with positive Chvostek and Trousseau signs, and it does not involve the

TABLE 21.1
Classification of the severity of tetanus (adapted from Ablett's classification[a])

Grade	Clinical features
I – mild	Mild or no respiratory involvement or dysphagia, no spasm
II – moderate	Moderate respiratory involvement, trismus, dysphagia and spasms
IIIA – severe	Severe respiratory involvement, generalized rigidity and major spasms, no autonomic involvement
IIIB – very severe	Severe manifestations as above with autonomic involvement

[a]Ablett (1967).

trunk muscles. Strychnine poisoning can closely resemble generalized tetanus but trismus is absent. Stiff-man syndrome has an insidious onset; hypertonia involves face and jaw muscles minimally and improves during sleep. Other differential diagnoses include Guillain–Barré syndrome (we have seen a child who initially had characteristic stimulation-induced opisthotonus and arching, mimicking tetanus). In neonates, birth asphyxia, hypoglycaemia, hypocalcaemic tetany, seizures and maple-syrup urine disease can sometimes cause confusion.

MANAGEMENT
The goals of management of tetanus are as follows.

1 Cessation of toxin production.
2 Neutralization of unbound toxin and eradication of the source of toxin.
3 Symptomatic treatment: control of rigidity, spasms and autonomic dysfunction.
4 Appropriate supportive management and avoidance of complications.

Neutralization of unbound toxin
The unbound toxin can be neutralized by rapid administration of human tetanus immunoglobulin (HTIG) or equine tetanus antiserum. Passive immunization shortens the course of disease and may reduce the severity of symptoms.

HTIG is the preparation of choice. It is given by intravenous infusion over 30 minutes. The recommended dose varies from 500–6000 IU; but 1500 IU is most commonly used. If HTIG is not available, equine immunoglobulin 500–1000 units/kg intramuscularly (maximum dose 20 000 units) may be used.

Intramuscular HTIG cannot arrest the axonal ascent of the bound toxin. It is suggested that intrathecal HTIG may neutralize the toxin released from motor neurons and act on the inhibitory interneurons preventing the release of GABA. Use of a combination of intrathecal and intramuscular HTIG has been shown to be superior to intramuscular HTIG alone; the former reduced the frequency and duration of spasms, length of hospital stay, and need for respiratory assistance in adult patients (Miranda-Filho Dde et al. 2004). In a meta-analysis of 942 patients included in 12 trials (484 treated intrathecally and 458 intramuscularly), the combined relative risk of mortality for the intrathecal group compared to the intramuscular group was 0.71 (95% confidence interval, 0.62–0.81). The superiority of intrathecal therapy also emerged when the analysis was performed in subcategories of both adults and neonates, and for high and low dose of intrathecal serotherapy (Kabura et al. 2006). Intrathecal anti-tetanus immunoglobulin in addition to the standard treatment improved the outcome of neonatal tetanus in terms of mortality and hospital stay (Ahmad et al. 2011).

Eradication of source of toxin
Wound debridement removes spores and thereby reduces germination and prevents further absorption of the neurotoxin.

Penicillin is the antibiotic of choice in tetanus. Metronidazole may be used as an alternative. Some authors prefer metronidazole because penicillin is believed to be a competitive GABA antagonist and could therefore cause CNS hyperexcitability at higher doses.

Control of rigidity and spasms

• *Benzodiazepines* (diazepam, midazolam, lorazepam) are the most commonly used agents for control of spasms and rigidity. Diazepam is often the initial choice. It is a sedative and muscle relaxant, has a wide margin of safety and can be given IV, orally or rectally. A diazepam bolus of 0.2mg/kg (diluted to 0.1mg/mL) by IV infusion over 15 minutes is given to terminate spasm. For subsequent control, diazepam or midazolam by continuous infusion is used. The dose is titrated according to the patient's clinical condition and response. At higher doses, diazepam can cause respiratory and myocardial depression and hyperosmolarity because of the propylene glycol used as solvent; the latter can increase the risk of haemolysis and myoglobinuria. Once spasms are adequately controlled, the patient can be shifted to enteral diazepam in 4–6 divided doses through nasogastric tube (Singhi et al. 2001). Midazolam has a relatively short duration of action and early reversibility of sedation, and can be given IM and by other routes, e.g. bucally.

• *Magnesium sulphate.* Magnesium is a physiological antagonist of calcium and causes depression of neuromuscular transmission. It inhibits the release of catecholamines and thus helps in controlling dysautonomia in tetanus. In adults, magnesium sulphate was shown to reduce the need for other drugs such as benzodiazepines and to improve cardiac stability but not to lessen the requirement for ventilation (Thwaites et al. 2006). Its use has not been established in children. The infusion should be titrated to maintain magnesium levels at 4–8mEq/L. In the absence of a facility to monitor magnesium levels, abolition of the patellar reflex may be used as the endpoint and positive Chvostek and Trousseau signs as evidence of hypocalcaemia. Magnesium should be avoided in the presence of renal failure.

• *Neuromuscular blocking agents* are needed in severe tetanus where benzodiazepines fail to control the spasms. Vecuronium is preferred as it has a short duration of action and does not cause cardiovascular instability. Pancuronium should be avoided as it worsens autonomic instability. Endotracheal intubation and mechanical ventilation become necessary once neuromuscular blocking agents are used. Paralysis should be induced with infusions of morphine and midazolam to minimize pain and anxiety.

• *Dantrolene* is a direct-acting muscle relaxant. It has been used for managing spasms and has the major benefit of not requiring artificial ventilation. The drug is expensive and is not recommended for routine use.

• *Baclofen* is a physiological GABA agonist that inhibits medullary reflexes. Intrathecal baclofen has been used to treat muscle rigidity and spasms in tetanus in children older than 1 year. Adverse effects include respiratory depression, coma, hypotension, bradycardia and meningitis (Boots et al. 2000).

Control of autonomic dysfunction (Table 21.2)
Several agents have been used for controlling autonomic dysfunction, including the following.

• *Beta blockers* – propranolol, labetalol and esmolol.
• *Morphine* – a centrally acting sedative with minimal cardiovascular effects.
• *Magnesium sulphate*. A randomized placebo-controlled trial of magnesium sulphate in adults with severe tetanus found a significant lowering of urinary adrenaline and elevated noradrenaline excretion following magnesium therapy (Thwaites et al. 2006).
• *Epidural blockade*. Epidural anaesthesia has been used to control cardiovascular in-stability. Encouraging results were seen with epidural bupivacaine and sufentanil using midazolam as an adjunct (Bhagwanjee et al. 1999).
• *Clonidine* – a centrally acting sympatholytic agent that acts as an anxiolytic and sedative (Gregorakos et al. 1997).
• *Other drugs*. Atropine, sodium valproate, angiotensin-converting enzyme inhibitors and adenosine have been used.

Supportive and other therapies

• *Airway and ventilation*. Securing the airway is the first priority. Patients with pharyngeal spasms and/or upper-airway obstruction are best managed with a tracheostomy; this avoids undue stimulation of the upper airway and prevents spasms and respiratory complications. In others, endotracheal intubation may be attempted. However, it can be very difficult. Tracheostomy is better if the recovery is likely to be slow. Mechanical ventilation is used if the spasms impair respiration and the risk of hypoxaemia and respiratory failure are high.

• *Enteral feeding*. Energy requirements of tetanus patients are high due to spasms. Enteral feeding should be started as early as possible.

• *Antibiotics*. Because associated bacteraemia and sepsis are not uncommon in the neonate,

TABLE 21.2
Pharmacological treatment of tetanus

Drug	Dose	Contraindication	Duration
Antibiotics			
Penicillin G	100 000–200 000 IU/kg IV in 4 divided doses	Hypersensitivity	7–10d
Metronidazole	30–40mg/kg/d IV every 6h; maximum 4g/d	Hypersensitivity	7–10d
Control of spasms: benzodiazepines			
Diazepam	0.2mg/kg initial dose through IV infusion, stepped up rapidly in increments until spasms are controlled; usually 1mg/kg/h. Change to enteral route in 4–6 divided doses through nasogastric tube; max. 2mg/kg/h	Shock, respiratory depression	Full doses for 2–3wks; then gradually tapered off over 2 weeks
Midazolam	0.1–0.3mg/kg/h as IV infusion	Shock	
Lorazepam	0.15mg/kg loading dose, followed by 1–2µg/kg/min	Hypotension, shock	
Neuromuscular blocking agents			
Vecuronium	Initial dose 0.08–0.1mg/kg; then as IV infusion 0.1mg/kg/h	Used cautiously in presence of hepatic or renal disease	Shortest possible
Atracurium	Initial dose 0.5mg/kg, followed by infusion of 4–12µg/kg/min	Safe in hepatic and renal disease	Shortest possible
Intrathecal baclofen	No definite guidelines. Average bolus dose for patients <55 years is 1000µg. Infusion through an epidural catheter placed in the L3–L4 space for prolonged therapy	Known hypersensitivity. Use with caution in presence of respiratory depression and altered consciousness	7–14d

TABLE 21.2
[continued]

Drug	Dose	Contraindication	Duration
Control of autonomic instability			
Propranolol	0.5–1mg/kg/d in 3–4 divided doses. Increased gradually every 3–5 days to 1–5mg/kg/d, max. 8mg/kg/d	Known asthma/chronic obstructive pulmonary disease, cardiogenic shock, bradycardia, pulmonary oedema	6–8wks
Labetalol	IV 0.2–0.5mg/kg/dose titrated to effect, max 20mg/dose. Oral 4mg/kg/d in 2 divided doses, max. 20mg/kg/d	Known asthma, cardiogenic shock, bradycardia, pulmonary oedema	6–8wks
Morphine	0.01–0.1 µg/kg/min as IV infusion or 0.1mg/kg IV every 4–6h	Use with caution in advanced liver and renal disease and in patients with asthma	7–10d
Magnesium sulphate	25–50mg/kg/dose IV as an hourly infusion, max. 2g/dose, repeated every 6h, depending on the clinical response and serum magnesium	Compromised renal function	Maintain serum magnesium at approximately 4–8mEq/L
Clonidine	Initial 5–10µg/kg/min in divided doses every 8–12h. Increase to 5–25µg/kg/min every 6h gradually		

additional broader-spectrum antibiotics are required. Nosocomial infections are also common, especially pneumonia, and need appropriate antibiotics. Gram-negative rods and *Staphylococcus aureus* are the common organisms causing secondary infections.

Good nursing care, with attention to suction to clear secretions from the airway, maintenance of adequate hydration, mouth hygiene, and regular turning of the patient to avoid orthostatic pneumonia and bedsores, will reduce complications.

A single, non-randomized trial from Bangladesh suggests that vitamin C (1g/d) may reduce mortality, although this finding needs confirmation (Hemila and Koivula 2008).

All patients should be monitored for oxygen saturation by pulse oximetry, blood glucose, urea and electrolytes, fluid input/output and caloric intake. In an intensive care unit, continuous electrocardiographic monitoring should be employed for early detection of arrhythmias and autonomic instability.

A stepwise plan for treatment of generalized tetanus is given in Table 21.3.

PROGNOSIS

Localized tetanus has a good prognosis; generalized forms are associated with the worst prognosis. The mortality rate is below 10% in mild generalized disease but goes up to 50% in the severe generalized form and to 90% in neonatal tetanus. Tetanus following penetrating injury has a higher mortality than infection following abrasions. Mortality is lower in otogenic tetanus. The usual causes of death are pneumonia, respiratory failure, sepsis and cardiovascular autonomic instability. The longer the period of onset, the milder the disease is and the better the outcome.

The prognosis for neonatal tetanus is poor, especially with a short incubation period (<7d) or with rapid evolution of symptoms. Afebrile patients have better chances of recovery. Fever is found in patients with brainstem involvement and secondary infections. Antitoxin may modify the disease if it is given during the incubation period or very early in the course of the illness. Recovery may take months and requires starting of new nerve terminals. Neonates who survive may have microcephaly and neurodevelopmental delay, possibly as a result of hypoxia (Barlow et al. 2001).

PREVENTION

Tetanus is entirely preventable with immunization with tetanus toxoid, which induces the formation of specific antitoxins to neutralize the toxin. Following administration of tetanus toxoid to the mother, antibodies pass to the fetus across the placenta to provide protection against neonatal tetanus. A serum antibody titre of 0.01U/mL or more is considered protective.

The primary schedule entails three doses at 4–6 weeks interval starting at 6 weeks of age, and two booster doses, at 18 months and 5 years of age. Thereafter, a booster dose is recommended every 10 years to ensure long-lasting protection. All pregnant women should receive two properly timed doses of tetanus toxoid in the last trimester.

Besides the wound debridement as indicated, wound management should include both

TABLE 21.3
A stepwise management of tetanus

Emergency stabilization

1 Assess, secure and maintain airway and ventilation: prepare for endotracheal intubation using rapid-sequence intubation technique, if generalized rigidity or spasm

2 Establish vital sign monitoring: connect to a multiparametric monitor

3 Establish an intravenous access for sampling and medication. Obtain blood samples for electrolytes, blood urea, creatinine, creatinine kinase

4 Control acute spasms and hypertonia: administer diazepam or midazolam IV, starting with 0.2mg/kg slowly, or 0.4mg/kg rectally if IV not possible. If this compromises the airway or ventilation, intubate using rapid sequence intubation technique

5 Administer human tetanus immunoglobulin (HTIG; 500 units IM) and tetanus toxoid (0.5mL IM), at two different sites

6 Consider intrathecal administration of HTIG (1000 IU)

7 Start crystalline penicillin (100 000 IU/kg/d, given 6 hourly IV) for 10–14d or metronidazole (50mg/kg, IV every 8 hours) for 7–10d

8 Debride and clean the wound under local anaesthesia

9 Transfer the patient to a dark isolated room in the paediatric intensive care unit (PICU)

Early care in PICU

1 Review airway management: plan and perform a tracheostomy if spasms produce any degree of airway compromise or difficulty in managing secretions

2 Start continuous monitoring of heart rate, oxygen saturation, blood pressure and cardiac rhythm

3 Establish a nasogastric tube for fluids, food and drugs: feed small amounts, ideally hourly

4 Control of spasms. Continue benzodiazepine infusion (in incremental doses as needed). If adequate control of spasm is not achieved, try magnesium sulphate infusion (to control muscle spasms and severe generalized rigidity without the need for deep sedation and mechanical ventilation). If still uncontrolled, initiate neuromuscular paralysis with vecuronium infusion. Continue benzodiazepine and morphine for sedation and analgesia

5 Continue antibiotics: crystalline penicillin (100 000 IU/kg/d, given 6 hourly IV) for 10–14d or metronidazole (50mg/kg, IV 8 hourly) for 7–10 days

6 Chart paracetamol 15mg 6 hourly for pain relief; if needed, oral or IV morphine

Continuing management in PICU: next 2–3 weeks

1 Control sympathetic hyperactivity with IV propranolol or labetalol if sustained bradycardia; atropine is useful; a pacemaker may be needed

2 Administer fluids, dopamine or norepinephrine as and when needed to maintain haemodynamic stability. Avoid diuretics and blood

3 Use water or air mattress, if possible, to prevent skin breakdown and pressure sores

4 Maintain benzodiazepines until neuromuscular junction blockade is no longer necessary, tapering the dose over 14–21d

5 Maintain serum magnesium, if used, until spasms are no longer present

Convalescent stage

1 Active physical therapy. Supportive psychotherapy

2 Administer another dose of the appropriate tetanus toxoid

passive immunization with tetanus immunoglobulin and active immunization with vaccine (tetanus–diphtheria–pertusis or tetanus–diphtheria).

Botulism

Botulism is caused by a neurotoxin produced by *Clostridium* species, which produces paralysis of the peripheral nervous system. It affects infants and older children and occurs in five different forms: infantile, food-borne, wound, inadvertent and iatrogenic (Zhang et al. 2010).

Epidemiology

Botulism occurs throughout the world, the spores being found in the soil and dust and in common foods such as honey. Hence, living in rural areas and having parents who work with the soil are recognized risk factors (Zhang et al. 2010). In infantile, wound and inadvertent botulism, the organism produces the toxin in the body. Food-borne botulism occurs with the ingestion of preformed toxins in contaminated (often tinned) foods, whilst iatrogenic botulism occurs following injection of the botulism toxin.

Infants appear to be susceptible due to normal gut flora changes caused by immaturity or changes in diet such as weaning from breast milk or the ingestion of honey. Wound botulism is rare in children and is associated with intravenous drug abuse in older children. Inadvertent botulism, where the *Clostridium* is found in the gastro-intestinal tract, is often associated with gastro-intestinal surgery and disease.

Pathogenesis

A number of species of *Clostridium* cause botulism, but *C. botulinum* is the most common. Clostridia are divided into seven serotypes, designated A–G, according to the neurotoxins that they produce; types A, B, E and F cause disease in humans (Zhang et al. 2010).

The clostridial neurotoxins block neurotransmitter release at the motor-nerve endplates causing paralysis. They inhibit acetylcholine release through cleavage of soluble N-ethylmaleimide-sensitive factor-attachment protein receptors (neurotoxins A and E) or synaptobrevin (neurotoxins B, D and F), which are involved in the exocytosis process of the neurotransmitters. It is this presynaptic blockade that leads to the incremental response on high-frequency repetitive nerve stimulation due to post-tetanic facilitation. Neurotoxins A and B bind irreversibly to nerve endings, but since this does not occur with other types, recovery from types E and F may be more rapid.

The different species of *Clostridium* may cause different clinical features. *C. baratii*, with production of neurotoxin type F, has an earlier age at onset without preceding constipation, and is characterized by development of severe disease, rapid progression to flaccid paralysis and respiratory failure, and a short duration.

Clinical Features

Infantile botulism usually presents after the first 2 weeks of age, although it has been recorded as early as 54 hours after birth (Fox et al. 2005). Constipation is one of the first signs, occurring before the other cholinergic signs such as hypotonia, flaccid paralysis and cranial nerve palsies. The paralysis descends from the cranial nerves to the extremities before affecting the diaphragm.

Food-borne botulism usually occurs 12–36 hours after ingestion of contaminated food, presenting with blurring of vision, diplopia, ptosis, ophthalmoplegia, dysarthria and dysphagia (Brook 2007, Zhang et al. 2010). Symmetrical weakness descends from the head, affecting the upper and lower limbs, and in severe cases causing paralysis of the respiratory muscles. Autonomic involvement presents as constipation, dry mouth, postural hypotension, urinary retention and pupillary abnormalities. Sensations are normal.

DIAGNOSIS

Electrophysiology is often the most rapid way to make a diagnosis, with electromyography usually showing increased insertional activity along with polyphasic motor units of small amplitude and short duration, with normal nerve-conduction studies. These findings are not specific for botulism and can be seen in axonal neuropathies or certain myopathies. Up to 15% of affected individuals do not show any abnormalities. The M-wave amplitude is usually small, and rapid repetitive nerve stimulation causes an incremental response. However, even in severe botulism findings can be relatively non-specific.

Clostridium species isolated from the stools of patients with infantile and inadvertent botulism, and in the tissue from wounds, is sufficient for the diagnosis. Neurotoxins can be detected in the blood (if taken within 2 days of ingestion of the food) or stool, but require mice bioassays which are often not available (Sobel 2005, Brook 2007).

MANAGEMENT

The main modalities of treatment are antitoxin immunoglobulin and supportive treatment.

Intravenous human botulism immunoglobulin administered to infants with botulism reduces duration of intensive care and hospital admission, and decreases the need for mechanical ventilation and nutritional support. Equine immunoglobulin to toxin types A, B and E is used in other types of botulism and in older patients, but is not recommended for infants because of the risk of hypersensitivity reactions and the shorter half-life (5–8 days), which may not be adequate to combat the ongoing intestinal absorption of toxin. Pooled human immunoglobulin is available, which is effective (Chalk et al. 2011), but it is expensive and difficult to obtain (Ramroop et al. 2012).

Supportive nursing care plays an important role while the motor endplates are replaced (Brook 2008). Aminoglycosides may aggravate the neuromuscular weakness. Early elective intubation reduces mortality.

PROGNOSIS

With appropriate supportive care, recovery is usual, although it may take weeks to months in severe cases. The case fatality is about 3%–5% in infantile botulism, usually from aspiration pneumonia or respiratory failure. It is unclear whether *Clostridium* is associated with sudden infant death syndrome. Residual weakness appears to be rare.

Botulism is prevented by avoiding contaminated foods, particularly those in tins and honey. Vaccinations do exist, but are not widely available and would preclude the use of botulinum toxin for medical conditions.

Diphtheria

Diphtheria is an acute infectious disease caused by exotoxin-producing *Corynebacterium* species, typically *C. diphtheriae* and rarely toxigenic strains of *C. ulcerans*.

EPIDEMIOLOGY

C. diphtheriae inhabits human mucosa and skin. It is an aerobic, pleomorphic, gram-positive bacillus. Four biotypes of *C. diphtheriae* (*mitis*, *intermedius*, *belfanti* and *gravis*) are known to cause diphtheria.

Diphtheria is worldwide in distribution. In warm climates, transmission takes place throughout the year; in temperate climates, it tends to occur during the colder months and spreads from person to person through respiratory droplets generated during coughing and sneezing and through close contact with a patient. Asymptomatic respiratory carriage is an important mode of transmission.

Diphtheria is uncommon. Although it affects people of all ages, it occurs most often in unimmunized children, as young infants are often protected by maternal antibodies. With the advent of the World Health Organization's Expanded Program on Immunization, the incidence has decreased. However, the low booster coverage and lack of routine vaccination has led to a shift in the age of patients and to the outbreak of epidemics.

PATHOGENESIS

The respiratory tract and skin can be infected by the toxigenic and non-toxigenic strains of diphtheria. The bacteria adhere to the mucosa via the antigens (K and O). The toxigenic strains produce a biologically active protein consisting of two functionally distinct polypeptides, A and B, linked by a disulphide bond; both fragments are necessary for cytotoxicity. Fragment B binds to specific receptors on susceptible cells and allows fragment A to enter into the cell. The toxin causes both local and systemic cell destruction. The toxic effect on the cells causes tissue necrosis, which enhances growth and production of more toxin.

The necrotic epithelial cells of the mucosa, leukocytes, red blood cells, fibrinous material, diphtheria bacilli and other bacteria from nasopharyngeal flora combine to form the typical membrane, which firmly adheres to the underlying mucosa (Fig. 21.1). The toxin also induces local inflammatory and exudative reaction and spreads haematogenously, causing renal tubular necrosis, thrombocytopenia, myocarditis and demyelination of nerves.

The disease is usually mild in previously vaccinated persons, because the vaccine-induced immunity decreases local tissue spread and necrosis. Vaccination does not prevent infection with toxigenic *C. diphtheriae*. The protective level of serum antitoxin is 0.01 IU/mL, but levels may decline with age.

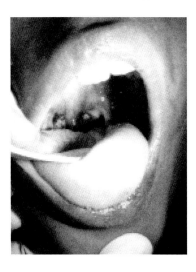

Fig. 21.1. Diphtheretic membrane in a 5-year-old male. A colour version of this figure is available in the plate section at the end of the book.

CLINICAL FEATURES

The typical incubation period is 2–4 days. Onset of symptoms may be insidious, ranging from a moderate sore throat to toxic life-threatening diphtheria involving the larynx or the upper and lower respiratory tracts. The presence of the characteristic thick and smooth, fibrinous, dull greyish pseudomembrane on the respiratory epithelium is pathognomonic. Attempts to remove it result in bleeding.

In a large study of 381 Thai children with clinical and bacteriological diagnoses of diphtheria (Pancharoen et al. 2002), the most common manifestations were a pseudomembrane (100%), fever (92.4%), upper respiratory tract infection (91.6%), upper-airway obstruction (42.3%), hoarseness (36.7%) and 'bull neck' (11.3%). The membrane involved the tonsils (91.9%), pharynx (55.9%) and larynx (27.8%). The major complications were upper-airway obstruction (42.3%), and cardiac (10.0%) and neurological problems (4.7%). The mortality rate was 5.8%. There were significant associations between death and the presence of bull neck, laryngeal patch, airway obstruction and cardiac complications.

The clinical manifestations depend upon the size and site of membrane, immunization status of the host, and production and distribution of the toxin.

Nasal diphtheria is a milder disease causing sore nose and lip, with minimal toxin production.

Pharyngotonsillar diphtheria is the most common form of infection. Initial symptoms are non-specific, such as anorexia, malaise, sore throat and low-grade fever. Within 24 hours, a patch of exudate or dirty white to grey-black membrane appears in the faucial area. In susceptible persons it may spread rapidly, and within 12–24 hours it extends beyond the tonsils and covers the anterior and posterior faucial pillars, the soft palate and the uvula. Cough and stridor are the presenting features in most children with an acute fulminant course. Hoarseness of voice and dysphagia may be evident in 30%–40% of patients (Pancharoen et al. 2002). A variable degree of tender cervical adenitis and, in severe cases, marked swelling causing a bull-neck appearance is characteristic.

Laryngeal diphtheria is usually an extension of the pharyngeal disease. The child presents with fever, hoarseness of voice and a barking cough. With increasing oedema and mechanical obstruction of the airway by the membrane, inspiratory stridor develops. Signs of toxaemia are minimal in primary laryngeal involvement because toxin is poorly absorbed from the mucous membrane of the larynx.

In milder cases, the membrane sloughs off between the 7th and 10th days and the patient has an uneventful recovery. In moderately severe cases, convalescence is slow, and is frequently complicated by myocarditis and neuritis. In severe cases, increasing toxaemia causes severe prostration, rapid thready pulse, stupor, coma, and death within 6–10 days.

Other forms of diphtheria (aural, conjunctival, cutaneous or vulvo-vaginal) are less common.

COMPLICATIONS

Airway obstruction is seen in nearly three-quarters of patients with 'severe disease' and is caused by extension of diphtheritic membrane into the larynx and tracheobronchial tree, worsened further by oedema and congestion. Sudden complete airway obstruction by a detached piece of membrane may cause sudden death. Dexamethasone may prevent tracheostomy in laryngeal diphtheria.

Toxic myocarditis is one of the most serious complications of diphtheria, occurring in 10%–25% of patients. In patients with severe and fulminant disease requiring intensive care, the incidence is much higher (66%); the development of myocarditis is an independent predictor of death (Kneen et al. 1998, Jayashree et al. 2006). Mortality is high in early-onset severe carditis that has progressed to ventricular dysrhythmias.

Neurological complications such as diphtheric neuritis appear after a variable latent period and resolve completely though there are reports of sequelae (Logina and Donaghy 1999). The severity depends on the severity of primary infection. In a series from Thailand, neurological complications were seen in 4.7% of hospitalized patients (Pancharoen et al. 2002).

Paralysis of the soft palate is the most common manifestation of diphtheritic neuritis. It occurs 2–3 weeks after the onset of illness, probably due to local absorption of the toxin. It is characterized by a nasal quality to the voice and nasal regurgitation. It may occur as early as in the first week after onset of illness and usually subsides completely within 1–2 weeks.

Ocular palsy causing paralysis of the muscles of accommodation usually occurs between the 3rd and 5th weeks. It is characterized by blurring of vision and sometimes strabismus.

Paralysis of the diaphragm may occur between the 5th and 7th weeks as a result of neuritis of the phrenic nerve. Death occurs if mechanical respiratory support is not provided.

Peripheral neuropathy involves both the sensory and motor nerves. Paraesthesiae are followed by weakness of the extremities and loss of deep tendon reflexes. Paralysis of limbs

314

occurs between the 5th and 10th weeks and is bilaterally symmetrical. Clinically it may resemble Guillain–Barré syndrome. Nerve-conduction studies show slowing of conduction, prolongation of distal-motor latency and, in severe cases, conduction block.

Other complications may include pneumonia, renal failure, encephalitis, cerebral infarction, pulmonary embolism, thrombocytopenia and coagulation abnormalities.

DIAGNOSIS

The diagnosis of diphtheria is based on clinical signs and symptoms plus laboratory confirmation. Children with sore throat, toxic appearance or symptoms of upper-airway obstruction including croup may have diphtheria. They should be examined for a tonsillo-pharyngeal membrane. The diagnosis is confirmed by the demonstration of *C. diphtheriae* cultured from a clinical specimen obtained from the site of infection, or fourfold or greater rise in serum antibody. In patients with suspected diphtheria, swabs should be obtained for bacterial culture from the nasopharynx, preferably from the edges and underneath the mucosal lesions. The laboratory should be asked to look for diphtheria, as routine cultures are not likely to identify the organism. Presumptive rapid diagnosis is usually obtained with Albert's methylene blue or Gram stain of pharyngeal smear. Diphtheria species that are normal commensals in the throat may yield a false-positive test. Isolated diphtheria species should be classified by biotype (*mitis*, *gravis*, *intermedius* or *belfanti*) and tested for toxigenicity. A polymerase chain reaction-based assay detecting the A and B subunit of the toxin gene has also been developed.

Additional investigations are needed to evaluate the extent of multisystem involvement and to support the presence of infection and detect complications. Serial electrocardiograms should be done in the second week of illness to detect early changes of myocarditis and monitor conduction abnormalities. Cardiac enzymes may be measured to detect myocarditis; lactate dehydrogenase and creatinine phosphokinase are elevated. Elevations in serum aspartate transaminase reflect the severity of myocarditis. A chest radiograph and echocardiography should be obtained to assess the cardiac size and contractility, respectively. Platelet counts to detect thrombocytopenia, serum electrolytes and blood urea nitrogen are obtained to assess renal injury.

DIFFERENTIAL DIAGNOSIS

The following differential diagnoses should be considered, depending on the site of infection.

- Nasal diphtheria may be confused with a foreign body in the nose.
- Pharyngotonsillar diphtheria may resemble acute streptococcal membranous tonsillitis, infectious mononucleosis, non-bacterial membranous tonsillitis, thrush and post-tonsillectomy faucial membrane. In all suspected cases, a swab should be obtained for smear examination and culture.
- In suspected laryngeal diphtheria, other causes of upper-airway obstruction such as infectious croup, spasmodic croup, epiglottis and foreign body in the larynx should be ruled out.

TABLE 21.4
Recommended doses of diphtheria antitoxin

Type of diphtheria	Dosage (units)
Anterior nasal	20 000
Tonsillar (localized)	20 000–40 000
Laryngeal	40 000
Pharyngeal or nasopharyngeal	60 000
Extensive disease of >3 days duration or any patient with brawny swelling of the neck	80 000–120 000

MANAGEMENT

Emergency care
A patient with suspected diphtheria with any signs of upper-airway compromise should immediately receive the following:

1 Oxygen by face mask: calm the child and do not attempt to look inside the mouth.
2 Airway management: attempts at endotracheal intubation should be avoided; early tracheostomy to establish emergency airway is advisable.
3 Dexamethasone, 0.6mg/kg IV.
4 Diphtheria antitoxin.
5 First dose of antibiotic – IV crystalline penicillin.
6 Send throat swab for Albert stain and culture to confirm the diagnosis.

Diphtheria antitoxin
Antitoxin should be administered as soon as a clinical diagnosis of diphtheria is made. It neutralizes the circulating toxin, but not the internalized toxin. Early use reduces local disease and decreases the incidence of systemic complications (Table 21.4).

The preferred route of administration is intravenous, though antitoxin may also be administered by IM injection. For intravenous therapy, antitoxin should be diluted in 250–500mL of normal saline and given by infusion over 90 minutes. The rate for the first 30 minutes should be very slow to allow for desensitization, because currently available diphtheria antitoxin is of equine origin and can result in an acute anaphylactic shock. History regarding previous horse-serum injections or possible allergy should be obtained, and the patient must be tested for hypersensitivity (by intradermal injection of 0.1mL of a 1:100 dilution of diphtheria antitoxin in normal saline). The patient must be carefully monitored during the infusion, and the infusion must be stopped if any signs of shock appear.

Antibiotics
The World Health Organization recommends either penicillin or erythromycin as follows.

- Crystalline penicillin 40 000 IU/kg 4–6 hourly until toxicity subsides, then procaine penicillin 25 000–50 000 IU/kg once daily for a total of 10–14 days.
- Oral erythromycin 40–50mg/kg/d 6 hourly for 10–14 days if child is sensitive to penicillin.

Antibiotic therapy treats localized infection and eradicates *C. diphtheriae*, stops toxin production, and prevents transmission of the organism to contacts. Untreated patients are infectious for 2–3 weeks; antibiotics usually render patients non-infectious within 24 hours.

In an open-label, randomized trial of Vietnamese children with diphtheria, penicillin therapy (IM benzyl penicillin 50 000U/kg/d for 5 days and then oral penicillin 50mg/kg/d for 5 days) resulted in an earlier clearance of fever than oral erythromycin (27 hours vs 46 hours, $p=0.0004$) (Kneen et al. 1998).

Supportive care
Patients with laryngeal diphtheria and any sign of airway obstruction require tracheostomy for securing the airway. Bed rest is required during the acute phase of disease (usually a couple of weeks) to prevent cardiac damage. Regular monitoring of cardiac function with electrocardiography should be performed; a cardiac pacemaker may be needed. Return to normal physical activity is guided by the degree of toxicity and cardiac involvement. Patients with palatal or bulbar paralysis need nasogastric feeding.

PROGNOSIS
The disease can be fatal; 5%–10% of hospitalized diphtheria patients die, even if properly treated. Fatal pseudomembranous diphtheria typically occurs in partially or unimmunized patients with non-protective antibody titres.

Risk factors for death include bull neck; virulence of the organism (*gravis* strain); age under 6 months; extensive pseudomembrane; laryngeal, tracheal or bronchial involvement; myocarditis with ventricular tachycardia; atrial fibrillation and complete heart block; and delay in antitoxin administration after the onset of symptoms (Pancharoen et al. 2002).

PREVENTION
Immunization with diphtheria toxoid produces antibodies that neutralize the toxin and prevent clinical disease. Individuals with an antitoxin titre below 0.01U/mL are at low risk of diphtherial disease. In populations where a majority of individuals have protective antitoxin titres, the carrier rate for toxigenic strains of *C. diphtheriae* decreases and the overall risk of diphtheria among susceptible individuals is reduced.

Prevention among contacts
Individuals in close contact with a diphtheria patient should undergo throat culture to determine whether they are carriers. After the samples for culture are obtained they should be treated immediately with antibiotics. Typical regimens are oral erythromycin, 40–50mg/kg/d 6 hourly for 7–10 days, and benzathine penicillin given as a single IM dose of 1.2 million units for children aged 6 years or older, or 600 000 units for children aged under 6 years.

The immunization status of close contacts should be assessed and managed accordingly to prevent repeat infection with the disease.

REFERENCES

Ablett JJL (1967) Analysis and main experience in 82 patients treated in the Leeds tetanus unit. In: Ellis M, ed. *Symposium on Tetanus in Great Britain.* Boston Spa, UK: National Lending Library, pp. 1–10.

Ahmad A, Qaisar I, Naeem M, et al. (2011) Intrathecal anti-tetanus human immunoglobulin in the treatment of neonatal tetanus. *J Coll Physicians Surg Pak* 21: 539–41.

Apte NM, Karnad DR (1995) Short report: the spatula test: a simple bedside test to diagnose tetanus. *Am J Trop Med Hyg* 53: 386–7.

Barlow JL, Mung'Ala-Odera V, Gona J, Newton CR (2001) Brain damage after neonatal tetanus in a rural Kenyan hospital. *Trop Med Int Health* 6: 305–8.

Bhagwanjee S, Bosenberg AT, Muckart DJ (1999) Management of sympathetic overactivity in tetanus with epidural bupivacaine and sufentanil: experience with 11 patients. *Crit Care Med* 27: 1721–5.

Boots RJ, Lipman J, O'Callaghan J, et al. (2000) The treatment of tetanus with intrathecal baclofen. *Anaesth Intensive Care* 28: 438–42.

Brook I (2007) Infant botulism. *J Perinatol* 27: 175–80.

Brook I (2008) Current concepts in the management of *Clostridium tetani* infection. *Expert Rev Anti Infect Ther* 6: 327–36.

Chalk C, Benstead TJ, Keezer M. (2011) Medical treatment for botulism. *Cochrane Database Syst Rev* 3: CD008123. doi: 10.1002/14651858.CD008123.pub2.

Cook TM, Protheroe RT, Handel JM (2001) Tetanus: a review of the literature. *Br J Anaesth* 87: 477–87.

Fox CK, Keet CA, Strober JB (2005) Recent advances in infant botulism. *Pediatr Neurol* 32: 149–54.

Gregorakos L, Kerezoudi E, Dimopoulos G, Thomaides T (1997) Management of blood pressure instability in severe tetanus: the use of clonidine. *Intensive Care Med* 23: 893–5.

Hemila H, Koivula TT (2008) Vitamin C for preventing and treating tetanus. *Cochrane Database Syst Rev* 2: CD006665.

Jayashree M, Shruthi N, Singhi S (2006) Predictors of outcome in patients with diphtheria receiving intensive care. *Indian Pediatr* 43: 155–60.

Kabura L, Ilibagiza D, Menten J, Van den EJ (2006) Intrathecal vs. intramuscular administration of human antitetanus immunoglobulin or equine tetanus antitoxin in the treatment of tetanus: a meta-analysis. *Trop Med Int Health* 11: 1075–81.

Kneen R, Pham NG, Solomon T, et al. (1998) Penicillin vs. erythromycin in the treatment of diphtheria. *Clin Infect Dis* 27: 845–50.

Logina I, Donaghy M (1999) Diphtheritic polyneuropathy: a clinical study and comparison with Guillain–Barré syndrome. *J Neurol Neurosurg Psychiatry* 67: 433–8.

Mitsui K, Mitsui N, Hase J (1982) Purification and some properties of tetanolysin. *Microbiol Immunol* 24: 575–84.

Miranda-Filho Dde B, Ximenes RA, Barone AA, et al. (2004) Randomised controlled trial of tetanus treatment with antitetanus immunoglobulin by the intrathecal or intramuscular route. *BMJ* 328: 615.

Pancharoen C, Mekmullica J, Thisyakorn U, Nimmannitya S (2002) Clinical features of diphtheria in Thai children: a historic perspective. *Southeast Asian J Trop Med Public Health* 33: 352–4.

Ramroop S, Williams B, Vora S, Moshal K (2012) Infant botulism and botulism immune globulin in the UK: a case series of four infants. *Arch Dis Child* 97: 459–60.

Singhi S, Jain V, Subramanian C (2001) Post-neonatal tetanus: issues in intensive care management. *Indian J Pediatr* 68: 267–72.

Sobel J (2005) Botulism. *Clin Infect Dis* 41: 1167–73.

Thwaites CL, Yen LM, Loan HT, et al. (2006) Magnesium sulphate for treatment of severe tetanus: a randomised controlled trial. *Lancet* 368: 1436–43.

World Health Organization (2012) Estimates of disease burden and cost-effectiveness (online: http://www.who.int/immunization/monitoring_surveillance/burden/estimates/en/index.html).

Zhang JC, Sun L, Nie QH (2010) Botulism, where are we now? *Clin Toxicol (Phila)* 48: 867–79.

22
POSTINFECTIOUS DISORDERS

John T Sladky and Hugh J Willison

This chapter considers disorders believed to have a postinfectious aetiology resulting from the immune response to the infectious agent, rather than a direct infectious effect. In some cases the infectious trigger is clear; however, in most series and in clinical practice, evidence of a preceding infection consists predominantly of the patient's recollection.

A number of acute neurological disorders have been described with distinct clinical presentations. The classic example of this process is chorea, an immune-mediated disorder shown to evolve after infection with type A beta-haemolytic streptococcus. Guillain–Barré syndrome (GBS) and acute disseminated encephalomyelitis (ADEM) are the two most common diagnostic categories among postinfectious diseases. Prior symptoms of an upper respiratory tract infection are the most commonly identified; other environmental encounters include other infections, immunizations, insect and animal bites, trauma and parturition.

The abundance of neurological diseases that fall under the broad rubric of postinfectious is daunting and it will be possible to deal with only a relatively thin representative cross-section of them in this chapter. Nor is there an entirely intellectually satisfying schema of classification that permits a consistent systematic approach to their explication. For the purposes of this discussion we have chosen to divide the group based on whether they affect primarily the central or peripheral nervous systems and whether they are most logically characterized as focal, disseminated or circuit disorders. These criteria are admittedly arbitrary; however, they provide a context in which to examine similarities and differences among these autoimmune diseases that provide insights into a mechanistic understanding of their pathogenesis (Table 22.1).

Pathogenesis

These disorders have final common pathways of tissue injury that consist principally of antibody- and T-cell-orchestrated, macrophage-mediated, cytokine- and complement-modulated epitope attack and cytolysis/proteolysis. While nuanced differences are apparent, there are no cogent reasons to believe that the immune system behaves differently in the brain than in the peripheral nerves. What is clear is that early on in the immunological cascade, an exquisitely precise targeting mechanism is activated that directs subsequent downstream events, resulting in focal tissue or cellular damage and neurological disease. In the most directly relevant examples, there are recognizable homologies between the infectious agent and constituents of the nervous system that reinforce the notion of cross-reactivity underpinning immune-mediated neurological injury, a process that has been termed

TABLE 22.1
Categories of postinfectious neurological disease

Central nervous system disease	
Disseminated disease	ADEM
Restricted disease	Optic neuritis
	Transverse myelitis
	Neuromyelitis optica
	Cerebellitis
	Brainstem encephalitis
Circuit disorders	Sydenham chorea
	PANDAS
	Acute idiopathic choreoathetosis
Antichemoreceptor disorders	Rasmussen syndrome
	Anti-NMDA receptor encephalitis
Peripheral nervous system disease	
Disseminated disease	Guillain–Barré syndrome
	AIDP
	AMSAN
Restricted disease	AMAN
	Miller Fisher syndrome
	Pandysautonomia
	Polyneuritis cranialis
	Brachial neuritis
	Idiopathic VIth nerve palsy
	Bell palsy
	Peroneal neuropathy

ADEM, acute disseminated encephalomyelitis; PANDAS, paediatric acute neuropsychological disorder after streptococcal infection; NMDA, N-methyl-D-aspartate; AIDP, acute inflammatory demyelinating polyneuropathy; AMSAN, acute motor and sensory axonal neuropathy; AMAN, acute motor axonal neuropathy.

'molecular mimicry'. This appears to be the case with *Campylobacter jejuni* and GBS, where epidemiological studies confirm a significant relationship between antecedent *Campylobacter* enteritis and subsequent peripheral neuropathy. There are compositional homologies between oligosaccharides expressed on the lipo-oligosaccharide membrane of the bacterium and neural membrane gangliosides from which oligosaccharide moieties protrude, where they are recognizable by immune surveillance mechanisms. Antibodies directed toward these surface epitopes can be demonstrated in many of these patients and almost certainly play a role in the pathogenesis of the disease. There are even stronger correlations between some GBS phenotypical subtypes in which discrete populations of peripheral axons and Schwann cells are under attack directed by antibodies against specific gangliosides, as has been persuasively demonstrated with anti-GQ1b antibody expression in patients with the Miller Fisher syndrome variant of GBS. Similarly in the acute motor axonal neuropathy variant of GBS, anti-GM1 or -GD1a ganglioside antibodies specifically target motor nerve axolemmal membranes.

The ability of this immune-targeting apparatus to make strikingly precise distinctions between motor and sensory axolemma within mixed peripheral nerves results in the subsequent, equally remarkable, meticulously restricted pattern of tissue injury. Widespread tissue necrosis observed in pathological studies can be explained by multiple antigenic species being targeted, secondary mechanisms such as antigenic spread widening the scope of epitopes coming under immune attack, or other mechanisms of injury such as ischaemia instigated by the initial inflammation. It is likely that the mechanism of tissue injury in these disorders is multifactorial. Perhaps unexpectedly, the immune system is able to accurately segregate neural constituents. Yet the spectrum of pathologies in these disorders ranges from scenarios where the immune system executes a precise and discrete attack to others where the primary target of the immune attack is obscured by inflammation and widespread haemorrhagic tissue coagulation necrosis within areas of injury that may not even respect grey–white matter demarcations in the brain.

Further to the puzzle, there often does not appear to be any rhyme or reason for the topography of injury within the brain or peripheral nervous system in ADEM or GBS. An acute episode of ADEM may consist of a solitary focus of inflammation and demyelination within cerebral white matter, or multifocal lesions with similar pathology, or they may be accompanied by inflammatory and necrotic lesions nested within white matter or even tumefactive regions within deep grey masses in the brain or brainstem. The majority of putative antigens that have been proposed as potential immunological targets for attack in ADEM or GBS, by contrast, are diffusely distributed throughout the nervous system rather than concentrated in multiple discrete foci as the patterns of injury in these diseases might suggest. The host factors that may influence the susceptibility of the individual to respond to a particular infection with a specific autoimmune disorder, the guidance systems determining the antigen(s) targeted for autoimmune attack, and the processes by which that target becomes visible to the immune surveillance system, the regulatory mechanisms governing the breadth and intensity of the attack and finally bringing the process to a close, are incompletely understood. This chapter is intended to paint a recognizable picture from a patchwork of images based on concepts we believe to be based on reliable evidence, whilst acknowledging that some of these snapshots represent speculative interpretations in order to fill gaps in the narrative fabric.

Disorders of the central nervous system (CNS)

ACUTE DISSEMINATED ENCEPHALOMYELITIS

The nosology of this group of disorders suffers from imprecision, due in part to inconsistent criteria employed in classification. ADEM appears to be more common in younger individuals extending from early infancy through early to middle adulthood, tapering off among the elderly. The estimated incidence is around 0.5–1/100 000 individuals below 19 years of age. The peak occurs at around 7 years, and it is relatively uncommon under 2 years. Similar to GBS, ADEM demonstrates a mild male preponderance, with a male:female ratio in the range of 1.2–1.4:1. Most authors have suggested that it has a seasonality, being more common in the winter and spring months, although this has not been a ubiquitous conclusion. At this point, there is no evidence that there are particular geographical correlates with disease phenotype or pathogenesis. By all accounts, it appears that the disease knows no racial, ethnic or geographical boundaries. One would anticipate that it occurs more frequently in regions where wild-type infections with the common childhood viral illnesses have not been controlled with widespread immunization programmes. Reliable data, however, on the worldwide distribution of these disorders is wanting (Leake et al. 2004, Tenembaum et al. 2007, Banwell et al. 2009).

Many large population-based studies have confirmed that about 70% of patients who develop ADEM have a history of antecedent events 6–16 weeks prior to the onset of neurological symptoms, most commonly upper respiratory complaints. Previous vaccine exposure accounts for a small fraction (2%–10%) of affected individuals. Because many of these studies take place in the wake of mass immunization campaigns, higher numbers of patients reporting prior immunization exposure may reflect a purely temporal association between vaccine and disease. Over the past five decades postvaccinal ADEM has been on the decline. This phenomenon may be related to progressive refinement in the vaccine manufacturing process, with the incorporation of recombinant technologies, and the trend away from culturing organisms in vital biological systems or live animals. Most recent surveys found that in general the incidence of antecedent immunization in children presenting with ADEM is not above background levels within the unimmunized population.

A striking exception to this observation, which in a sense proves the rule, is rabies vaccine. In order to fully appreciate the significance of this point it is necessary to be familiar with the historical role that rabies immunization played in our attempts to understand the pathogenesis of ADEM. The first successful experimental primate model of ADEM in humans was developed in the 1930s by Rivers and Schwentker (1935) who performed serial injections of sterile rabbit brain homogenates into monkeys. Some of these animals developed a clinical disease with clinical and pathological features closely resembling cases of postvaccinal encephalomyelitis in patients treated with the Semple rabies vaccine. The brains of affected animals demonstrated widespread, patchy perivascular inflammation along with contiguous regions of axonal demyelination, features virtually indistinguishable from those in human postvaccinal encephalomyelitis. This model became the prototype of 'experimental allergic encephalomyelitis' (EAE), which has been recapitulated in multiple mammalian species using different protocols to induce the autoimmune phenomenon and has become a linchpin approach employed in laboratories worldwide for the study of acute autoimmune diseases of the CNS such as ADEM, transverse myelitis and multiple sclerosis (Noorbakhsh et al. 2008). The work of Rivers and Schwentker suggested quite plainly that the viral component of the immunization might be a relatively innocent bystander in the pathogenesis of postvaccinal encephalomyelitis, which appeared to be induced by sensitization to myelin and perhaps other fractions in the whole-brain homogenates.

The Semple vaccine is produced by homogenizing tissue from live mammalian brains in which the rabies virus is grown, inactivating the virus and injecting a crude sterilized preparation of the homogenate. This vaccine is no longer in use in most resource-rich countries where newer preparations employing recombinant strategies are routinely in place. In some regions where the disease is endemic and public health resources are limited, the Semple preparation continues in use because of its minimal cost. In addition to the inoculation of the patient with a whole-brain homogenate, the vaccine must be administered in multiple sequential injections. This treatment schedule was the likely model for Rivers and Schwentker's protocol for inducing EAE in experimental animals. Given the homologies between rabies immunization and EAE induction, it comes as no surprise that some patients given sequential injections of the Semple vaccine developed neurological complications including ADEM and GBS along with overlap syndromes. In fact, the incidence of serious neurological complications with the Semple vaccine is roughly one in every 200 patients treated for rabies. More recently, the Semple vaccine has been supplanted by formulations that employ recombinant techniques avoiding the administration of neural tissue components; the incidence of adverse neurological events has subsequently diminished dramatically and now approaches the combined incidence of ADEM and GBS in the unimmunized general population. A similar lesson was learned from the massive rubella immunization campaigns of the 1960s and 1970s when there was a relatively high incidence of rheumatological and neurological complications when the vaccine was produced in monkey kidney and duck embryo tissue culture substrates. Later when the virus was produced in human diploid cell culture media, the incidence of these complications too fell dramatically. In the case of both rabies and rubella the virus administered in the vaccine remained essentially unchanged over time. The marked reduction in the complication rates of these vaccines was related to modification of the vehicle, not the infecting organism (Agmon-Levin et al. 2009).

A number of pathogens appear to be capable of eliciting an autoimmune response. As noted above, common childhood epidemic viral illnesses are notoriously neurotropically immunogenic, and measles and mumps in particular have some of the highest frequencies of meningoencephalitis-like complications. Numerous other viral species carry the potential to instigate an immunological reaction, as defined by an increase in the incidence of autoimmune neurological disease among infected individuals compared to the general population. A selection of bacterial and fungal pathogens also share this capacity. Some of the more commonly reported infectious substrates for autoimmune disorders of the CNS are listed in Table 22.2.

Clinical features

The clinical presentation in children with ADEM can be striking, but often not distinctive. Constitutional symptoms such as fever, headache and malaise are nearly ubiquitous. Ataxia, choreoathetosis or pyramidal tract involvement are present in the majority of children. Most parents will also describe altered cognitive status ranging from excessive somnolence to encephalopathy. The latter has been described as a major diagnostic criterion, especially for research purposes. Visual complaints occur in about one in three children, caused by diplopia secondary to cranial nerve involvement, optic neuritis or optic pathway involvement. Seizures

TABLE 22.2
Infections associated with acute disseminated encephalomyelitis

Viral infections	Non-viral infections
Measles	Group A β-haemolytic streptococcus
Rubella	*Mycoplasma pneumoniae*
Mumps	*Legionella pneumonophilia*
Varicella-zoster virus	*Salmonella typhi*
Influenza	Leptospirosis
Hepatitis A	*Plasmodia falciparum*
Hepatitis C	*Rickettsii rickettsii*
Epstein–Barr virus	*Borrelia burgdorferi*
Herpes simplex virus	
Enterovirus 73	

as a presenting feature are seen in roughly one-fifth of children with ADEM, possibly more common and more frequently associated with status epilepticus in younger children (Tenembaum et al. 2002).

Initial laboratory investigations are directed toward identifying potentially treatable illnesses, primarily infections. Routine blood studies frequently reveal reactive changes consistent with an inflammatory process. Spinal fluid examination may be normal but more typically will demonstrate a modest cellular pleocytosis with a mononuclear predominance. The spinal fluid protein concentration may be elevated, reflecting blood–brain barrier breakdown with consequent transudation of serum proteins into the CSF. It may also indicate evidence of intrathecal synthesis of immunoglobulin G (IgG), which could be present with direct invasion of the CNS by the infectious organism or because of an autoimmune-mediated injury to neural tissue. The IgG index measures organism-specific IgG, which is synthesized within the intrathecal space. When an immunization is suspected, an elevated IgG index coupled with the absence of evidence of direct invasion by the organism itself by virtue of a negative culture or the failure to identify its genome via polymerase chain reaction (PCR) techniques strongly buttresses the argument that the relationship is causal and not merely coincidence. Oligoclonal bands on cerebrospinal fluid (CSF) immuno-electrophoresis may be transiently and rarely found in ADEM but more frequently during an acute attack of multiple sclerosis (Banwelli et al. 2007a,b).

The key to establishing the diagnosis is magnetic resonance imaging (MRI), although, ironically, none of the findings that may be present are, in themselves, diagnostic because of the diversity in the nature and location of the lesions. Computed tomographic (CT) images are often normal in the absence of blood products or significant oedema. Most abnormalities are best seen in T2-weighted or fluid-attenuated inversion recovery (FLAIR) spin-echo sequences on MRI. Typical findings reveal patchy, ill-defined areas of increased signal intensity diffusely distributed, predominantly involving white matter although central grey matter structures are commonly involved. Multiple punctate lesions involving the periventricular white matter are frequently noted, and this region appears to be affected in more than half of the children with ADEM. Similar lesions may be present in the brainstem, cerebellum and spinal cord. Occasionally, large confluent areas of increased signal with distinct margination, perilesional oedema and mass effect are discovered. Enhancement on T1 sequences after intravenous contrast administration is atypical for the smaller amorphous regions of increased T2 signal; however, these larger discrete, so-called 'tumefactive' lesions frequently demonstrate contrast enhancement reflecting blood–brain barrier incontinence and regions of perilesional oedema. Some of these types of lesions may exhibit partial or complete ring enhancement mimicking tumour or abscess. Other patterns of enhancement include patchy, punctate, nodular, gyral or, less frequently, linear meningeal enhancement. A small portion of children (<5%) will develop a more severe clinical syndrome frequently associated with haemorrhagic lesions on MRI. This syndrome has been termed acute haemorrhagic encephalomyelitis (AHEM) and carries considerably greater short- and long-term morbidity and mortality (Banwell et al. 2007a,b; Marin and Callen 2013).

Like the clinical neurological deficits of the disease, the lesions illustrated on MRI are dynamic in nature and frequently change over time. Most of the lesions that accompany the clinical presentation of ADEM are transient. In some series one-half to three-quarters of MRI scans normalize after treatment and recovery on follow-up examinations. Some have proposed that normalization of the MRI scan within 6 months be a sine qua non for the diagnosis of ADEM as opposed to multiple sclerosis (Anlar et al. 2003, Banwell et al. 2007a, Dale and Pillai 2007, Alper et al. 2009).

Relapse

For the most part, ADEM is a monophasic illness with a relatively rapid pace of progression from onset to nadir and from initiation of treatment to the beginning of recovery. The rate of progress early in recovery can also be remarkably rapid, with some children achieving nearly complete return to normal within a matter of days. Alternatively slow, gradual improvement may continue more than a year after the acute illness. The literature suggests that 5%–20% of children with ADEM will sustain a relapse within the first 6 months. These estimates are compromised by the absence of clear clinical criteria to define relapse. They likely overestimate the real incidence by including exacerbations related to weaning of treatment. ADEM is a relatively rare disease in childhood, and the number of centres with extensive experience in managing the disorder is limited: blinded, controlled treatment trials and standardized treatment protocols are difficult to realize. Most children receive corticosteroids at some time during the course of illness and are then tapered off of these drugs according to idiosyncratic schedules. Recurrence of clinical symptoms may occur when corticosteroids are rapidly lowered, possibly owing to recurrence of oedema or intensification of the attenuated inflammatory process. A more accurate estimate of the rate of recurrent ADEM may be 5% or even less (Anlar et al. 2003, Divekar et al. 2007).

The International Pediatric Multiple Sclerosis Study Group has promulgated a set of definitions (Table 22.3) that seem appropriate to allow clinicians to develop a shared nomenclature (Krupp et al. 2007, Dale et al. 2009). The primary distinction between 'recurrent

TABLE 22.3
Definitions of acute disseminated encephalomyelitis (ADEM)[a]

ADEM	First clinical event
	Presumed inflammatory or demyelinating
	Multifocal
	Includes encephalopathy and at least one other symptom
	Event is followed by improvement – clinical, MRI or both
	No prior demyelinating event clinically or on MRI
	No other aetiologies can explain the event
	New or fluctuating symptoms or MRI lesions occurring within months of onset are considered part of the initial event
Recurrent ADEM	Recurrence of original symptoms or signs ≥3 months after first event
	No new areas of involvement by clinical or MRI criteria
	Patient not on steroids and at least 1 month after completing therapy
Multiphasic ADEM	ADEM followed by new clinical event meeting criteria for ADEM but involving new anatomic areas of the central nervous system
	Event occurs at least 3 months after initial event and 1 month after treatment
	Symptoms or signs differ from initial event but include encephalopathy
	Magnetic resonance imaging shows new lesions with complete or partial resolution of prior lesions

[a]Krupp et al. (2007), Dale et al. (2009).

ADEM' and 'multiphasic ADEM' has to do with the fact that the latter involves the dissemination of the inflammatory process to affect new regions of the CNS as opposed to a recapitulation of the process in previously targeted areas of injury. Some authors have given considerable weight to this distinction in terms of whether the second episode foreshadows the emergence of multiple sclerosis. Data in children are limited, as is the duration of follow-up in most of the largest series; hence, it is difficult to know whether the distinction has, in fact, any predictive value. The hope is that these terms will become incorporated into the vocabulary and thought processes of those clinicians who routinely care for children with acute and chronic demyelinating diseases, and will help to standardize the nosology for future multicentre initiatives.

Therapy
As alluded to above, there are no extant blinded, randomized, controlled therapeutic trials in ADEM in children. Perusal of a number of series of children with ADEM reveals that most who have developed significant neurological disability have been treated, the majority with corticosteroids, some with intravenous immunoglobulin, plasmapheresis or all three. Treatment strategies in children have largely been extrapolated from trials in adults. The most internally consistent and intellectually satisfying arguments can be made in favour of high-dose parenteral corticosteroids. The severely ill child with ADEM presents a scenario where it is difficult to advocate for restraint in terms of the dosage since acute side-effects

can be monitored and managed in the hospital setting. A regimen of methylprednisolone, 30mg/kg/d up to a maximum of 1g depending on the size of the child, given intravenously in three or four divided doses seems appropriate. The drug can be continued for 3 days or longer, depending on the clinical response, followed by a change to an oral regimen equivalent to 2–3mg/kg/d for sufficiently long to be confident that there is no clinical deterioration. The drug should then be slowly tapered over 10–12 weeks to avoid recrudescence of symptoms.

Prognosis

In general, the prognosis is good. Lesions vary in both number and size, their topography is apparently random, and the pathology of individual lesions fluctuates from site to site. Clearly it is impossible to define a consistent starting point to correlate with a later outcome. The situation is further complicated because of relapsing or recurrent disease and rarely may be the sentinel event heralding the later development of multiple sclerosis. In three series from the post-MRI era in which patients were not routinely treated, children demonstrated gradual improvement over several weeks after the illness and 50%–75% appeared to achieve complete recovery. There appeared to be a relationship between the severity of changes on MRI and the nature of antecedent infection and outcome. More extensive white matter injury was associated with incomplete recovery, and ADEM after wild-type measles or rubella infection had a more severe course and worse outcome than post-varicella illness (Tenembaum et al. 2007, Donmez et al. 2009). Treatment has limited if any effect on long-term outcome, but may hasten clinical improvement. Mortality is quite rare.

Acute disseminated encephalomyelitis and multiple sclerosis

Childhood onset of multiple sclerosis is fortunately a rare occurrence. It is estimated that roughly 0.5% of patients with multiple sclerosis have their first episode under 10 years of age and 3%–4% before the age of 16. By contrast, ADEM is more common in childhood. The likelihood that a child who develops ADEM will later be diagnosed with multiple sclerosis is, for various reasons, difficult to characterize with accuracy. A fundamental issue is the lack of a consistent definition of terms that have been incorporated into the larger studies. A second issue is the limited follow-up in many well-designed studies. Looking at a range of studies performed on different continents over the past decade, it appears that roughly 25% of children who present with an ADEM-like illness at the initial encounter will accrue subsequent clinical episodes that establish a definite diagnosis at some point in the future. There are no diagnostic linchpins that permit reliable predictive information regarding subsequent multiple sclerosis in children. This is unfortunate as such information would be useful for counselling and early intervention. Clinical features that weight the odds, either in favour of or against developing multiple sclerosis, are listed in Table 22.4.

RESTRICTED DISEASE

Transverse myelitis

Transverse myelitis is an uncommon disorder, especially in childhood. Despite its rarity, it

TABLE 22.4

Clinical features that influence the risk of developing multiple sclerosis after acute disseminated encephalomyelitis

Increased risk	First event at ≥10 years
	Magnetic resonance imaging showing features of multiple sclerosis[a]
	Optic nerve lesion on magnetic resonance imaging
Decreased risk	Myelitis at onset
	Severe encephalopathy
	Negative oligoclonal bands in cerebrospinal fluid

[a]Presence of multiple well-circumscribed lesions at grey–white junctions and in periventricular white matter.

has perhaps received a disproportionate amount of attention in the neurological literature over the past century or more. Childhood myelitis has been the subject of treatises by several of the more august practitioners of child neurology of the 19th and 20th centuries including Bernard Sachs, Frank Ford and Richmond Paine. Some current authors eschew the term transverse myelitis in favour of the more generic transverse myelopathy. We prefer the former because we believe it has cogency both in terms of its nosological context and also because of important historical connotations. The term itself evolved, at least in part, as a practical imperative. The clinical and pathological features of epidemic poliomyelitis were enumerated in the mid-19th century by Charcot and colleagues at the Salpetrière at a time when the highly transmissible nature of the disease was well recognized and the infectious aetiology postulated. Although 'epidemic myelitis' and the emerging entity 'transverse myelitis' shared many features, it was noted that with the exception of pain, sensory disturbances, especially dense sensory deficits, were rare in infectious poliomyelitis. The term transverse myelitis emphasized the importance of a relatively symmetrical, although not necessarily congruent sensory and motor deficit that helped to distinguish the disorder from the highly infectious viral disease that may herald an impending epidemic. The diagnosis therefore had considerable practical implications for managing the patient, quarantining family and contacts, and taking appropriate public health precautions.

Transverse myelitis has a worldwide distribution without appreciable racial or ethnic predispositions. The incidence in childhood is difficult to quantify. Most series that include patients of all ages estimate the incidence to be between one and four persons per million, or about one-tenth the incidence of ADEM or GBS in the general population. The age distribution is bimodal, with peaks occurring in the teens and in the fourth decade. About 20% of individuals with transverse myelitis are less than 18 years old at the time of their disease. There are approximately 300 new cases annually in the population under 18 years of age in the USA. A recent large series of children observed a separate bimodal pattern in age of presentation under age 18 years, with the first peak in the 1–3 year age group, and the second around 14–16 years. The experience in most tertiary referral centres that care for children with transverse myelitis is that cases tend to cluster in time, and experienced clinicians observe considerable variation in the annual rate of admissions from one year to the next.

Given the polyfactorial nature of the pathogenesis of the disease, it is difficult to know how to account for these fluctuations over time. It is also true that the characteristics of a disease such as antecedent events, clinical severity or response to treatment may be location specific. Snapshots taken simultaneously at different geographic locations may result in quite different clinical images of transverse myelitis.

• *Clinical features.* A history of an antecedent event recognizable to the patient or family, most commonly an upper respiratory tract infection, is obtained in roughly two-thirds of patients in the 12 weeks preceding the onset of symptoms. In the large series from Johns Hopkins just under a third of the children reported receiving an immunization in the 30 days prior to the onset (Pidcock et al. 2007). The bulk of these children were in the 3 years and under age group, which is the most highly immunized segment in childhood. No coherent pattern emerged to suggest a causal link between immunization and transverse myelitis.

By definition, clinical symptoms are confined to dysfunction of spinal cord segmental levels and those sensory and motor modalities traversing long tracts that pass through the affected regions. General malaise, fever and headache are less frequent than in ADEM, while back and leg pain is more common (Kahloon et al. 2007, Pidcock et al. 2007, Yiu et al. 2009).

Characterizing the extent of the disease process within the cord can be difficult on the basis of the clinical examination, even in older children who are able to understand and cooperate. Children with transverse myelitis generally present with a history of dysaesthesiae followed by segmental weakness and back pain. This scenario, acute onset of symptoms of myelopathy, is a true medical emergency, and it is imperative to mobilize the necessary resources to exclude potentially treatable causes that might require urgent surgical intervention. MRI studies will be able to exclude spinal cord compression, mass lesions, haemorrhage or significant trauma. At this point, the differential diagnosis is extensive; transverse myelitis may be most difficult to distinguish from GBS because of the propensity of deep tendon reflexes to be diminished or absent in the acute phases of the illness and because MRI may be normal early in the disease course. Table 22.5 represents a meta-analysis of several previous series describing the clinical features of transverse myelitis in children. The data from the different studies were amalgamated to create an equivalent mean, although the data were incomplete in that some measures of particular variables were not included in all of the series, or the data were not generalizable (Paine 1953, Dunne et al. 1986, Knebusch et al. 1998, Defresne et al. 2003, Pidcock et al. 2007, Kalra et al. 2009, Yiu et al. 2009).

The single most useful diagnostic finding at the bedside is the demonstration of a segmental level of dysfunction on examination. Classically, this consists of demonstrating a 'level' of sensory loss corresponding to the somatotopical geography of the lesion. This may include tactile reflexes. There is often discordant sensory loss when the lesion does not homogeneously affect the entire cross-sectional area of the cord. There may be disproportionate involvement of those sensory modalities located in predominantly ventral or dorsally positioned tracts within the cord. MRI studies are essential to appreciate the true boundaries of inflammation within the cord parenchyma. If myelitis presents as the salient manifestation

TABLE 22.5
Clinical features of transverse myelitis in children[a]

Age	7.4 years
Male:female ratio	0.97:1
Preceeding infection	Average time between symptoms of infection and onset of transverse myelitis, 10 days
Pain of any sort	78%
Back pain	51%
Progressive phase	3 days
Plateau phase	7.5 days
Weakness	92%
Upper-extremity weakness	42%
Sensory loss or numbness	85%
Sensory level	
Cervical	17%
Thoracic	63%
Lumbosacral	9%
Uncertain	9%
Positive sensory phenomena	60%
(dysaesthesiae, Lhermitte sign)	
Sphincter dysfunction	91%
Chair- or bed-dependent at clinical nadir	87%
Mortality	3%

[a]The data in this table represent an amalgamation of multiple series culled from the literature over a half century epoch. It is not meant to represent a statistical analysis, but instead a 'best possible fit' of phenomenological observations in so far as information from several sources could be amalgamated (Paine 1953, Altrocchi 1963, Dunne et al. 1986, Knebusch et al. 1998, Defresne et al. 2003, Pidcock et al. 2007, Kalra et al. 2009, Yiu et al. 2009).

of ADEM, cranial MRI may often provide evidence of subclinical involvement of the cerebral hemispheres. As many as 10%–20% of patients with transverse myelitis will have a normal MRI scan in the early stages of the disease. The MRI may later become abnormal as the disease pathology progresses (Table 22.6). The most common abnormalities are abnormal signal characteristics on T2-weighted, FLAIR and diffusion-weighted spin-echo sequences. Swelling of the cord is the next most frequent finding, seen in about half of the MRI examinations in children with transverse myelitis, followed by signal attenuation on T1-weighted sequences. Most studies demonstrating tissue swelling will also indicate evidence of inflammation or blood–brain barrier breakdown in the form of focal enhancement after injection of intravenous contrast medium. CSF examination is abnormal in around 70% of patients, with elevations of the cell count with a predominantly lymphocytic pleocytosis or total protein concentration or both. Oligoclonal bands are present in approximately 6%, while measures for evidence of intrathecal IgG synthesis are typically normal. Studies to exclude infection should be performed routinely, including the application of

TABLE 22.6
Magnetic resonance imaging features
of transverse myelitis in childhood

Normal study	10%
Abnormal study	90%
Increased T2 signal	
Cervical	50%
Thoracic	40%
Lumbosacral	7%
Holocord	6%
Cord swelling	51%
Hypointense T1 signal	37%
Contrast enhancement	70%

antibody- and PCR-based techniques. Demonstration of specific intrathecal antibody synthesis, however, can be very useful for confirmation when a particular antecedent infection or immunization is suspected as the causative agent.

• *Treatment.* The first line of therapy in transverse myelitis is corticosteroids. Methylprednisolone at a dose of 30mg/kg/d IV to a maximum of 1g/d for 3–5 days is usually recommended (Defresne et al. 2003, Yiu et al. 2009). This is followed with a fairly prolonged tapering regimen of oral steroids in order to avoid a relapse due to precipitous withdrawal. Some small case series and uncontrolled studies report successful treatment with intravenous immunoglobulin or plasmapheresis. The data are insufficient to support specific therapeutic recommendations in children. The majority of patients have some degree of bladder dysfunction early in the course of their illness that requires immediate attention at admission and appropriate intervention and management during recovery. Early institution of physical and occupational therapy is essential to optimized recovery and outcome.

• *Prognosis.* In general, the prognosis is good. It is certainly better among children than in adult populations. The disease is, however, capable of producing devastating outcomes, and different observers have come away from the issue with quite different perspectives. Two relatively recent reports of comparatively large series of children with transverse myelitis, one from a well-known institute for paediatric rehabilitation in the USA and the other from a tertiary children's hospital in Australia, show the potential differences in observation. In the first instance, patients were referred for evaluation after treatment of the acute episode of transverse myelitis, in some instances up to 35 years earlier (Pidcock et al. 2007). In the second, patients were referred for acute treatment (Yiu et al. 2009). The long-term outcome of patients seen in the US rehabilitation facility proved to be a cautionary tale, with only 36% of patients able to ambulate 30ft (9.1m) independently. By contrast, 82% of patients followed up 12 months after treatment at the Australian children's hospital were either completely recovered (50%) or independently ambulatory. Possible explanations for these remarkable differences in outcome include the referral patterns to the rehabilitation facility or differences in the acute management of the disease. All patients reported from Australia were treated acutely between 1997 and 2004 with a protocol including high-dose intravenous corticosteroids, whereas the US series included a far more heterogeneous group seen over a more protracted time interval; many did not receive specific treatment during acute illness. Most studies show that children generally do well. The characteristics associated with poor outcome are: very young age, flaccid paresis below the level of the lesion at the time of presentation, high cervical involvement and respiratory failure requiring mechanical support (Dunne et al. 1986, Defresne et al. 2003, Miyazawa et al. 2003, Tanaka et al. 2006, Banwell 2007, Hamnik et al. 2008, Yiu et al. 2009).

Acute transverse myelitis and multiple sclerosis
In comparison to older populations, the risk of developing chronic autoimmune neurological disease after an episode of transverse myelitis in childhood, in the form of either multiple sclerosis or neuromyelitis optica (NMO), is surprisingly low. There are a number of clinical features that appear to correlate with an increased likelihood of having relapsing disease in adulthood. One of the stronger associations is the presence on MRI of longitudinally extensive disease, defined by evidence of MRI signal abnormalities involving multiple adjacent levels in the spinal cord, which carries with it an enhanced risk of recurrence and/or progression to clinical multiple sclerosis. This finding on MRI is also indicative of increased risk of developing NMO and testing positive for the anti-aquaporin 4 antibody, thought to be a highly reliable marker for the disease. By comparison, the risk of recurrence in children is very low, in the order of 5%, as is the future risk of developing multiple sclerosis, testing positive for the aquaporin-4 antibody or going on to a clinically confirmed diagnosis of NMO.

Optic neuritis
Optic neuritis is characterized largely by the company it keeps. Much of the impact of the disease is related to what it may bode for the future predominantly as a symptom of a more widespread autoimmune disorder, either with multiorgan involvement such as systemic vasculitis or one confined to the nervous system, multiple sclerosis or NMO. When the diagnosis of idiopathic optic neuritis is made in an adult, it is predicated on exclusion of other aetiologies. The spectre of multiple sclerosis and NMO persists, however, because one of these entities may surface at a later date. In childhood it is more often possible to identify major risk factors in the early stages of the disease and to reassure the patient and family regarding the prognosis and the potential risk for other autoimmune neurological complications.

The typical presenting complaint is visual loss, often accompanied by eye pain that may be exacerbated by eye movement. The visual disturbance can be unilateral or bilateral. The ratio of unilateral to bilateral disease varies from series to series, but reports range from around 40:60 to 60:40. Among patients below 18 years of age the mean age at onset is around 10 years, although this observation appears to be influenced by the population from which the patients are identified: those culled from multiple sclerosis clinics tend to be slightly older. The male:female ratio is similarly influenced by the ascertainment process but, on the whole, appears to be roughly equal. The classic clinical findings include an inflamed optic disk, anterior distribution visual loss and an afferent papillary defect in affected eyes. The pattern of visual loss can be quite protean including enlarged scotomata, visual field defects or complete visual loss. The degree of visual loss in the acute phase is often more severe in children than in adults, and is in the severe range in 60%–70% of eyes. About 25%–30% of optic disks will appear normal in children with optic neuritis, hence the term retrobulbar neuritis implying that swelling and inflammation are occurring proximal to the optic nerve head and are not apparent during ophthalmoscopy. Abnormalities can be visualized in the optic nerves or chiasm in somewhat more than half of patients on MRI in terms of abnormal signal intensity, swelling of the nerve or contrast enhancement. Patchy changes in white matter within the cerebral hemispheres is also present in about half of children with acute optic neuritis, especially bilateral optic neuritis, which can be considered as a form of ADEM. Visual evoked potential studies can be useful as adjunctive diagnostic investigations and are abnormal in 80%–90% of affected eyes (Wilejto et al. 2006, Alper and Wang 2009, Banwell et al. 2009).

• *Treatment.* High-dose intravenous corticosteroids is the widely accepted first-line therapy for acute optic neuritis in both adults and children (Kaufman et al. 2000, Toker et al. 2003, Wilejto et al. 2006). The usual protocol prescribes methlyprednisolone at a dose of 30mg/kg/d up to a maximum dose of 1g/d for 3 days followed by a prolonged tapering-off period using oral preparations.

• *Prognosis.* The prognosis for recovery of visual function is generally excellent. Almost irrespective of the degree of visual loss, roughly 75% of eyes achieve a full recovery. Somewhere in the order of 25%–30% of children with optic neuritis will go on to develop multiple sclerosis at some point later in life. In most but not all of those cases, cranial MRI will demonstrate signal changes. In a smaller fraction of children the initial episode of optic neuritis will be the first manifestation of NMO. Acute bilateral optic neuritis with a completely normal MRI scan carries a low risk for future multiple sclerosis (Toker et al. 2003, Alper and Wang 2009, Cakmakli et al. 2009).

Neuromyelitis optica
The description of the disease is credited to Eugene Devic and his graduate student Fernand Gault in 1894 and classically the diagnosis requires presentation with acute optic neuritis along with transverse myelitis either sequentially or in combination with a subsequent chronic and relapsing or progressive course. There has been a century of contention around the issue of whether and how this disease differs from multiple sclerosis because, as the disease progresses, cerebral hemispheric involvement is almost inevitable. The argument was refined by the publication from a group at the Mayo Clinic showing that the disease in large measure is apparently mediated by antibodies directed toward aquaporin-4, the most

important water transport channel in the brain, also present in other organs, prominently in gut and kidney. The aquaporin-4 protein is highly concentrated in astrocyte foot processes especially on the abluminal surfaces of cerebral blood vessels. This autoantibody, termed NMO-IgG, is present in 75%–80% of patients with clinically defined NMO but may also be found in a minority of patients with multiple sclerosis (Magana et al. 2009, Saini et al. 2010). There is also a strong correlation among adults with longitudinally extensive myelitis defined as those patients in whom spinal cord lesions extend up to and beyond three vertebral segments on MRI and which portend high risk of relapse or progression to clinically definite NMO. This association has not been observed in children. In adults there is a strong female preponderance, and this may also be the case, although to a much lesser extent, among children with the disease. Although familial cases have been reported, there are no reports of multigenerational occurrences in kinships.

An unanswered question that frequently arises is why should the pathology localize to optic nerve and spinal cord when the aquaporin-4 protein is widely distributed in the brain and other tissues? First, this distribution appears to be more tightly correlated among adults than children. Approximately 60% of adults with chronic relapsing NMO have lesions of the cerebral hemispheres on MRI. My own anecdotal experience (JTS) is that it is closer to ubiquitous among children with a decade of disease. Unlike in patients with relapsing and remitting multiple sclerosis, the recovery after an attack of NMO is less complete and there is a stepwise pattern of cumulative disability over time (Hamnik et al. 2008, Saini et al. 2010).

Histopathologically the lesions of NMO are typically in perivascular locations, which corresponds to the distribution of the aquaporin protein within the glia limitans of astrocytes around blood vessels. The inflammatory infiltrates more frequently contain prominent numbers of neutrophils and eosinophils as opposed to the typical lymphocytic inflammation seen in multiple sclerosis. In addition, compared to the acute lesions in multiple sclerosis, which are characterized by evidence of demyelination with axonal sparing, those of NMO are more apt to be associated with coagulation necrosis of affected tissues resulting in encephalomalacia. Many of the drugs that are mainstays of treatment in multiple sclerosis are ineffective in NMO. Treatment relies on immunosuppression using corticosteroids, azathioprine, cyclosporine, or even cyclophosphamide. Both plasmapheresis and intravenous immunoglobulin are thought to be efficacious for acute attacks, although controlled trials are wanting even among adults with this disease, let alone children. There are isolated reports of other immunosuppressant regimens showing promise. One can hope for more effective, less toxic therapies in the future; however, the current prognosis is rather bleak and appears to correlate inversely with the age at onset.

Cerebellitis

Postinfectious ataxia is generally a benign disorder, which for nearly a century has been recognized as a relatively common sequel to varicella infection. It garnered the appellation 'cerebellitis' because of the apparently discrete involvement of cerebellar pathways in the syndrome and because of the frequency of aseptic CSF with evidence of lymphocytic inflammatory features on lumbar puncture. Affected children typically develop axial greater than appendicular ataxia around 7–14 days after the vesicular eruptions of varicella have resolved. While this infection has largely disappeared from the list of commonly encountered, epidemic viral infections of childhood following the introduction of the varicella vaccine, not so the clinical entity of presumed postinfectious cerebellitis. It is difficult to know just how common this entity is. The clinical semiology has become part of the pattern recognition repertoire of general paediatricians who are by and large comfortable making the diagnosis and following the patient without referral. In a fraction of cases there may be a history of antecedent symptoms attributable to an infection but rarely any as striking and memorable as a case of chickenpox. It seems reasonable to assume that if varicella is capable of instigating this clinical syndrome, other organisms might also act as immune triggers for the disorder. Treatment is purely supportive. The outcome is almost invariably a complete recovery; however, rare instances of permanent ataxia do occur (Adams et al. 2000, Nussinovitch et al. 2003). More importantly, in the differential diagnosis the physician should consider posterior fossa tumours, paraneoplastic manifestations of neuroblastoma and drug intoxications, all of which present with similar symptoms in the same age group.

CIRCUIT DISORDERS

Sydenham chorea
Sydenham chorea is one of the earliest-recognized disorders in child neurology. The term is attributed to Paracelsus in the 16th century when the disease was colloquially described as St Vitus dance after the patron saint of dancers because of the relatively acute onset of dramatic, involuntary movements intensified with excitement. The striking semiology was reemphasized by Sydenham a century later and subsequently reclaimed attention as one of the major criteria for the diagnosis of rheumatic fever, perhaps the archetypal postinfectious autoimmune disease. In addition to the involuntary movements, behavioural alterations were recognized as prominent features of the disease by Sir William Osler in the late 19th century (Walker et al. 2006).

Chorea appears as the main symptom sometimes months after group A beta-haemolytic streptococcal infection. This gram-positive bacterium is astonishingly immunoreactive and capable of presenting an abundance of biologically significant epitopes resulting in auto-antibodies directed toward multiple tissue targets within multiple organs. One of the most thoroughly investigated and securely established examples of molecular mimicry, the group A streptococcal M protein plays a critical role in rheumatic heart disease and is an integral player in the process of generating auto-antibodies cross-reacting to host α-helical proteins including myosin, tropomyosin, keratin, vimentin and laminin. The M protein may also play a role in the pathogenesis of chorea, but the principle actor in the neurological disorder appears to be the group A carbohydrate moiety, which harbours the epitope N-acetyl-β-D-glucosamine (GlcNAc), which produces auto-antibodies that cross-react with lysoganglioside G_{M1}. Multipotent antibodies derived from humans with Sydenham chorea can be shown to bind simultaneously to neurons at two sites: within the neuropil where they bind to the α-helical structural protein tubulin, and also to the external cell membrane where they are capable of activating calcium-calmodulin-dependent protein kinase II in human neuronal precursor cells in vitro (Martino and Giovannoni 2004, Teixeira et al. 2005a, Kirvan et al. 2007). The precise binding site on the cell surface has yet to be characterized. These antibodies are, therefore, potentially capable of altering circuit function by modifying neuronal activity or by neuronolysis, causing transient functional perturbations or permanent transformation of dynamic striatal circuitry respectively, affecting movements, mood, affect and attention.

The typical presentation is in childhood, usually the second half of the first decade. There may be a female preponderance. The hyperkinetic movement disorder is typically the herald manifestation of the disease but it may be antedated by alterations in mood, affect or behaviour. Unlike more indolently evolving movement disorders, the accessory movements are initially obvious to parents as new phenomena. These are usually perceived as 'clumsiness' as the non-volitional movements often result in upset objects, loss of balance or falls. The movements themselves are rarely confined to chorea and almost invariably include athetoid and ballistic components that engender the most salient motor symptoms. The movements are less prominent at rest and can be brought out by asking the patient to perform complex volitional tasks. Maintaining a stationary posture or activity may invoke dystonic postures and motor impersistence: the classic finding is the so-called 'milkmaid's grip'. Observing the patient's gait can be very informative as the athetoid movements of the legs impose an obvious impairment of coordination and tendency to stumble. Less commonly, speech may be affected in the form of disturbed modulation of phonation (Swedo et al. 1993, Bonthius and Karacay 2003, Walker et al. 2006, Cardoso 2008).

Because of the stereotypical nature of the movement disorder, it is understandable that focus should have been on disturbances affecting the basal ganglia, and autoantibodies directed toward epitopes related to synaptic function of neuronal populations in those regions have been described including the globus pallidus, putamen and subthalamic nucleus (Martino and Giovannoni 2004, Teixeira et al. 2005a). It is difficult, if not impossible, however, to interrupt the functional integrity of neurotransmitter systems within these deep regulatory centres without altering behaviour in multiple cortico-thalamo-striatal feedback pathways that more widely impact neurological function. Hence, the cogency of the term circuit disorder to describe these types of neurological disease. Although the hyperkinetic movement disorder is the most obvious, and may be the sole neurological manifestation of the disease, it is often not the most disabling or disturbing to the child and family. Frequently, emotional lability, attentional disturbances and profound affective symptoms including obsessive/compulsive ideations, anxiety and depression are present. In concert, these factors impair both the patient's desire and capability to participate in social activities and daily life (Swedo et al. 1989, 1993).

As with other postinfectious autoimmune diseases, Sydenham chorea is usually a self-limited disorder. The peak of the illness generally lasts several weeks with gradual attenuation in the frequency and amplitude of the accessory movements. The psychiatric manifestations similarly wane over time. Traditionally, it was thought that in most cases recovery is complete within 6–9 months; however, in some series as many as half of the children have psychological disturbances that persist for 2 years or more. Reports of an exacerbation of symptoms after repeat episodes of streptococcal pharyngitis are common, as are frank relapses triggered by recurrent infection (Walker et al. 2006, Tumas et al. 2007, Cardoso 2008).

• *Treatment.* This has traditionally been symptomatic. Although only a relatively small fraction of children with Sydenham chorea have evidence of cardiac involvement, prophylaxis against recurrent streptococcal infection is indicated and may be helpful in guarding against relapses of the neurological condition, although that issue remains unresolved. Sedatives and anxiolytics are often helpful along with stimulant medications for attention problems and antidepressants. The movement disorder tends to be only marginally responsive to drugs such as tranxene, valproate, tetrabenazine and dopamine agonists. For reasons that are intuitively obvious, many clinicians have been reluctant to employ aggressive immunomodulatory strategies in managing this disease. Clearly, the risk:benefit equation must be reviewed with the patient and family, but in some circumstances disability is quite profound and there is accumulating evidence that corticosteroids, intravenous immunoglobulin and plasmapheresis may be of benefit in these more severe cases (Teixeira et al. 2005b, Paz et al. 2006).

• *Prognosis.* Whether, in some cases, there are persistent neurological sequelae from this disease, and whether streptococcal infection could engender or exacerbate chronic neuropsychiatric diseases such as Tourette syndrome, attention deficit disorder, obsessive–compulsive disorders (OCD) and depression are active arenas of current research. Over the past two decades there has been vigorous debate regarding the boundaries of the spectrum of poststreptococcal neuropsychiatric disorders. Some of the most strident opinions have surrounded the issue of the entity of PANDAS, a rather awkward acronym for the equally clumsy descriptive term, paediatric acute neuropsychological disorder after streptococcal infection (see below). In light of what is known and widely accepted regarding Sydenham disease, it seems gratuitously obdurate to object to the notion that subsets of symptoms will dominate the clinical landscape in particular individuals, resulting in apparently diverse semiologies in what are collectively derivative manifestations of the parent disease. It is also certain that there are genetic components that determine or influence disease susceptibility and expression in rheumatic fever, Tourette syndrome, attention deficit disorder, depression and OCD (Ramasawmy et al. 2007).

The concept that rheumatic fever is primarily a genetic disorder with an obligate environmental component has gained increasing acceptance. In the face of a pathogen as nearly ubiquitous as streptococcus it seems plausible that in predisposed individuals it is only a matter of time before the genetic switch is tripped. In that context, the questions are, how long can an autoimmune process persist, and can a transient autoimmune disease induce persistent abnormalities in cerebral circuitry resulting in chronic neuropsychiatric disease (Sallakci et al. 2005, Ramasawmy et al. 2007)?

Paediatric acute neuropsychological disorder after streptococcal infection (PANDAS)
The entity of PANDAS came into focus after an outbreak of streptococcal pharyngitis was

TABLE 22.7
Clinical criteria for the diagnosis of paediatric acute neuropsychological disorder after streptococcal infection (PANDAS)

1 Presence of obsessive–compulsive disorder and/or tics
2 Paediatric (prepubertal) onset
3 Episodic course with abrupt onset and dramatic exacerbations (frequently explosive)
4 Association with group A streptococcal infection
5 Association with neurological abnormalities such as adventitious movements, motor hyperactivity or choreiform movements

associated with a tenfold increase in the incidence of motor tics among children in Rhode Island in the 1980s. These were not associated with chorea, carditis or other manifestations of acute rheumatic fever (Swedo et al. 1998). A striking feature was the abrupt onset of symptoms including tics and/or features of OCD, often thought to have evolved overnight. Exacerbation or relapse of symptoms was noted in association with subsequent recurrent streptococcal infections. Choreiform hyperkinetic involuntary movements could be present, at least at some point in the illness. The proposed diagnostic criteria for this disorder are included in Table 22.7.

The existence of the entity of PANDAS has been vigorously debated since the nosology was first proposed by Swedo and colleagues. There have been several arguments against the concept of PANDAS as a discrete clinical disease (Kurlan 2004, Singer et al. 2005, Dale et al. 2006, Gilbert and Kurlan 2009, Swedo et al. 2010). One obvious concern is the clear overlap of features with those of Sydenham chorea. It seems intuitive to assume that these patients are a subgroup of children with rheumatic fever in whom the tic/OCD components are more prominent than others. While this may prove to be true, echocardiographic studies of groups of children with PANDAS have found virtually no evidence of cardiac involvement in these patients. By contrast, roughly 30% of patients with Sydenham chorea have evidence of carditis on echocardiogram. A reasonable interpretation of these observations is that Sydenham chorea is a manifestation of an organism-wide, multi-organ, systemic illness while PANDAS appears to involve exclusively the brain, based on genetic susceptibility. A second problem is the difficulty in establishing a relationship between streptococcal infection and the emergence or recurrence of PANDAS symptoms. The presence of the bacterium in the oropharynx is not evidence of systemic infection and random measures of satellite markers like antistreptolysin O or anti-DNAase provide only limited information. More recent studies have relied on longitudinal correlations of clinical symptoms with serological markers of an antistreptococcal immune response to provide confirmation of a temporal relationship between infection and disease expression. Using these approaches, investigators have been able to illustrate a clear association between streptococcal infection and neuropsychiatric symptoms typical of PANDAS (Church et al. 2003, Murphy et al. 2007, da Rocha et al. 2008, Ridel et al. 2010). Attempts to establish a nexus between streptococcal infection and chronic neuropsychiatric disorders such as Tourette syndrome, OCD, attention deficit disorder and depression have yielded more tenuous results.

Antichemoreceptor disorders

The classic antibody-mediated antineurotransmitter receptor disease is myasthenia gravis, where antibodies directed toward the postsynaptic acetylcholine receptor alter the efficiency of cholinergic transmission at the neuromuscular junction. It should come as no surprise that similar phenomena directed at alternative receptor systems would come to light (Rogers et al. 1994). Perhaps the longest standing and most widely clinically recognized of these is Rasmussen encephalitis. This disorder has been recognized for a generation as a progressive, malignant epilepsy syndrome that can begin insidiously as an idiopathic seizure disorder or explosively as intractable focal seizures, a presentation also referred to as epilepsia partialis continua. Affected individuals develop progressive hemiparesis with chronic inflammation and progressive sclerosis of the cerebral hemisphere where the seizures began. Because of the intractable nature of the epilepsy, these children have frequently undergone surgical excision or functional isolation of the affected hemisphere or its cortical elements, often with excellent results in terms of seizure control and neurological function. Pathological examination of the excised cerebral cortex revealed perivascular collections of mononuclear cells without evidence of vasculitis or infection. For reasons that are entirely unclear, the disease remains confined predominantly to that single cerebral hemisphere where it originally set up housekeeping.

Circulating antibodies to subunit 3 of the neuronal glutamate/AMPA (α-amino-3-hydroxy-5-methyl-4-isoxazole propionic acid) receptor (GluR3) have been demonstrated in some children with typical clinical features of Rasmussen encephalitis. There are also reasons to believe that the disease may be related to direct infection with several neurotropic viruses of the herpes family including cytomegalovirus and Epstein–Barr virus, possibly interlinked with underlying cortical dysplasia. Anti-GluR3 antibodies are found in other populations of children with epilepsy, although their relationship to preceding or concomitant infections is even less clear.

Paediatric cases of encephalitis associated with antibodies to the NR1 subunit of the N-methyl-D-aspartate receptor (NMDAR) are being increasingly recognized. The syndrome was first identified in 2007, often as a paraneoplastic syndrome in patients with ovarian teratoma, and is one of an expanding spectrum of autoimmune disorders involving specific neuronal membrane proteins (Dalmau et al. 2008). Around half of the cases are not associated with tumours, more so in young patients. It thus remains possible that some cases may represent a postinfectious syndrome, as prodromal infectious symptoms and elevated mycoplasma titres have been identified in some young patients, although their causal significance remains unknown. Patients as young as 2 years have been described, and the clinical picture in children includes psychiatric and behavioural symptoms, seizures, movement disorders, autonomic instability and central hypoventilation. Investigations reveal a sterile, lymphocytic CSF, often with oligoclonal bands, an abnormal electroencephalogram and normal or mildly abnormal MRI. The diagnosis is made on anti-NMDAR antibody testing.

The differential diagnosis is of other causes of acute or subactue encephalitis, and treatment is with immunotherapy.

Disorders of the peripheral nervous system: Guillain–Barré syndrome and variants
GBS includes a spectrum of acquired immune-mediated disorders causing dysfunction or degeneration in peripheral nerves, spinal sensory and motor nerve roots, and occasionally cranial nerves. The hallmark clinical picture is that of a previously well individual who develops ascending paralysis that evolves acutely or subacutely and is associated with loss of tendon stretch reflexes. A history of antecedent infectious illness, trauma, surgery or parturition can be obtained in one- to two-thirds of patients. Typically, weakness progresses over several days/weeks followed by a more prolonged period of stabilization, and finally by gradual recovery. The diagnosis is based on clinical and laboratory examination of the CSF. Electrodiagnostic studies provide ancillary evidence to support or refute the diagnosis. For decades, we have conceptualized these diseases as inflammatory disorders with myelin-related antigens as the primary targets of autoimmune attack. Hence, the evolution of the terms acute inflammatory demyelinating polyneuropathy (AIDP) to denote GBS-like syndromes and chronic inflammatory demyelinating polyneuropathy (CIDP) to refer to more chronic or relapsing sensorimotor neuropathies. However myelin is not the only immunological target in these disorders. One of these GBS look-alikes, acute motor axonal neuropathy (AMAN), appears to affect predominantly children, presenting as an acute paralytic illness. In contradistinction to GBS, motor axons are selectively targeted by the immune response in this disorder while sensory axons are almost entirely spared (McKhann et al. 1993, Griffin et al. 1995). It is likely that the primary antigenic targets in these diseases represent a spectrum including those related exclusively to constituents of the myelin sheath and others directed toward axolemmal-related moieties. Recently neurofascin at nodes of Ranvier has been shown as a target antigen for a small proportion of AIDP cases (Ng et al. 2012). Consequently, any neural network with either executive or reporter functions that relies on peripheral axons for communication could be affected, resulting in constellations of symptoms that either conform to the typical clinical picture of GBS or reside on the peripheral boundaries of our concept of what constitutes a GBS phenotype. Furthermore, depending on the primary site of targeted immune attack, the course of the illness could be a relatively brief period of neurological dysfunction, reflecting the time-frame for remyelination and resolution of conduction block, or a severe and prolonged illness with the tempo and quality of recovery dependent on the pace and completeness of regeneration of interrupted axonal projections.

GUILLAIN–BARRÉ SYNDROME: THE CLINICAL SPECTRUM (Table 22.8)

Acute inflammatory demyelinating polyneuropathy
AIDP is the traditionally recognized, hallmark phenotype of GBS. It is the most common clinical presentation among affected children in Western nations (Paradiso et al. 1999, Jones 2000, Hung et al. 2004, Hughes and Cornblath 2005). It is customarily conceived of as an

TABLE 22.8
Variants of immune-mediated acute and chronic demyelinating and axonal disorders seen in children

Guillain–Barré syndrome subtype	Description
Acute inflammatory demyelinating polyneuropathy (AIDP)	Acute onset of ascending weakness and hyporeflexia with elevated CSF protein and EMG showing demyelinating neuropathy; triphasic course, usually with good recovery
Acute motor and sensory axonal neuropathy (AMSAN)	Acute onset of ascending weakness and hyporeflexia with elevated CSF protein with reduction of CMAP; triphasic course and EMG showing axonal involvement more often with limited recovery
Acute motor axonal neuropathy (AMAN)	Clinical syndrome similar to AIDP or AMSAN; elevated CSF protein; electrophysiological and histopathological evidence of degeneration strictly limited to sensory axons
Miller Fisher syndrome	Acute onset of ophthalmoplegia, hyporeflexia, and ataxia with elevated CSF protein and subsequent recovery
Polyneuritis cranialis	Acute onset of multiple cranial neuropathies (usually bilateral VII and sparing of II) with elevated CSF protein, slowing of motor conduction velocities and often incomplete recovery
Acute sensory neuropathy	Acute onset of sensory loss, areflexia, elevated CSF protein, variable slowing of motor conduction velocities and eventual recovery
Acute pandysautonomia	Acute onset of multiple dysautonomic symptoms with limited or no motor involvement, CSF protein elevation, and good recovery

CMAP, compound motor unit action potentials; CSF, cerebrospinal fluid; EMG, electromyography.

acquired, immune-mediated disorder with activated T cells and antibody responses directed at Schwann cell and myelin epitopes within spinal roots and peripheral nerves, characterized by inflammatory infiltration with concomitant macrophage-mediated vesicular demyelination along the course of sensory and motor axons. These pathological features are accompanied by physiological correlates including multifocal slowing of saltatory conduction and conduction block (Asbury 1981, Sumner 1981, Brown and Snow 1991). The functional consequences of these processes are determined by the location and severity of conduction block, and degree of concomitant axonal degeneration.

Acute motor and sensory axonal neuropathy (AMSAN)
Also termed axonal GBS, this entity occurs relatively infrequently within the spectrum of neuropathies encompassed by the term GBS. The clinical presentation is indistinguishable from AIDP; however, electrophysiological testing reveals markedly diminished compound motor action potential (CMAP) amplitudes and sensory evoked potential amplitudes with evidence of severe, widespread denervation on electromyography and relatively preserved

motor and sensory nerve conduction velocities when evoked potentials are elicitable. The histopathological features are indicative of severe degeneration of motor and sensory axons. As noted above, distinction from severe AIDP may not be a trivial exercise.

Acute motor axonal neuropathy

AMAN was originally described in a Southern Mexican population, then more recently among children from rural Northern China. The clearly distinct nature of the disorder from AIDP has been appreciated. This is a seasonal syndrome that is highly correlated with antecedent *Campylobacter jejuni* enteritis resulting in a pure motor axonal neuropathy. The clinical phenotype closely resembles that of AIDP but has unique characteristics on electrophysiological testing: (1) diminished compound motor action potential amplitudes, (2) preserved motor nerve conduction velocities, (3) denervation on EMG testing, and (4) normal sensory nerve conduction studies (Griffin et al. 1995, Paradiso et al. 1999). Autopsy and sural nerve biopsy studies on children confirmed the discrete involvement of peripheral motor axonal projections with sparing of dorsal spinal nerve roots and peripheral sensory axons. Typical histopathological features include inflammatory mononuclear endoneural infiltrates with macrophage-mediated phagocytosis of motor axons. Despite the fact that the axon appears to be the primary immunological target in this disorder, the clinical course is very similar to that of AIDP. This observation invites speculation that distal axonal segments may be preferentially affected rather than proximal injury at the level of ventral spinal nerve roots, or that the autoimmune insult is capable of inducing a transient, relatively prolonged functional disturbance without physically abolishing axonal integrity.

Fisher (Miller Fisher) syndrome

Originally reported in 1956, this GBS variant is characterized by the triad of ophthalmoparesis, ataxia and areflexia (Fisher 1956). Some authors consider bulbar weakness to be within the spectrum of the syndrome while others consider additional functional disturbances exclusionary. This syndrome shares with AIDP the finding of albumino-cytological dissociation on CSF examination. Abnormalities on electrophysiological testing should be confined to sensory axonal populations, although exceptions abound in the literature and there is no unanimous consensus. Many children who present initially with features consistent with Miller Fisher syndrome will exhibit evidence of slowing of motor and sensory nerve conduction or go on to develop appendicular and axial weakness as the disease process evolves. Recovery from the Miller Fisher variant is generally complete and parallels the time course of mild to moderate AIDP. The syndrome has been shown to correlate with evidence of circulating IgG and IgM antibodies to the ganglioside GQ1b, a glycolipid that is expressed on the axolemmal membrane (Yuki 2009).

Polyneuritis cranialis

This is one of the least often encountered phenotypes within the spectrum of acquired immune-mediated radiculoneuropathies. Bilateral facial neuropathy is the most common manifestation, which more typically occurs in the evolution of a syndrome of ascending paralysis with other clinical features of AIDP. Rarely, facial and bulbar weakness present with dysphagia and dysphonia and only minimal, if any, appendicular weakness. These children generally have diminished or absent tendon stretch reflexes and spinal-fluid examination discloses typical features encountered in AIDP. Visser et al. (1996) suggested that cranial nerve involvement may be seen more commonly in GBS patients in whom the disease was preceded by cytomegalovirus infection. The disorder in these patients was also associated with prominent sensory symptoms and a more severe and prolonged clinical course. Multiple cranial nerve involvement may be associated with serological evidence of antibody response to gangliosides GT1a and GQ1b. Many patients who may present initially with isolated cranial-nerve involvement later develop clinical features that overlap with those of AIDP (Kusunoki et al. 1999, Willison 2001, Hughes and Cornblath 2005, Kusunoki et al. 2008, Yuki 2009).

INCIDENCE

GBS is a relatively rare disorder with an incidence of between 0.5 and 1.5 cases per 100 000 in the population under 18 years of age (Rantala et al. 1991, Olive et al. 1997). In nations where immunization programmes are widespread and poliomyelitis nearly eliminated, GBS remains the most common cause of acute paralysis in childhood and therefore a significant contributor to morbidity. GBS is a well-recognized entity around the world and appears to affect all ethnic groups. There is some variability among estimates in the incidence of the disease in different countries. Whether this represents a difference in genetic susceptibility, in potential pathogens, or in case reporting systems is unclear. The disease is frequently associated with a history of antecedent infection. Viral pathogens are the most commonly associated organisms, including Epstein–Barr virus, cytomegalovirus, hepatitis, varicella and other herpesviruses (Kusunoki et al. 1995, Rees et al. 1998, Jacobs et al. 2008). *Mycoplasma pneumoniae* and *Campylobacter* gastroenteritis may antedate or present concurrently with the onset of GBS. Immunizations are frequently but anecdotally implicated for a causal role in the pathogenesis of GBS. The incidence of GBS increased among individuals who received the vaccine during the nationwide swine flu immunization programme that was implemented in the USA (Asbury 1990, 2000; Safranek et al. 1991). A biologically plausible, causal relationship between immunization and the development of GBS has been hypothesized, but never convincingly established.

CLINICAL FEATURES AND DIAGNOSIS

The salient clinical features from a personal (JTS) series of 49 children with GBS are summarized in Table 22.9. These characteristics are similar to those reported in adults and in other series of children with the disorder (Jones 1995, 2000; Korinthenberg and Monting 1996; Korinthenberg et al. 2007). Although weakness was the most common presenting feature in this group of patients, pain was often the most prominent (Ropper and Shahani 1984, Mikati and DeLong 1985, Khatri and Pearlstein 1997, Moulin et al. 1997, Nguyen et al. 1999, Jones 2000). Other series of children and adults with GBS have estimated the incidence of significant pain early in the course of GBS at between 50% and 80%. This fact is especially important in young children who may be unable to articulate a complaint of

TABLE 22.9
Clinical features in children with
Guillain–Barré syndrome[a]

Mean age	7.1 years
Male:female ratio	1.2:1
Weakness	73%
Pain	55%
Ataxia	44%
Paraesthesiae	18%
Dysautonomia	18%
Cranial neuropathy	15%
Miller Fisher triad	5%
Shortness of breath	4%

[a]Data from 49 children under 18 years of age.

weakness, and in whom distinguishing muscle weakness from a reluctance to move due to pain may be nearly impossible. In the clinic, pain may be attributed to musculoskeletal sources such as synovitis, and weakness and diminished reflexes may be overlooked. The paediatric neurologist is often the second or third specialist to see the child for leg or back pain, after orthopaedic and rheumatological causes have been thought to be less likely. Another prominent feature occurring in about one-half of the children with GBS is axial or gait ataxia that appears to be an admixture of cerebellar dysfunction and sensory ataxia. In some cases proximal muscle weakness presenting with clumsiness and frequent falls can be misinterpreted as ataxia. Paraesthesiae are present in around 20% and transient urinary retention in 10%–15% of children early in the course of GBS.

The diagnosis is based on the presence of a constellation of clinical features including weakness, sensory disturbances and loss of tendon stretch reflexes that, in aggregate, strongly support GBS. Differential diagnosis can include disorders involving the CNS, neuromuscular junction and muscle.

Lumbar puncture may be helpful for both inclusionary and exclusionary purposes. Although polio immunization campaigns have largely eradicated that virus, other enteroviruses, notably enterovirus 71 or West Nile virus, can produce acute paralysis due to infection of anterior horn cells (Alexander et al. 1994, Sejvar et al. 2005, Kelly et al. 2006). The typical findings of an elevated spinal fluid protein concentration in the absence of a cellular pleocytosis strongly reinforces the clinical diagnosis of GBS. Electrophysiological testing can also be very helpful in confirming the diagnosis and in providing some insights into prognosis. Sensory and motor nerve conduction studies can characterize the primary pathological process as demyelination or axonal degeneration. The hallmark electrophysio-logical features of GBS include evidence of non-uniform slowing of saltatory conduction along motor and sensory axons and the presence of conduction block. These features include prolongation of distal latencies or F-wave latencies, differences in conduction velocity of more than 5m/s among comparable nerve segments and dispersion of proximally evoked compound motor action potentials. The presence of conduction block may be difficult to document with confidence because of the inability to confirm supramaximal stimulation in proximal nerve segments. In AMAN, electrodiagnostic testing can document axonal degeneration as profound reduction in compound motor action potential amplitudes. The relatively more severe outcome described for axonal GBS in adults has not been observed in children (Cornblath 1990, Lee et al. 2008). If the primary site of demyelination, accompanied by conduction block, is in terminal segments of motor axons, predominantly in intramuscular regions, it may not be possible to distinguish this situation from extensive axonal degeneration in the electrophysiology laboratory. Prognostic implications of severely reduced compound muscle action potential (CMAP) amplitudes must therefore be interpreted with caution. When severely diminished CMAP amplitudes are present in the company of evidence of severe acute denervation on electromyography, prognostic conclusions can be drawn with greater security.

PATHOGENESIS

The immunological mechanisms have been extensively studied in human autopsy and biopsy materials, in population studies and in experimental models. There is ongoing debate as to whether the primary effector mechanism of autoimmune injury is mediated via antibody or T-cell pathways. Whatever the mechanism of axonal and Schwann cell injury, a sequence of events must take place that eventually leads to autoimmune-mediated tissue injury (Hartung et al. 1995, 2001; Dalakas 1995; van der Meché 1996; Hughes 2000; Hughes and Cornblath 2005; Willison 2005; Cornblath and Hughes 2009).

The initial step in this process is breakdown of tolerance. Antecedent infection or other immune-activating event may act through molecular mimicry, superantigen mechanisms or cytokine stimulation to activate T cells to recognize autoantigens. The second phase elicits antigen recognition by T-cell receptors and antigen processing through major histocompatibility complexes. The activated T cells and antibody must gain access to their targeted autoantigens in endoneurial contents: the myelin, or the axon, or both. This process requires traversing the blood–nerve barrier maintained by the tissue microvasculature at the level of endothelial cell tight junctions within capillary beds. The blood–tissue barrier is less restrictive in dorsal root ganglia. Activated T cells migrate into the endoneurium, generally through a pathway of adhesion molecules including selectins and leukocyte integrins and their counter-receptors on endoneurial vascular endothelial cell walls. The blood–nerve barrier can also be broached by trauma, toxins, endoneurial denervation or any mechanism that disrupts endothelial cell tight junctions. A number of non-specific antecedent events could cause disruption of the blood–nerve barrier, expose endoneurial molecules to immune-surveillance mechanisms and result in the initial breakdown of tolerance. The endpoint in this cascade of events occurs when activated T cells and autoantibody enter the endoneurium along with macrophages where both antibody and T-cell targeting mechanisms identify autoantigens on Schwann cell and/or axonal constituents and result in tissue injury and phagocytosis (Hartung et al. 1995a,b, 1996, 2001, 2002; van der Meché and van Doorn 2000; van Doorn 2009).

The classic autopsy study by Asbury et al. (1969) characterized the hallmark histopathological features of the disorder including mononuclear endoneurial inflammatory infiltrates,
variable degrees of Wallerian degeneration and macrophage-mediated segmental demyelination. Subsequent investigations on human biopsy material have confirmed these observations,
which are consonant with an antibody-directed, macrophage-executed attack on myelin-
related antigens (Hughes et al. 1992; Griffin et al. 1996a,b; Hafer-Macko et al. 1996).

In a parallel vein, many studies have attempted to correlate serological evidence of antibody responses to gangliosides with clinical features of GBS and related radiculoneuropathies. The strongest association between expression of antiganglioside antibodies and
clinical manifestations is in the Miller Fisher syndrome. There is a high-level correlation in
these patients with IgG1 antibodies that react with ganglioside GQ1b. This association
appears to be relatively specific as these antibodies are not detected in comparison children
and have otherwise been reported almost exclusively in GBS spectrum radiculoneuropathies
that share clinical features with the Miller Fisher syndrome (Willison and Veitch 1994,
Willison et al. 1997, Susuki et al. 2001, Yuki et al. 2001, Yuki 2009). Serological evidence
of antibody response is more likely to have pathological relevance with the primary pathogenic process directed toward populations of axons. Gangliosides are a common constituent
within, and on the surface of, neuronal and axolemmal membranes (Oomes et al. 1995; Rees
et al. 1995; Chiba et al. 1997; Kuwabara et al. 1998, 2004; Kuwabara 2007). By contrast,
they are comparatively infrequent on the surface of Schwann cells and myelin. In clinical
series, the most commonly reported antibody populations are those directed against ganglioside GM1. Studies of patients with AIDP and AMSAN have demonstrated that a significant
proportion of these patients have an IgG1 antibody against GM1. In the largest series of
patients with AMAN, serological evidence of an association with an antibody response to
ganglioside GD1a has been reported (Ho et al. 1999, Ogawara et al. 2003). Many of these
patients also express reactivity to GM1, and less commonly to other ganglioside species.
Clearly, these antibody responses are not specific for GBS subtypes, and antibody–target
and clinical correlations have been loose, with overlaps of both antibody cross-reactivities
and the spectrum of clinical features. Earlier studies focused on the presence of antibodies
to peripheral nerve myelin that, in one series, were detected in more than 90% of blood
samples from patients with GBS (Koski et al. 1989). It is unlikely that these circulating antibodies, to gangliosides or myelin-related antigens measured in sera from patients with these
disorders, play an important role in the pathogenesis of GBS and related acute radiculoneuropathies. It seems more plausible that they represent components of a polyclonal antibody response that is directed toward more specifically targeted (and relevant) peripheral
nervous system antigens.

T-cell-mediated pathways are clearly also critically involved in orchestrating the autoimmune injury to peripheral nerves in GBS and related syndromes. Reactive T cells can be
induced by immunization using peripheral myelin, whole constituent myelin proteins or even
protein constituent fragments in rodent models of experimental allergic neuritis (EAN). This
procedure also elicits an antibody response to the protein or protein fragment used as an
immunogen. The disease can be induced by passive transfer, with intravenous injection of

CD4+ T cells from animals with EAN into naive syngenic animals, indicating that activated T cells are capable of directing macrophages to Schwann cell targets and inducing segmental demyelination, more severe when targeting antibodies act synergistically with T cells.

Levels of circulating proinflammatory cytokines are elevated in serum: their precise role in modulating the macrophage-mediated ingestion of endoneurial contents is poorly characterized (Sivieri et al. 1997, Creange et al. 1999). Measures that diminish the levels of proinflammatory cytokines or enhance anti-inflammatory molecules may modulate the severity of acute immune-mediated demyelinating disorders (Koski 1997; Lisak et al. 1997; Redford et al. 1997; Zhu et al. 1997, 1998; Di Marco et al. 1999; Dalakas 2002).

TREATMENT

Any child who is suspected of having GBS requires hospitalization until the maximal degree of clinical disability can be established. The disease can proceed in a fulminant fashion and respiratory failure can develop rapidly, so careful monitoring of respiratory function is essential. Substantial, disabling pain is nearly ubiquitous among the more severely affected children, particularly those requiring mechanical ventilation. Surveys of patients with GBS reveal that their painful symptoms were either not treated, in part because of concerns of depressing respiratory drive, or, according to the perception of the patient, notably undertreated. Opioid analgesics are often a necessary and integral part of managing the painful symptoms in children with GBS (Jackman and Klig 1998, Wong et al. 1998). Dysautonomic symptoms can be life threatening because of cardiovascular instability and arrhythmias (McLeod 1993; Murwani and Armati 1998; Previtali et al. 1998; Dalakas 2002, 2004; Kieseier et al. 2008).

Attention to nutritional requirements in these critically ill children, more so in the presence of bulbar weakness, will prevent muscle becoming the prime donor of amino acids and other metabolic substrates. In severely affected children, especially those in the intensive care unit requiring mechanical ventilatory support, joint contractures and trophic skin changes over areas subjected to excessive pressure can develop remarkably rapidly. The importance of early introduction of physical and occupational therapy for mobilization of joints and splinting to maintain maximal functional motility with careful attention to skin care cannot be overemphasized. Because of the pain associated with limb mobilization in some cases, coordinating pain management strategies with physical therapy sessions is much appreciated by the patients.

Treatment strategies targeting autosensitization and tissue inflammation have reduced severity of tissue injury in experimental models. Targeted stages are (1) antigen recognition of T-cell activation, (2) co-stimulatory pathways, (3) cytokine activity, (4) access of activated T cells and autoantibody to target tissues, (5) activated lymphocyte sub-populations through cytotoxic T-cell receptor ligands, and (6) macrophage targeting or lysosomal activity at antigen recognition sites within the endoneurium (Murwani and Armati 1998; Previtali et al. 1998; Dalakas 2002, 2004; Kieseier et al. 2008). The biological mechanisms through which plasmapheresis or intravenous immunoglobulin (IVIg) infusion act to attenuate tissue injury in GBS are not clearly understood. It appears likely that a principle effect of plasmapheresis is to reduce levels of circulating autoantibodies, possibly also circulating proinflammatory cytokines or cell adhesion molecules. The dominant mechanism of action of IVIg may be binding anti-idiotypic antibodies, downregulating B-cell-mediated antibody production, or complement binding. Other mechanisms may include blockade of activated T-cell receptors, augmentation of suppressor T-cell activity or inhibition of lymphocyte proliferation.

There are no well-designed, prospective, randomized treatment trials in childhood GBS. A number of reports on both plasmapheresis and human IVIg are merely descriptive, while others have attempted to use historical controls from their institutions for statistical comparison purposes. Reports of the effect of plasmapheresis and IVIg document significant shortening of hospitalization (Shahar et al. 1990, Abd-Allah et al. 1997). The numbers of children in the literature are insufficient to come to any conclusions regarding the effect of treatment on the need for mechanical ventilatory support or the duration of mechanical ventilation. Comparison of the natural history of GBS in adults and children suggests that children tend to have a faster recovery than adults, with a lower incidence of significant neurological residua. There is currently no evidence that treatment during the acute illness changes the long-term outcome.

The optimal dose and dosage schedules for plasmapheresis and IVIg have not been determined in childhood GBS. At this point in time, most child neurologists would reserve treatment for those children with more severe GBS: those who, by virtue of weakness or ataxia, had lost the ability to ambulate, or those with bulbar involvement resulting in significant dysphagia or aspiration. The ability to utilize plasma exchange in the therapeutic repertoire may be limited by difficulty with vascular access or by the child's size. Plasmapheresis is generally safe in children who weigh 10kg or more; however, not all centres have equipment designed to accommodate the procedure in patients with small intravascular volumes and some set the cut-off limit at 15 or 20kg. The optimal exchange protocol also has not been determined. As a rule, children with sufficiently severe symptoms to justify treatment should receive a series of exchanges with a cumulative total of approximately 250mL/kg volume exchange or roughly a triple volume exchange. There is no clear consensus on whether the total exchange should be accomplished over three, five or more sessions, although patients do not accrue further functional benefit from more than four single volume plasma exchanges. The conventional dose of IVIg is a total of 2g/kg administered over 5 days. Others have suggested 0.5mg/kg/d for 4 days or 1.0g/kg/d for 2 days. Some centres have advocated serial treatments alternating plasmapheresis with IVIg administration. This approach is unsupported by any objective data and flies in the face of a rational interpretation of our understanding of the biology of treatment strategies in autoimmune disease. The Plasma Exchange/Sandoglobulin Guillain–Barré Syndrome Trial Group (1997) compared plasmapheresis with IVIg alone and pheresis followed by IVIg in adults with GBS, and found no significant difference. It is likely that there is a very finite temporal window for intervention in the active phase of the autoimmune process and that outside of that period, additional therapeutic measures are ineffective. There does not appear to be a viable role for the use of corticosteroids in the treatment of children with GBS, and studies in adults have documented worse outcomes in those patients with GBS treated with corticosteroids.

COURSE AND PROGNOSIS

Acknowledging the protean manifestations of this syndrome, the clinical course of GBS typically conforms to a triphasic model.

(1) The first phase comprises the onset and progression of symptoms, evolving to a maximum level of disability. In a majority of instances the evolution is rapid, sometimes progressing from mild symptoms to mechanical ventilation over a matter of hours. A substantial majority of children reach a nadir within 2 weeks with only a small group progressing up to 4 weeks (Korinthenberg and Monting 1996, Korinthenberg et al. 2007). This phase represents the period of the active immune-mediated attack.

(2) The progressive phase is followed by a plateau phase of variable duration. This plateau in clinical function probably reflects the transition period, as the pace of immune-mediated damage to peripheral nerve tissues slows and the dysimmune process comes under control. At the same time, regenerative processes within peripheral nerves begin to repair damaged myelin and injured axons.

(3) The third phase of recovery occurs over a more prolonged period, requiring weeks or months. The severity of disability at the clinical nadir is quite variable. I (JTS) have person-ally seen a number of children in whom the diagnosis was made during the recovery phase, and I am sure that many mild cases of GBS go undiagnosed. In most series of hospitalized children the mean maximal disability grade is 3.5–4 based on the Hughes clinical grading scale. Roughly 45% of hospitalized children will develop a maximum disability score of 2 or 3: able to ambulate 5m independently (grade 2) or able to walk 5m with a walker or equivalent support (grade 3). Approximately 40% of children become bed- or wheelchair-dependent (grade 4) during their admission. Approximately 15% of children require mech-anical ventilatory support (grade 5). Fortunately, with high-quality supportive management, the mortality from this potentially lethal disorder in children is rare: for the most part, independent of therapeutic intervention, 90%–95% of children make a complete recovery within 6–12 months. In most series, those who have not recovered completely are ambulating independently with only minor neurological residua.

FUTURE DIRECTIONS

As our understanding of the pathogenesis of autoimmune inflammatory neuropathies expands and is enhanced by experimental models of these disorders, our refinement of approaches at therapeutic intervention in human diseases remains woefully crude. Experimental models of these disorders have indicated the potential to interfere with the immunopathological process at multiple stages in the evolution of the disease. In humans, many of these stages occur before the appearance of any symptoms of the disease and are therefore unlikely to produce viable treatment strategies. There is ample evidence that modulating the expression of endoneurial and circulating cytokines may influence the course of the illness. Strategies for selective targeting of activated T cells have been shown to be effective in the laboratory and may have applications to human disease. Additionally, attempts to modify the expression of cell adhesion molecules or other effector mechanisms (Willison et al. 2008, Cornblath and Hughes 2009, Zhang et al. 2009) also appear to provide fertile ground for basic and translational research.

REFERENCES

Abd-Allah SA, Jansen PW, Ashwal S, Perkin RM (1997) Intravenous immunoglobulin as therapy for pediatric Guillain–Barré syndrome. *J Child Neurol* 12: 376–80.
Adams C, Diadori P, Schoenroth L, Fritzler M (2000) Autoantibodies in childhood post-varicella acute cerebellar ataxia. *Can J Neurol Sci* 27: 316–20.
Agmon-Levin N, Kivity S, Szyper-Kravitz M, Shoenfeld Y (2009) Transverse myelitis and vaccines: a multi-analysis. *Lupus* 18: 1198–204.
Alexander JP Jr, Baden L, Pallansch MA, Anderson LJ (1994) Enterovirus 71 infections and neurologic disease—United States, 1977–1991. *J Infect Dis* 169: 905–8.
Alper G, Wang L (2009) Demyelinating optic neuritis in children. *J Child Neurol* 24: 45–8.
Alper G, Heyman R, Wang L (2009) Multiple sclerosis and acute disseminated encephalomyelitis diagnosed in children after long-term follow-up: comparison of presenting features. *Dev Med Child Neurol* 51: 480–6.
Altrocchi PH (1963) Acute transverse myelopathy. *Trans Am Neurol Assoc* 88: 186–8.
Anlar B, Basaran C, Kose G, et al. (2003) Acute disseminated encephalomyelitis in children: outcome and prognosis. *Neuropediatrics* 34: 194–9.
Asbury AK (1981) Diagnostic considerations in Guillain–Barré syndrome. *Ann Neurol* 9 Suppl: 1–5.
Asbury AK (1990) Guillain–Barré syndrome: historical aspects. *Ann Neurol* 27 Suppl: S2–6.
Asbury AK (2000) New concepts of Guillain–Barré syndrome. *J Child Neurol* 15: 183–91.
Asbury AK, Arnason BG, Adams RD (1969) The inflammatory lesion in idiopathic polyneuritis. Its role in pathogenesis. *Medicine* 48: 173.
Banwell B, Ghezzi A, Barr-Or A, et al. (2007a) Multiple sclerosis in children: clinical diagnosis, therapeutic strategies, and future directions. *Lancet Neurol* 6: 887–902.
Banwell B, Krupp L, Kennedy J, et al. (2007b) Clinical features and viral serologies in children with multiple sclerosis: a multinational observational study. *Lancet Neurol* 6: 773–81.
Banwell B, Kennedy J, Sadovnick D, et al. (2009) Incidence of acquired demyelination of the CNS in Canadian children. *Neurology* 72: 232–9.
Banwell BL (2007) The longitudinally extensive and the short of it: transverse myelitis in children. *Neurology* 68: 1447–9.
Bonthius DJ, Karacay B (2003) Sydenham's chorea: not gone and not forgotten. *Semin Pediatr Neurol* 10: 11–9.
Brown WF, Snow R (1991) Patterns and severity of conduction abnormalities in Guillain–Barré syndrome. *J Neurol Neurosurg Psychiatry* 54: 768–74.
Cakmakli G, Kurne A, Güven A, et al. (2009) Childhood optic neuritis: the pediatric neurologist's perspective. *Eur J Paediatr Neurol* 13: 452–7.
Cardoso F (2008) Sydenham's chorea. *Curr Treat Options Neurol* 10: 230–5.
Chiba A, Kusunoki S, Obata H, et al. (1997) Ganglioside composition of the human cranial nerves, with special reference to pathophysiology of Miller Fisher syndrome. *Brain Res* 745: 32–6.
Church AJ, Dale RC, Lees AJ, et al. (2003) Tourette's syndrome: a cross sectional study to examine the PANDAS hypothesis. *J Neurol Neurosurg Psychiatry* 74: 602–7.
Cornblath DR (1990) Electrophysiology in Guillain–Barré syndrome. *Ann Neurol* 27 Suppl: S17–20.
Cornblath DR, Hughes RA (2009) Treatment for Guillain–Barré syndrome. *Ann Neurol* 66: 569–70.
Creange A, Sharshar T, Planchenault T, et al. (1999) Matrix metalloproteinase-9 is increased and correlates with severity in Guillain–Barré syndrome. *Neurology* 53: 1683–91.
Dalakas MC (1995) Basic aspects of neuroimmunology as they relate to immunotherapeutic targets: present and future prospects. *Ann Neurol* 37 Suppl 1: S2–13.
Dalakas MC (2002) Mechanisms of action of IVIg and therapeutic considerations in the treatment of acute and chronic demyelinating neuropathies. *Neurology* 59 Suppl 6: S13–21.

Dalakas MC (2004) Intravenous immunoglobulin in autoimmune neuromuscular diseases. *JAMA* 291: 2367–75.

Dale RC, Pillai SC (2007) Early relapse risk after a first CNS inflammatory demyelination episode: examining international consensus definitions. *Dev Med Child Neurol* 49: 887–93.

Dale RC, Church AJ, Candler PM (2006) Serum autoantibodies do not differentiate PANDAS and Tourette syndrome from controls. *Neurology* 66: 1612; author reply 1612.

Dale RC, Brilot F, Banwell B (2009) Pediatric central nervous system inflammatory demyelination: acute disseminated encephalomyelitis, clinically isolated syndromes, neuromyelitis optica, and multiple sclerosis. *Curr Opin Neurol* 22: 233–40.

Dalmau J, Gleichman AJ, Hughes EG, et al. (2008) Anti-NMDA-receptor encephalitis: case series and analysis of the effects of antibodies. *Lancet Neurol* 7: 1091–8.

da Rocha FF, Correa H, Teixeira AL (2008) Obsessive–compulsive disorder and immunology: a review. *Prog Neuropsychopharmacol Biol Psychiatry* 32: 1139–46.

Defresne P, Hollenberg H, Husson B, et al. (2003) Acute transverse myelitis in children: clinical course and prognostic factors. *J Child Neurol* 18: 401–6.

Di Marco R, Khademi M, Wallstrom E, et al. (1999) Amelioration of experimental allergic neuritis by sodium fusidate (fusidin): suppression of IFN-gamma and TNF-alpha and enhancement of IL-10. *J Autoimmun* 13: 187–95.

Divekar D, Bhosale S, Divate P (2007) Recurrent acute disseminated encephalomyelitis. *Indian Pediatr* 44: 138–40.

Donmez FY, Aslan H, Koskun M (2009) Evaluation of possible prognostic factors of fulminant acute disseminated encephalomyelitis (ADEM) on magnetic resonance imaging with fluid-attenuated inversion recovery (FLAIR) and diffusion-weighted imaging. *Acta Radiol* 50: 334–9.

Dunne K, Hopkins IJ, Shield LK (1986) Acute transverse myelopathy in childhood. *Dev Med Child Neurol* 28: 198–204.

Fisher CM (1956) An unusual variant of acute idiopathic polyneuritis (syndrome of ophthalmoplegia, ataxia and areflexia). *N Engl J Med* 255: 57–65.

Gilbert DL, Kurlan R (2009) PANDAS: horse or zebra? *Neurology* 73: 1252–3.

Griffin JW, Li CY, Ho TW, et al. (1995) Guillain–Barré syndrome in northern China. The spectrum of neuropathological changes in clinically defined cases. *Brain* 118: 577–95.

Griffin JW, Li CY, Ho TW (1996a) Pathology of the motor-sensory axonal Guillain–Barré syndrome. *Ann Neurol* 39: 17–28.

Griffin JW, Li CY, Macko C, et al. (1996b) Early nodal changes in the acute motor axonal neuropathy pattern of the Guillain–Barré syndrome. *J Neurocytol* 25: 33–51.

Hafer-Macko CE, Sheikh KA, Ho TW, et al. (1996) Immune attack on the Schwann cell surface in acute inflammatory demyelinating polyneuropathy. *Ann Neurol* 39: 625–35.

Hamnik SE, Hacein-Bey L, Biller J, et al. (2008) Neuromyelitis optica (NMO) antibody positivity in patients with transverse myelitis and no visual manifestations. *Semin Ophthalmol* 23: 191–200.

Hartung HP, Pollard JD, Harvey GK, Toyka KV (1995a) Immunopathogenesis and treatment of the Guillain–Barré syndrome—Part I. *Muscle Nerve* 18: 137–53.

Hartung HP, Pollard JD, Harvey GK, Toyka KV (1995b) Immunopathogenesis and treatment of the Guillain–Barré syndrome—Part II. *Muscle Nerve* 18: 154–64.

Hartung HP, Kiefer R, Gold R, et al. (1996) Autoimmunity in the peripheral nervous system. *Baillieres Clin Neurol* 5: 1–45.

Hartung HP, Kieseier BC, Kiefer R (2001) Progress in Guillain–Barré syndrome. *Curr Opin Neurol* 14: 597–604.

Hartung HP, Willison HJ, Kieseier BC (2002) Acute immunoinflammatory neuropathy: update on Guillain–Barré syndrome. *Curr Opin Neurol* 15: 571–7.

Ho TW, Willison HJ, Nachamkin I, et al. (1999) Anti-GD1a antibody is associated with axonal but not demyelinating forms of Guillain–Barré syndrome. *Ann Neurol* 45: 168–73.

Hughes R, Atkinson P, Coates P, et al. (1992) Sural nerve biopsies in Guillain–Barré syndrome: axonal degeneration and macrophage-associated demyelination and absence of cytomegalovirus genome. *Muscle Nerve* 15: 568–75.

Hughes RA (2000) Pathogenesis and treatment of inflammatory demyelinating polyradiculoneuropathy. *Acta Neurol Belg* 100: 167–70.

Hughes RA, Cornblath DR (2005) Guillain–Barré syndrome. *Lancet* 366: 1653–66.

Hung PL, Chang WN, Huang LT, et al. (2004) A clinical and electrophysiologic survey of childhood Guillain–Barré syndrome. *Pediatr Neurol* 30: 86–91.

Jackman NL, Klig JE (1998) Lower extremity pain in a three year old: manifestations of Guillain–Barré syndrome. *Pediatr Emerg Care* 14: 272–4.

Jacobs BC, Koga M, van Rijs W, et al. (2008) Subclass IgG to motor gangliosides related to infection and clinical course in Guillain–Barré syndrome. *J Neuroimmunol* 194: 181–90.

Jones HR Jr (1995) Guillain–Barré syndrome in children. *Curr Opin Pediatr* 7: 663–8.

Jones HR Jr (2000) Guillain–Barré syndrome: perspectives with infants and children. *Semin Pediatr Neurol* 7: 91–102.

Kahloon AA, Arif H, Khawaja MR, Baig M (2007) Characteristics of acute transverse myelitis at Aga Khan University Hospital, Karachi. *J Pak Med Assoc* 57: 215–8.

Kalra V, Sharma S, Sahu J, et al. (2009) Childhood acute transverse myelitis: clinical profile, outcome, and association with antiganglioside antibodies. *J Child Neurol* 24: 466–71.

Kaufman DI, Trobe JD, Eggenberger ER, Whitaker JN (2000) Practice parameter: the role of corticosteroids in the management of acute monosymptomatic optic neuritis. Report of the Quality Standards Subcommittee of the American Academy of Neurology. *Am J Ophthalmol* 130: 541.

Kelly H, Brussen KA, Lawrence A, et al. (2006) Polioviruses and other enteroviruses isolated from faecal samples of patients with acute flaccid paralysis in Australia, 1996–2004. *J Paediatr Child Health* 42: 370–6.

Khatri A, Pearlstein L (1997) Pain in Guillain–Barré syndrome. *Neurology* 49: 1474.

Kieseier BC, Meyer Zu Hörste G, Lehmann HC, et al. (2008) Intravenous immunoglobulins in the treatment of immune neuropathies. *Curr Opin Neurol* 21: 555–62.

Kirvan CA, Cox CJ, Swedo SE, Cunningham MW (2007) Tubulin is a neuronal target of autoantibodies in Sydenham's chorea. *J Immunol* 178: 7412–21.

Knebusch M, Strassburg HM, Reiners K (1998) Acute transverse myelitis in childhood: nine cases and review of the literature. *Dev Med Child Neurol* 40: 631–9.

Korinthenberg R, Monting JS (1996) Natural history and treatment effects in Guillain–Barré syndrome: a multicentre study. *Arch Dis Child* 74: 281–7.

Korinthenberg R, Schessl J, Kirschner J (2007) Clinical presentation and course of childhood Guillain–Barré syndrome: a prospective multicentre study. *Neuropediatrics* 38: 10–7.

Koski CL (1997) Mechanisms of Schwann cell damage in inflammatory neuropathy. *J Infect Dis* 176 Suppl 2: S169–72.

Koski CL, Chou DK, Jungalwala FB (1989) Anti-peripheral nerve myelin antibodies in Guillain–Barré syndrome bind a neutral glycolipid of peripheral myelin and cross-react with Forssman antigen. *J Clin Invest* 84: 280–7.

Kurlan R (2004) The PANDAS hypothesis: losing its bite? *Mov Disord* 19: 371–4.

Krupp LB, Banwell B, Tennenbaum S, et al. (2007) Consensus definitions proposed for pediatric multiple sclerosis and related disorders. *Neurology* 68 Suppl 2: S7–S12.

Kusunoki S, Chiba A, Hitoshi S, et al. (1995) Anti-Gal-C antibody in autoimmune neuropathies subsequent to mycoplasma infection. *Muscle Nerve* 18: 409–13.

Kusunoki S, Chiba A, Kanazawa I (1999) Anti-GQ1b IgG antibody is associated with ataxia as well as ophthalmoplegia. *Muscle Nerve* 22: 1071–4.

Kusunoki S, Kaida K, Ueda M (2008) Antibodies against gangliosides and ganglioside complexes in Guillain–Barré syndrome: new aspects of research. *Biochim Biophys Acta* 1780: 441–4.

Kuwabara S (2007) Guillain–Barré syndrome. *Curr Neurol Neurosci Rep* 7: 57–62.

Kuwabara S, Yuki N, Koga M, et al. (1998) IgG anti-GM1 antibody is associated with reversible conduction failure and axonal degeneration in Guillain–Barré syndrome. *Ann Neurol* 44: 202–8.

Kuwabara S, Ogawara K, Misawa S, et al. (2004) Does *Campylobacter jejuni* infection elicit "demyelinating" Guillain–Barré syndrome? *Neurology* 63: 529–33.

Leake JA, Albani S, Kao AS, et al. (2004) Acute disseminated encephalomyelitis in childhood: epidemiologic, clinical and laboratory features. *Pediatr Infect Dis J* 23: 756–64.

Lee JH, Sung IY, Rew IS (2008) Clinical presentation and prognosis of childhood Guillain–Barré syndrome. *J Paediatr Child Health* 44: 449–54.

Lisak RP, Skundric D, Bealmear B, Ragheb S (1997) The role of cytokines in Schwann cell damage, protection, and repair. *J Infect Dis* 176 Suppl 2: S173–9.

Magana SM, Pittock SJ, Lennon VA, et al. (2009) Neuromyelitis optica IgG serostatus in fulminant central nervous system inflammatory demyelinating disease. *Arch Neurol* 66: 964–66.

Marin SE, Callen DJA (2013) The magnetic resonance imaging appearance of monophasic acute disseminated encephalomyelitis: an update post application of the 2007 consensus criteria. *Neuroimag Clin N Am* 23: 245–66.

Martino D, Giovannoni G (2004) Antibasal ganglia antibodies and their relevance to movement disorders. *Curr Opin Neurol* 17: 425–32.

McKhann GM, Cornblath DR, et al. (1993) Acute motor axonal neuropathy: a frequent cause of acute flaccid paralysis in China. *Ann Neurol* 33: 333–42.

McLeod JG (1993) Autonomic dysfunction in peripheral nerve disease. *J Clin Neurophysiol* 10: 51–60.

Mikati MA, DeLong GR (1985) Childhood Guillain–Barré syndrome masquerading as a protracted pain syndrome. *Arch Neurol* 42: 839.

Miyazawa R, Ikeuchi Y, Tomomasa T, et al. (2003) Determinants of prognosis of acute transverse myelitis in children. *Pediatr Int* 45: 512–6.

Moulin DE, Hagen N, Feasby TE, et al. (1997) Pain in Guillain–Barré syndrome. *Neurology* 48: 328–31.

Murphy TK, Snider LA, Mutch PJ, et al. (2007) Relationship of movements and behaviors to Group A *Streptococcus* infections in elementary school children. *Biol Psychiatry* 61: 279–84.

Murwani R, Armati P (1998) Peripheral nerve fibroblasts as a source of IL-6, TNFalpha and IL-1 and their modulation by IFNgamma. *J Neurol Sci* 161: 99–109.

Ng JK, Malotka J, Kawakami N, et al. (2012) Neurofascin as a target for autoantibodies in peripheral neuropathies. *Neurology* 79: 2241–8.

Nguyen DK, Agenarioti-Belanger S, Vanasse M (1999) Pain and the Guillain–Barré syndrome in children under 6 years old. *J Pediatr* 134: 773–6.

Noorbakhsh F, Johnson RT, Emery D, Power C (2008) Acute disseminated encephalomyelitis: clinical and pathogenesis features. *Neurol Clin* 26: 759–80, ix.

Nussinovitch M, Prais D, Volovitz B, et al. (2003) Post-infectious acute cerebellar ataxia in children. *Clin Pediatr (Phila)* 42: 581–4.

Ogawara K, Kuwabara S, Koga M, et al. (2003) Anti-GM1b IgG antibody is associated with acute motor axonal neuropathy and *Campylobacter jejuni* infection. *J Neurol Sci* 210: 41–5.

Olive JM, Castillo C, Castro RG, de Quadros CA (1997) Epidemiologic study of Guillain–Barré syndrome in children <15 years of age in Latin America. *J Infect Dis* 175 Suppl 1: S160–4.

Oomes PG, Jacobs BC, Hazenberg MP, et al. (1995) Anti-GM1 IgG antibodies and *Campylobacter* bacteria in Guillain–Barré syndrome: evidence of molecular mimicry. *Ann Neurol* 38: 170–5.

Paine RBR (1953) Transverse myelopathy in childhood. *Am J Dis Child* 28: 198–204.

Paradiso G, Tripoli J, Galicchio S, Fejerman N (1999) Epidemiological, clinical, and electrodiagnostic findings in childhood Guillain–Barré syndrome: a reappraisal. *Ann Neurol* 46: 701–7.

Paz JA, Silva CA, Marques-Dias MJ (2006) Randomized double-blind study with prednisone in Sydenham's chorea. *Pediatr Neurol* 34: 264–9.

Pidcock FS, Krishnan C, Crawford TO, et al. (2007) Acute transverse myelitis in childhood: center-based analysis of 47 cases. *Neurology* 68: 1474–80.

Plasma Exchange/Sandoglobulin Guillain-Barré Syndrome Trial Group (1997) Randomised trial of plasma exchange, intravenous immunoglobulin, and combined treatments in Guillain–Barré syndrome. *Lancet* 349: 225–30.

Previtali SC, Archelos JJ, Hartung HP (1998) Expression of integrins in experimental autoimmune neuritis and Guillain–Barré syndrome. *Ann Neurol* 44: 611–21.

Ramasawmy R, Fae KC, Spina G, et al. (2007) Association of polymorphisms within the promoter region of the tumor necrosis factor-alpha with clinical outcomes of rheumatic fever. *Mol Immunol* 44: 1873–8.

Rantala H, Uhari M, Niemela M (1991) Occurrence, clinical manifestations, and prognosis of Guillain–Barré syndrome. *Arch Dis Child* 66: 706–8; discussion 708–9.

Redford EJ, Smith KJ, Gregson NA, et al. (1997) A combined inhibitor of matrix metalloproteinase activity and tumour necrosis factor-alpha processing attenuates experimental autoimmune neuritis. *Brain* 120: 1895–905.

Rees JH, Gregson NA, Hughes RA (1995) Anti-ganglioside antibodies in patients with Guillain–Barré syndrome and *Campylobacter jejuni* infection. *J Infect Dis* 172: 605–6.

Rees JH, Thompson RD, Smeeton NC, Hughes RAC (1998) Epidemiological study of Guillain–Barré syndrome in south east England. *J Neurol Neurosurg Psychiatry* 64: 74–7.

Ridel KR, Lipps TD, Gilbert DL (2010) The prevalence of neuropsychiatric disorders in Sydenham's chorea. *Pediatr Neurol* 42: 243–8.

Rivers TM, Schwentker FF (1935) Encephalomyelitis accompanied by myelin destruction experimentally produced in monkeys. *J Exp Med* 61: 689–702.

Rogers SW, Andrews PI, Gahring LC, et al. (1994) Autoantibodies to glutamate receptor GluR3 in Rasmussen's encephalitis. *Science* 265: 648–51.

Ropper AH, Shahani BT (1984) Pain in Guillain–Barré syndrome. *Arch Neurol* 41: 511–4.

Safranek TJ, Lawrence DN, Kurland LT, et al. (1991) Reassessment of the association between Guillain–Barré syndrome and receipt of swine influenza vaccine in 1976–1977: results of a two-state study. Expert Neurology Group. *Am J Epidemiol* 133: 940–51.

Saini H, Fernandez G, Kerr D, Levy M (2010) Differential expression of aquaporin-4 isoforms localizes with neuromyelitis optica disease activity. *J Neuroimmunol* 221: 68–72.

Sallakci N, Akcurin G, Köksoy S, et al. (2005) TNF-alpha G-308A polymorphism is associated with rheumatic fever and correlates with increased TNF-alpha production. *J Autoimmun* 25: 150–4.

Sejvar JJ, Bode AV, Marfin AA, et al. (2005) West Nile virus-associated flaccid paralysis. *Emerg Infect Dis* 11: 1021–7.

Shahar E, Murphy EG, Roifman CM (1990) Benefit of intravenously administered immune serum globulin in patients with Guillain–Barré syndrome. *J Pediatr* 116: 141–4.

Singer HS, Hong JJ, Yoon DY, Williams PN (2005) Serum autoantibodies do not differentiate PANDAS and Tourette syndrome from controls. *Neurology* 65: 1701–7.

Sivieri S, Ferrarini AM, Lolli F, et al. (1997) Cytokine pattern in the cerebrospinal fluid from patients with GBS and CIDP. *J Neurol Sci* 147: 93–5.

Sumner AJ (1981) The physiological basis for symptoms in Guillain–Barré syndrome. *Ann Neurol* 9 Suppl: 28–30.

Susuki K, Yuki N, Hirata K (2001) Fine specificity of anti-GQ1b IgG and clinical features. *J Neurol Sci* 185: 5–9.

Swedo SE, Rapoport JL, Cheslow DL, et al. (1989) High prevalence of obsessive–compulsive symptoms in patients with Sydenham's chorea. *Am J Psychiatry* 146: 246–9.

Swedo SE, Leonard HL, Schapiro MB, et al. (1993) Sydenham's chorea: physical and psychological symptoms of St Vitus dance. *Pediatrics* 91: 706–13.

Swedo SE, Leonard HL, Garvey M, et al. (1998) Pediatric autoimmune neuropsychiatric disorders associated with streptococcal infections: clinical description of the first 50 cases. *Am J Psychiatry* 155: 264–71.

Swedo SE, Schrag A, Gilbert R, et al. (2010) Streptococcal infection, Tourette syndrome, and OCD: is there a connection? PANDAS: horse or zebra? *Neurology* 74: 1397–8; author reply 1398–9.

Tanaka ST, Stone AR, Kurzrock EA (2006) Transverse myelitis in children: long-term urological outcomes. *J Urol* 175: 1865–8; discussion 1868.

Teixeira AL Jr, Guimaraes MM, Romano-Silva MA, Cardoso F (2005a) Serum from Sydenham's chorea patients modifies intracellular calcium levels in PC12 cells by a complement-independent mechanism. *Mov Disord* 20: 843–5.

Teixeira AL Jr, Maia DP, Cardoso F (2005b) Treatment of acute Sydenham's chorea with methyl-prednisolone pulse-therapy. *Parkinsonism Relat Disord* 11: 327–30.

Tenembaum S, Chamoles N, Fejerman N (2002) Acute disseminated encephalomyelitis: a long-term follow-up study of 84 pediatric patients. *Neurology* 59: 1224–31.

Tenembaum S, Chitnis T, Ness J, Hahn JS (2007) Acute disseminated encephalomyelitis. *Neurology* 68 (16 Suppl 2): S23–36.

Toker E, Yenice O, Yilmaz Y (2003) Isolated bilateral optic neuropathy in acute disseminated encephalomyelitis. *J Pediatr Ophthalmol Strabismus* 40: 232–5.

Tumas V, Caldas CT, Santos AC, et al. (2007) Sydenham's chorea: clinical observations from a Brazilian movement disorder clinic. *Parkinsonism Relat Disord* 13: 276–83.

van der Meché FG (1996) The Guillain–Barré syndrome; pathogenesis and treatment. *Rev Neurol (Paris)* 152: 355–8.

van der Meché FG, van Doorn PA (2000) Guillain–Barré syndrome. *Curr Treat Options Neurol* 2: 507–16.

van Doorn PA (2009) What's new in Guillain–Barré syndrome in 2007–2008? *J Peripher Nerv Syst* 14: 72–4.

Visser LH, van der Meché FG, Meulstee J, et al. (1996) Cytomegalovirus infection and Guillain–Barré syndrome: the clinical, electrophysiologic, and prognostic features. Dutch Guillain–Barré Study Group. *Neurology* 47: 668–73.

Walker K, Lawrenson J, Wilmshurst JM (2006) Sydenham's chorea—clinical and therapeutic update 320 years down the line. *S Afr Med J* 96: 906–12.

Wilejto M, Shroff M, Buncic JR, et al. (2006) The clinical features, MRI findings, and outcome of optic neuritis in children. *Neurology* 67: 258–62.

Willison HJ (2001) Fine specificity of anti-GQ1b antibodies and clinical features. *J Neurol Sci* 185: 1–2.

Willison HJ (2005) The immunobiology of Guillain–Barré syndromes. *J Peripher Nerv Syst* 10: 94–112.

Willison HJ, Veitch J (1994) Immunoglobulin subclass distribution and binding characteristics of anti-GQ1b antibodies in Miller Fisher syndrome. *J Neuroimmunol* 50: 159–65.

Willison HJ, O'Hanlon G, Paterson G, et al. (1997) Mechanisms of action of anti-GM1 and anti-GQ1b ganglioside antibodies in Guillain–Barré syndrome. *J Infect Dis* 176 Suppl 2: S144–9.

Willison HJ, Halstead SK, Beveridge E, et al. (2008) The role of complement and complement regulators in mediating motor nerve terminal injury in murine models of Guillain–Barré syndrome. *J Neuroimmunol* 201–202: 172–82.

Wong BL, deGrauw T, Fogelson MH (1998) Pain in pediatric Guillain–Barré syndrome: case report. *J Child Neurol* 13: 184–5.

Yiu EM, Kornberg AJ, Ryan MM, et al. (2009) Acute transverse myelitis and acute disseminated encephalomyelitis in childhood: spectrum or separate entities? *J Child Neurol* 24: 287–96.

Yuki N (2009) Fisher syndrome and Bickerstaff brainstem encephalitis (Fisher–Bickerstaff syndrome). *J Neuroimmunol* 215: 1–9.

Yuki N, Susuki K, Hirata K (2000) Ataxic Guillain–Barré syndrome with anti-GQ1b antibody: relation to Miller Fisher syndrome. *Neurology* 54: 1851–3.

Yuki N, Odaka M, Hirata K (2001) Acute ophthalmoparesis (without ataxia) associated with anti-GQ1b IgG antibody: clinical features. *Ophthalmology* 108: 196–200.

Zhang ZY, Zhang Z, Fauser U, Schluesener HJ (2009) Improved outcome of EAN, an animal model of GBS, through amelioration of peripheral and central inflammation by minocycline. *J Cell Mol Med* 13: 341–51.

Zhu J, Bai XF, Mix E, Link H (1997) Cytokine dichotomy in peripheral nervous system influences the outcome of experimental allergic neuritis: dynamics of mRNA expression for IL-1 beta, IL-6, IL-10, IL-12, TNF-alpha, TNF-beta, and cytolysin. *Clin Immunol Immunopathol* 84: 85–94.

Zhu J, Mix E, Link H (1998) Cytokine production and the pathogenesis of experimental autoimmune neuritis and Guillain–Barré syndrome. *J Neuroimmunol* 84: 40–52.

INDEX

Page numbers in *italics* refer to material in figures while numbers in **bold** refer to material in tables. Abbreviations used: ADHD, attention-deficit–hyperactivity disorder; AIDS, autoimmune deficiency syndrome; CMV, cytomegalovirus; CNS, central nervous syndrome; CSF, cerebrospinal fluid; CT, computerized tomography; EEG, electroencephalography; ELISA, enzyme-linked immunosorbent assay; FLAIR, fluid-attenuated inversion recovery; HIV, human immunodeficiency virus; HSV, herpes simplex virus; ICP, intracranial pressure; MRI, magnetic resonance imaging; PANDAS, paediatric acute neuropsychological disorder after streptococcal infection; SIADH, syndrome of inappropriate secretion of antidiuretic hormone; TORCH, *Toxoplasma gondii*, rubella, cytomegalovirus and herpesviruses; vs refers to differential diagnoses.

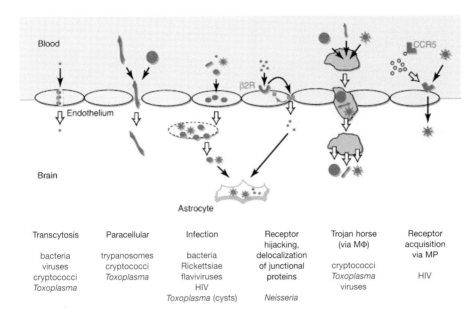

Transcytosis	Paracellular	Infection	Receptor hijacking,	Trojan horse (via MΦ)	Receptor acquisition via MP
bacteria	trypanosomes	bacteria	delocalization		
viruses	cryptococci	Rickettsiae	of junctional	cryptococci	
cryptococci	*Toxoplasma*	flaviviruses	proteins	*Toxoplasma*	HIV
Toxoplasma		HIV		viruses	
		Toxoplasma (cysts)	*Neisseria*		

Plate 1. (Figure 2.1, p. 9) Mechanisms by which pathogens cross the brain endothelial monolayer. The various biological mechanisms that can be used by pathogens to cross the blood–brain barrier are shown in black text, and examples of some pathogens implementing these mechanisms are shown in red text. The β2 adrenergic receptor (β2R) and the chemokine receptor, CCR5, are given as examples; several other receptors are known to serve as tools for central nervous system invasion. MΦ, macrophages; MP, microparticles. (Reproduced by permission from Combes et al. 2012.)

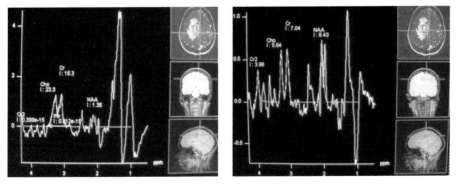

Plate 2. (Figure 4.14, p. 60) Multi-voxel magnetic resonance spectroscopy images of pyogenic abscess at echo times of (left) 30ms and (right) 135ms show peaks of lipid lactate (1.3ppm), acetate (2.3ppm) and succinate (2.5ppm).

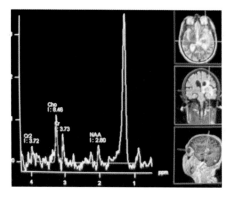

Plate 3. (Figure 4.15, p. 61) Tuberculoma. Magnetic resonance spectroscopy at echo time 30ms showing lipid peak at 1.3ppm.

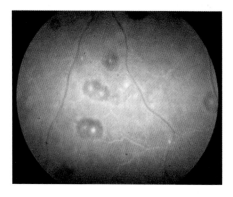

Plate 4. (Figure 16.1, p. 237) Retina in a 3-year-old child with cerebral malaria showing haemorrhages, white exudates and changes in the colour of the vessels. (Reproduced by courtesy of Nick Beare.)

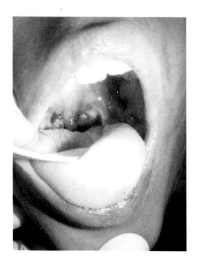

Plate 5. (Figure 21.1, p. 313) Diphtheretic membrane in a 5-year-old male.

International Review of Child Neurology Series

Published for the International Child Neurology Association by Mac Keith Press www.mackeith.co.uk

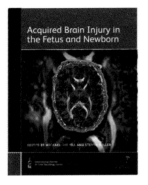

Acquired Brain Injury in the Fetus and Newborn
Michael Shevell and Steven Miller (Eds)

2012 ▪ 330pp ▪ Hardback ▪ 978-1-907655-02-9
£128.00 / €153.00 / US$199.00

Given the tremendous advances in the understanding of acquired neonatal brain injury, this book provides a timely review for the practising neurologist, neonatologist and paediatrician. The editors take a pragmatic approach, focusing on specific populations encountered regularly by the clinician. They offer a 'bench to bedside' approach to acquired brain injury in the preterm and term newborn infant. The contributors, all internationally recognized neurologists and scientists, provide readers with a state-of-the art review in their area of expertise.

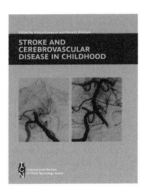

Stroke and Cerebrovascular Disease in Childhood
Vijeya Ganesan, Fenella Kirkham (Eds)

2011 ▪ 248pp ▪ Hardback ▪ 978-1-898683-34-6
£145.00 / €174.00 / US$209.95

The field of stroke and cerebrovascular disease in children is one in which there has been much recent research activity, leading to new clinical perspectives. This book for the first time summarizes the state of the art in this field. A team of eminent clinicians, neurologists and researchers provide an up-to-the-minute account of all aspects of stroke and cerebrovascular disease in children, ranging from a historical perspective to future directions, through epidemiology, the latest neuroimaging techniques, neurodevelopment, comorbidities, diagnosis, and treatment.

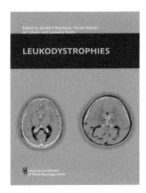

Leukodystrophies
Gerald V. Raymond, Florian Eichler, Ali Fatemi and Sakkubai Naidu (Eds)

2011 ▪ 240pp ▪ Hardback ▪ 978-1-907655-09-8
£81.95 / €98.40 / US$129.00

This book is the only up-to-date, comprehensive text on leukodystrophies. Its purpose is to summarize for the reader all aspects of the inherited disorders of myelin in children and adults. After a comprehensive overview of myelin and the role of oligodendrocytes, astrocytes and microglia in white matter disease, chapters are then devoted to individual disorders, covering their biochemical and molecular basis, genetics, pathophysiology, clinical features, diagnosis, treatment, and screening. The final chapters address therapeutic approaches in leukodystrophies and present a clinical approach to diagnosing leukoencephalopathies in children and adults.

International Review of Child Neurology Series

Published for the International Child Neurology Association by Mac Keith Press www.mackeith.co.uk

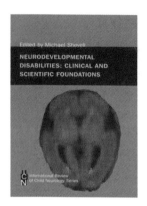

Neurodevelopmental Disabilities: Clinical and Scientific Foundations

Michael Shevell (Ed)

2009 ▪ 504pp ▪ Softback ▪ 978-1-898683-67-4
£75.00 / €90.00 / US$129.95

This book takes a comprehensive approach to addressing the challenges of neurodevelopmental disabilities in child health, with a special focus on global developmental delay and developmental language impairment. It presents the scientific basis of these disorders and their underlying causes. Issues related to medical management, rehabilitation, and eventual outcomes are also addressed in detail. The book has wide appeal to those in paediatrics, developmental paediatrics, child neurology, and paediatric rehabilitation. Some chapters are devoted to the particular issues faced in underdeveloped countries. The book also provides extensive information in a single source relating to often-overlooked areas such as medical management, rehabilitation, public policy, and ethics.

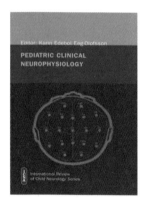

Pediatric Clinical Neurophysiology

Karin Edebol Eeg-Olofsson (Ed)

2007 ▪ 264pp ▪ Hardback ▪ 978-1-898683-48-3
£75.00 / €90.00 / US$119.95

This book introduces clinical neurophysiology and its applications to the paediatric neurologist. It does not aim at being a textbook of either clinical neurophysiology or paediatric neurology, but at bridging these two fields, as a handbook for the clinician. The focus is on the methods applied in the setting of a clinical neurophysiological laboratory. Particularly valuable are the examples and reference values for nerve conduction studies, EMG, evoked potentials, autonomic testing, EEG, and transcranial magnetic stimulation. The book will stimulate readers' interest in paediatric clinical neurophysiology in their daily clinical work.

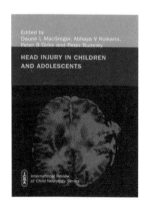

Head Injury in Children and Adolescents

Daune L. MacGregor, Abhaya V. Kulkarni, Peter B. Dirks and Peter Rumney (Eds)

2007 ▪ 272pp ▪ Hardback ▪ 978-1-898683-50-6
£60.00 / €72.00 / US$120.00

This is a comprehensive framework for the care needed by children and their families following a traumatic brain injury. The contributors review the long-term cognitive and behavioural disabilities of both severe and mild traumatic head injuries, and provide an overview of new treatments for children who have had traumatic brain injury, such as neuroprotective strategies, advanced treatment in neurointensive settings ,and new rehabilitation techniques. They demonstrate that preventative measures, with the regulatory and legislative strength of governments, hold the key to reduction in the incidence of traumatic brain injury.